Human
Plasma Proteins

The Author

J. W. KEYSER
M.Sc., Ph.D. (Lond.), F.R.I.C., F.R.C.Path.

Reader in Chemical Pathology in the University of Wales, at The Welsh National School of Medicine; Honorary Consultant in Biochemistry, South Glamorgan Health Authority; Director, Supraregional Protein Reference Unit (Cardiff)

Sometime Visiting Associate Professor of Clinical Chemistry, University of Pennsylvania

Library of Congress Cataloging in Publication Data:

Keyser, James William.
Human plasma proteins.

'A Wiley–Interscience publication.'
Includes index.
1. Blood protein disorders—Diagnosis. 2. Blood proteins—Analysis. I. Title.
RC647.B6K47 616.1′5 79-1089

ISBN 0 471 27598 0

Photoset at Thomson Press (India) Limited, New Delhi
and printed in Great Britain by The Pitman Press, Bath, Avon.

Human Plasma Proteins

Their Investigation in Pathological Conditions

J. W. KEYSER

A Wiley-Interscience Publication

JOHN WILEY & SONS

Chichester · New York · Brisbane · Toronto

To my wife Jean
and
Andrew and Debbie

Contents

Preface

In the preface to his *History of Western Philosophy* Bertrand Russell wrote: 'A few words of apology and explanation are called for if this book is to escape even more severe censure than it doubtless deserves.'

I feel in much the same position. In a book of this type, covering a wide area, specialists on the various topics will inevitably find much to criticize; it may be felt that certain topics have been over-emphasized, and that other topics might have been included. I can only plead that selection is unavoidable if such a book is to be kept to a reasonable size, and that in the circumstances the author's personal interests and experience must to a large degree influence the choice of content.

No attempt has been made to deal with every type of plasma protein of clinical significance. In particular, the blood coagulation proteins have, with a few exceptions, been excluded from consideration, as have the peptide hormones. Otherwise, the term 'plasma protein' has been liberally interpreted, so as to include the proteins of other body fluids, such as cerebrospinal fluid and urine.

I have had valuable help and advice from numerous correspondents: Dr. D. Burnett (Birmingham); Dr. D. Cramp (London); Dr. W. A. Coward (Cambridge); Dr. D. Goldie (Bristol); Prof. J. Hardwicke (Birmingham); Dr. J. Kohn (London); Dr. A. Koj (Krakow); Prof. O. W. Neuhaus (Vermillion, S. Dakota); Prof. K. Peters (London); Dr. D. N. Raine and Dr. G. Evans (Birmingham); Dr. M. K. Schwartz (New York); Dr. E. J. Thompson (London); Dr. R. A. Thompson (Birmingham); Dr. N. Wald (Oxford); Dr. A. M. Ward (Sheffield); Dr. H. E. Weimer (Los Angeles); Dr. J. Whicher (Bristol); Dr. R. H. Whitehead (Melbourne); Dr. C. Wilde (Doncaster). Many of these have read chapters, or sections of chapters, and I am grateful to all for their criticisms and advice. I am also grateful to my colleague Dr. R. Fifield, who kindly read the Appendices and made valuable suggestions for their improvement; to Dr. M. Davies and Dr. J. T. Whicher for Figures 4.2 and App. 6.1 respectively; to Dr. T. Takeoka for the original photographs for Figure 10.1; and to numerous authors, editors, and publishers for permission to reproduce material from published works.

I wish also to thank Mrs. Dorothy Jones and Mrs. Ann Edwards for typing the manuscript; Mr. P. Langham for many of the figures and photographs;

Dr. J. Gibson for the preparation of the index; the staff of the Library of The Welsh National School of Medicine for their unfailing help; Dr. Howard Jones of John Wiley and Sons Ltd. for his advice and help; and, last but not least, my wife and children for their patience during the long preparation of the book.

Cardiff
December, 1978

J. W. K.

CHAPTER 1

Immunodeficiency

A number of disorders of immunoglobulin and specific antibody production are seen in clinical medicine. A diffuse hyperglobulinaemia, evident as a general increase in the electrophoretic γ-globulin fraction, is found in a wide variety of disorders. This type of increase is discussed in later chapters. A different type of over-production is found in conditions associated with the presence of *monaclonal immunoglobulins*, and these are discussed in the next chapter. The phenomenon of *autoantibody production*, in which antibodies are present, in serum, having an affinity for some human tissue component, represents yet another abnormality of immunoglobulin production (Chater 7). Finally, a *diminished production* of immunoglobulin occurs in a number of immunological deficiency diseases, and these form the subject of the present chapter.

An entirely satisfactory classification of the various forms of immunological deficiency diseases is difficult to frame. A preliminary division can be made on the basis of whether the disease is due to a genetically determined abnormality affecting the development of the immune system, in which case it is termed a *primary* immunological deficiency disease, or whether, as in the *secondary* types, it results from the effect of some other disease or condition upon a fully mature immunological system. Secondary deficiencies are much commoner than primary, but in general the latter are the more severe.

Before discussing primary and secondary deficiencies it is necessary to mention briefly the normal, physiological hypogammaglobulinaemia that occurs in early infancy.

NORMAL HYPOGAMMAGLOBULINAEMIA OF INFANCY

The newborn child has a plasma concentration of between about 9 and 12 g of γ-globulin per litre. This consists almost entirely of IgG, derived *in utero* from the maternal circulation. The concentration of γ-globulin falls steadily over the next few months to a value of about 3.5–4.5 g/l at the 3rd to 4th month of post-natal life, after which there is a slow rise, corresponding to the production of γ-globulin by the infant. Adult concentrations may be reached by the 5th year (West *et al.*, 1962). The lowest concentrations of IgG occur at around 8–10 weeks after birth, and adult concentrations are reached by the age of about 3 years. IgM, which at birth is normally present in amounts not much exceeding 200 mg/l, rises more rapidly, to reach adult values within the first year. IgA

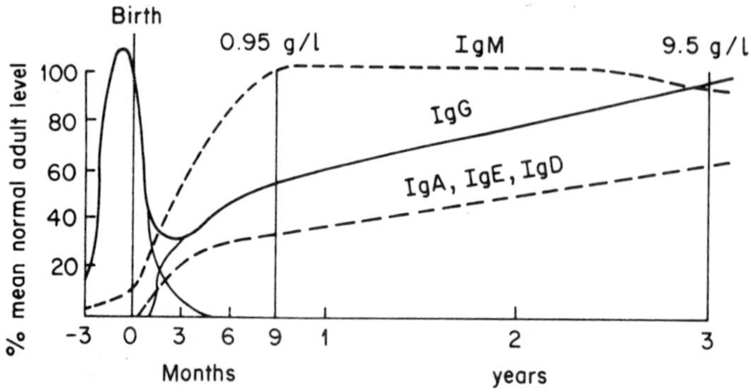

Figure 1.1. The normal development of serum immunoglobulin concentrations. Maturation for IgM occurs within 9 months, and for IgG by 3 years, but for IgA, IgD, and IgE is not complete till puberty. Prematurity of more than 3 months will result in inadequate maternal transfer of IgG, with dangerously low serum concentrations in the baby for the first 3 months of life. (After J. R. Hobbs, *Developmental Immunology* (Ed. M. Adinolfi), Spastics International Press, London, 1969, p. 114, by permission of Spastics International Medical Publications and Prof. Hobbs.)

concentrations rise more slowly and reach adult values at the age of 10–15 years. Figure 1.1 shows the pattern of IgG, IgA, and IgM production in the normal infant.

There have been several reports on the concentrations of the four IgG subclasses in maternal and cord blood (Wang *et al.*, 1970; Hay *et al.*, 1971; Morell *et al.*, 1971, 1972). It would appear that all four subclasses pass through the placenta but that for each subclass there is a different age of onset and speed of synthesis by the infant, leading to the attainment of adult concentrations at different times (Morell *et al.*, 1972). The relatively steep fall in the concentration of IgG_3 during the first month after birth is consistent with the observation made in adults that IgG_3 is the most rapidly catabolized of the subclasses (Spiegelberg *et al.*, 1968; Morell *et al.*, 1970).

Transference of the mother's IgG across the placenta occurs largely in the last trimester of pregnancy (Hobbs and Davis, 1967). Consequently many premature babies will either have, or in due course develop, severe hypogammaglobulinaemia (Yeung and Hobbs, 1968). This is regarded as a form of secondary immunoglobulin deficiency.

PRIMARY IMMUNOLOGICAL DEFICIENCY

In 1952 Bruton described a syndrome in a young boy that was characterized by recurrent infections and a lack of serum γ-globulins as shown by electrophoretic analysis. The condition, originally called agammaglobulinaemia, is often now referred to as hypogammaglobulinaemia, since more sensitive methods of analysis, developed since Bruton's report was published, have demonstrated the presence of small amounts of γ-globulin in the serum of such patients.

Infantile sex-linked agammaglobulinaemia

This is sometimes known as Bruton's disease, and is confined almost entirely to boys. After the disappearance of the antibodies derived from the mother's circulation, the child shows a marked susceptibility to bacterial infection. This usually takes the form of recurrent attacks of sinusitis, septicaemia, meningitis, and pulmonary infections. The basic defect in the disease is an absence of plasma cells from the lymph nodes, spleen, intestine, and bone marrow (Craig *et al.*, 1954; Good, 1955). The patient is unable to synthesize immunoglobulins in any but the smallest amounts, and plasma concentrations of IgG are usually well below 1 g/l and IgA and IgM below 30 mg and 10 mg/l respectively. Electrophoretic analysis of the serum proteins will indicate a virtual absence of γ-globulin, and measurement of the small amounts of immunoglobulins that are present demands the use of sensitive techniques such as that of Mancini and his colleagues (1965). Although reliable diagnosis of the condition by estimation of the immunoglobulins is not possible until the maternal IgG has fallen to a sufficiently low value (i.e. when the child is about 6–9 months old), it may be suspected even at the age of about 4 months if analysis indicates an absence of IgA and IgM.

Since the original studies of Bruton a host of investigators have described a variety of diseases associated with primary deficiency of immunoglobulins. In some of these the deficiency is confined to a single immunoglobulin class, while in others all the three main classes are affected. In yet other types of primary immune deficiency the serum immunoglobulin concentrations are normal (see below). Various attempts at classification have been made, based upon pathogenic mechanisms, genetic control of the synthesis of immunoglobulin polypeptide chains, and clinical findings. Probably the most useful of all the systems is that proposed by Seligmann and his colleagues (Seligmann *et al.*, 1968) and adopted, in all its essentials, by an expert committee of the World Health Organization (Allison *et al.*, 1968). This classification (Table 1.1) is based upon an analysis of each syndrome in terms of measurable cellular, immunological, and functional deficiencies, as well as upon pathological characteristics (with special reference to the thymus and peripheral lymphoid tissues), associated disorders, and genetic or aetiological considerations.

The first group in Seligmann's classification, *viz.* infantile sex-linked agammaglobulinaemia, has already been discussed. The main features of each of the other groups will now be described briefly, with particular reference to the immunoglobulins. It will be noted that the various diseases differ in the extent to which cell-mediated immune mechanisms and immunoglobulin synthesis are deficient. Thus in 'Swiss-type agammaglobulinaemia' both mechanisms are deficient, and the disease therefore represents a most serious form of immunological deficiency.

Table 1.1. Classification of immunological deficiency diseases. (Reproduced by permission of World Health Organization, from *Wld. Hlth. Org. Tech. Rep. Ser.*, 1968, **402**)

Syndrome	Pathological characteristics			Number of circulating lympho-cytes	Immuno-globulin deficiencies	Immunological defects		Genetics	Comments
	thymus	plasma cells	others			humoral antibody	cell-mediated responses		
Infantile sex-linked recessive agammaglobulinaemia[1] (Gitlin *et al.*, 1959)	Normal	Absent		Normal	All classes extremely deficient	Absent or extremely deficient to all antigens	Normal	X-linked	Recurrent infections with extra-cellular pyogenic pathogens
Selective Ig deficiency IgA (West *et al.*, 1962; Rockey *et al.*, 1964; Cattan *et al.*, 1966; Crabbé and Heremans, 1967)	Normal	IgA-producing plasma cells absent		Normal	Both secretory and serum IgA absent. Other Ig levels usually normal	Normal except for IgA antibodies	Normal	Unknown. Some may be autosomal recessive	Bronchitis, sinusitis, exudative enteropathy. Some such subjects are still perfectly healthy
Transient hypogammaglobulinaemia of infancy[2] (Janeway *et al.*, 1953)	?	Deficient		Normal	IgG primarily depressed	Antibody responses usually low or absent	Normal	Familial ? Genetic	May have low or low normal IgG later in life
Non-sex-linked primary immunoglobulin deficiency of variable onset and expression (primary immunoglobulin aberrations)[3] (Good *et al.*, 1962; Barandun *et al.*, 1959; Rosen and Janeway, 1966; Comings, 1965; Giedion and Scheidegger, 1957; Barth	?	Usually deficient but variable	Reticulum hyperplasia; tonsillar hyperplasia; infrequently giant follicular hyperplasia in nodes and spleen	Usually normal	Immunoglobulin deficit and abnormality invariably present but class involved, degree, and direction of change variable	Deficient responses to most antigens but not others (constant)	Deficient responses to some antigens but not others (inconstant)	Possibly autosomal recessive in some (Fudenberg *et al.*, 1967). Possibly multifactorial	This is possibly a large group from which specific forms may be removed as they are defined in aetiological or genetic terms

Thymoma with agammaglobulinaemia[4] (Good and Zak, 1956; Jeunet and Good, 1968)	Thymic enlargement of stromal epithelial spindle-cell type	Deficient or absent		Low and progressive decline often to extremely low level	All markedly reduced	Deficient responses to all antigens (constant)	Deficient responses to all antigens (constant)	May possibly be genetic factor	Eosinophils regularly absent or grossly deficient in blood and marrow. Associated pure red cell aplasia in some cases
Immune deficiency with thrombopaenia and eczema[5] (Stiehm and McIntosh, 1967; Cooper *et al.*, 1968)	Normal	Normal	Lymphocytes in thymus-dependent paracortical regions: progressive deficiency	Low and progressive decline	Immunoglobulin deficit invariably present but class, degree, and direction of change variable (Low IgM and high IgA frequent)	Deficient responses to some antigens but not others (Isohaemagglutinins absent and failure to respond to carbohydrate membrane antigens)	Deficient responses to some but not all antigens (inconstant)	X-linked recessive	Associated disorders: eczema and central thrombocytopaenia
Ataxia-telangiectasia[6] (Peterson *et al.*, 1966; Epstein *et al.*, 1966; Meshaka *et al.*, 1966)	Embryonic type lacking cortical and medullary organization. No Hassall's corpuscles	Variable	Lymphocytes deficient in thymus-dependent area	Slight decrease	Ig deficit usually present but classes involved and direction of changes variable. Often involves IgA (inconstant)	Deficient responses to some antigens and not to others (inconstant)	Deficient responses to some antigens but not to others (constant)	Autosomal recessive	Associated disorders: progressive cerebellar ataxia, ovarian dysgenesis in females, telangiectasia in all tissues when present. May appear late

Table 1.1. *(Contd.)*

Syndrome	Pathological characteristics			Number of circulating lympho-cytes	Immuno-globulin deficiencies	Immunological defects		Genetics	Comments
	thymus	plasma cells	others			humoral antibody	cell-mediated responses		
Hereditary lymphopaenic immunological deficiency (Gitlin and Craig, 1963; Hoyer *et al.*, 1968)	Thymus hypoplastic. Gross deficiency of lymphoid cells and Hassall's corpuscles	Variable	Lymphocytes in tissues grossly deficient but foci of lymphocytes present in spleen and lymph nodes	Low but variable	Ig deficit and abnormality invariably present, but class and direction of change variable	Deficient responses to some antigens but not to others (constant)	Deficient responses to some antigens but not to others (constant)	X-linked recessive or autosomal recessive	Often die of fungal or viral infection in early childhood.
Autosomal recessive alymphocytic agammaglobulinaemia[7] (Glanzmann and Riniker, 1950; Tobler and Cottier, 1958; Hitzig and Willi, 1961; Kadowaki *et al.*, 1965)	Thymus hypoplastic, often undescended; lacks lymphoid cells and Hassall's corpuscles	Absent	Absence of lymphocytes in tissues	Very low	All extremely deficient	Absent or extremely deficient to all antigens (constant)	Deficient responses to all antigens (constant)	Autosomal recessive	Do not survive infancy
Autosomal recessive lymphopaenia with normal plasma cells[8] and immunoglobulins (Nezelof *et al.*, 1964; Fulginiti *et al.*, 1966a)	Thymus hypoplastic, lacks lymphoid cells and Hassall's corpuscles	Present	Lymphocytes in tissues markedly deficient	Low	All normal	Antibodies present but responses not yet well studied	Decreased or absent responses to all antigens (constant)	Autosomal recessive	May be considered a disease entity but may be syndrome above + chimerism

Thymic aplasia[9] (Di George, 1965)	Failure of development of epithelium of 3rd and 4th pharyngeal pouch. No thymus	Present	Absence of parathyroid. Lymphocytes lacking in thymus-dependent paracortical areas. Germinal centres present	Low but variable. Sometimes in normal range	All normal	Not yet well studied but many apparently deficient responses	Absent responses to all antigens (constant)	No evidence of genetic mechanism	Usually recognized in neonatal period as tetany of the newborn

[1] Bruton's disease.
[2] See footnote, page 9.
[3] This group includes 'acquired' primary deficits, dysgammaglobulinaemias and 'congenital' non-sex-linked forms of previous nomenclatures.
[4] Good's syndrome.
[5] Wiskott–Aldrich syndrome.
[6] Mrs. Louis Barr's syndrome.
[7] Glanzmann and Riniker's lymphocytophthisis (Swiss-type agammaglobulinaemia).
[8] Nezelof's syndrome.
[9] Di George's syndrome.

Such disorders, in which cell-mediated mechanisms and immunoglobulin synthesis are both deficient, are referred to as combined immune deficiency disorders. In another type of deficiency state only the cell-mediated immune mechanisms are affected (e.g. Di George's syndrome), while in the condition discovered by Bruton the cell-mediated responses are normal and it is the production of immunoglobulins that is defective. For a discussion of the modern concepts of antibody production and of humoral and cell-mediated immunity the reader is referred to standard textbooks on immunology.

Immunodeficiency and adenosine deaminase activity

It has been shown that some forms of combined immunodeficiency disease are associated with a deficiency of adenosine deaminase activity in the red blood cells (Giblett *et al.*, 1972; Dissing and Knudsen, 1972; Pollara *et al.*, 1973). The causal relationships involved are not at present clear. The subject has recently been reviewed (Meuwissen *et al.*, 1975; *Lancet*, 1976). A screening test for adenosine deaminase deficiency, using a drop of blood, has been described (Moore and Meuwissen, 1975).

Selective inability to synthesize IgA or IgM

A well documented example of a selective inability to synthesize a single class of immunoglobulin involves IgA, which is absent from both circulation and secretions. The serum concentrations of IgG and IgM are usually normal. The condition can be associated with steatorrhoea and a form of malabsorption syndrome (Crabbé and Heremans, 1967), but the deficiency of IgA is thought to a primary defect and not a result of the malabsorption (Crabbé and Heremans, 1966, 1967). In the absence of secretory IgA, which is probably necessary for the defence of the gut against infection, bacteria may invade the upper portion of the gut and interfere with absorption. Although recurrent bacterial infections of the sinuses, middle ear, and respiratory system have been reported in patients with IgA deficiency, surveys have revealed a large number of healthy IgA-deficient subjects (*Lancet*, 1975); and in a study by Koistinen (1975) no significant difference was found between IgA-deficient and normal blood-donors in respect of the frequency of sinopulmonary infection.

A significant proportion of patients with other forms of hypogammaglobulinaemia suffer from chronic diarrhoea and a syndrome resembling sprue. It is important, therefore, if the diagnosis of selective IgA deficiency is to be established, to show that IgA is absent not only from the plasma but also from secretions (e.g. tears, saliva) and that in the humoral antibody response IgA is not produced.

A selective deficiency of IgA can be found in a very small proportion of apparently healthy persons (Rockey *et al.*, 1964; Bachmann, 1965).

Severe selective IgM deficiency

This is arbitrarily defined by serum concentrations of 10 per cent or less of the normal mean value for the patient's age and sex, and has been described in a few cases (Hobbs *et al.*, 1967; Stoelinga *et al.*, 1969; Faulk *et al.*, 1971; Ross and Thompson, 1976). This type of deficiency was previously known as Type V dysgammaglobulinaemia.

Transient hypogammaglobulinaemia of infancy*

This is similar in many features to infantile sex-linked agammaglobulinaemia, and was described by Janeway and his colleagues in 1953 (see also Janeway and Gitlin, 1957, and Rosen and Janeway, 1966). This condition appears to be due to an abnormally prolonged delay in the onset of γ-globulin synthesis by the infant. It is found equally in males and females. Although recovery usually occurs between the ages of 9 and 15 months, infants with transient hypogammaglobulinaemia may be unduly susceptible to infections of the skin, lungs, meninges, or respiratory tract. Depression of immunoglobulin synthesis affects chiefly IgG, the plasma concentration of which in some patients remains permanently low, as does that of IgM.

Non-sex-linked primary immunoglobulin deficiency with variable onset and expression

This group, which was described by Seligmann and his collaborators as the 'waste basket' of their system, includes 'acquired' primary deficiencies, 'dysgammaglobulinaemias' and 'congenital' non-sex-linked forms of previous systems of classification. As more information is acquired it should be possible to distinguish more precisely the various conditions comprised in this group. Attempts have been made to classify some of them on the basis of serum immunoglobulin patterns. The shortcomings of this approach are discussed below.

As indicated in Table 1.1, there is always a deficiency of immunoglobulins, but the class affected and the degree of change are variable.

Agammaglobulinaemia with thymoma

A proportion of patients diagnosed as having 'acquired idiopathic agammaglobulinaemia' were found to have a thymoma in addition to the gross deficiency or absence of eosinophils in the blood. In this class of primary

*Strictly speaking, transient hypogammaglobulinaemia of infancy is not a primary immunological deficiency disease, being secondary most often to prematurity or delayed maturity; however, neither does it fall in the group of secondary deficiency diseases, as defined above, since it does not result from the effect of some other disease or condition upon a fully mature immunological system. It is usually grouped together with the primary immunological deficiencies.

immune deficiency there is typically a marked reduction in the plasma concentrations of IgG, IgA, and IgM, the two latter usually being virtually absent.

Immunological deficiency with thrombocytopaenia and eczema

In this condition (the Wiskott–Aldrich syndrome) the characteristic immunoglobulin deficiency is one of IgM, the concentration of IgG usually being normal and that of IgA usually high. Patients have recurrent otitis media, thrombocytopaenic purpura, and eczema, and generally die in early childhood.

Ataxia-telangiectasia

Children with this disease (sometimes called the Louis-Barr syndrome) show progressive ataxia accompanied by arterial telangiectases of the bulbar conjunctivae and of exposed areas of the skin. There is poor development of the thymus and, possibly for this reason, an increased incidence of lymphoreticular malignancies. Recurrent respiratory infections, especially pneumonia, occur. Serum IgA is usually absent, the concentration of IgG may be low and that of IgM is usually normal. The interesting finding of raised serum concentrations of α-fetoprotein in patients with ataxia-telangiectasia (Waldmann and McIntire, 1972) suggests that a primary abnormality in this condition is a defect in tissue differentiation.

Primary lymphopaenic immunological deficiency

This condition (Gitlin's syndrome) is characterized by persistent lymphopaenia, deficiency of immunoglobulins, and a striking hypoplasia of the thymus. Infections start at about the age of 3 months and death occurs in early infancy. Although, as stated above, there is a deficiency of immunoglobulins, the class involved is variable.

Autosomal recessive alymphocytic agammaglobulinaemia

Children with this disease, which is known as Swiss-type agammaglobulinaemia, suffer from an almost complete absence of lymphoid tissue in the body. There is an extreme deficiency of the major immunoglobulin classes and of antibodies, and an inability to develop delayed (cell-mediated) hypersensitivity reactions. Progressive bacterial and/or viral infections lead to death, usually within 2 years of birth.

Several investigators have reported an association between Swiss-type agammaglobulinaemia and a skeletal disorder similar to achondroplasia. This association is now believed to have a genetic basis, and the condition is known as immunodeficiency with short-limbed dwarfism (Gatti *et al.*, 1969). There is abnormal cellular immunity and the serum immunoglobulin concentrations are low. A variety of short-limbed dwarfism has been described in which the serum immunoglobulin concentrations are normal or raised (Lux *et al.*, 1970).

Autosomal recessive lymphopaenia with normal immunoglobulins (Nezelof's syndrome)

In contrast to the Swiss-type agammaglobulinaemia, in Nezelof's syndrome there are normal serum concentrations of immunoglobulins. The thymus is, however, hypoplastic and lacking in lymphoid cells and Hassall's corpuscles (Nezelof *et al.*, 1964).

Thymic aplasia (Di George's syndrome)

In this condition also the plasma immunoglobulin concentrations are normal; however, the production of specific antibodies as a result of antigenic stimulation is low. There is complete aplasia of the thymus; and, since the parathyroids are usually absent, affected children tend to suffer from hypocalcaemia and neonatal tetany in addition to being unduly susceptible to infections.

SECONDARY IMMUNOLOGICAL DEFICIENCY

Secondary (or acquired) deficiencies of the immunological mechanisms can occur in a number of diseases, such as multiple myeloma, Hodgkin's disease, leukaemia, and lymphosarcoma, which affect the lymphoid tissues. A deficiency of immunoglobulins can also result from excessive loss of protein, either through diseased kidneys, as in the nephrotic syndrome, or via the intestine in protein-losing enteropathy. Certain agents used in therapy, such as irradiation, radiomimetic drugs, antimetabolic drugs, and so on, can also depress the immune system. As with primary immunological deficiencies, the result is an increased susceptibility to infections.

Secondary immunological deficiencies are much commoner than primary, on account of the number of diseases that can affect the immune system. According to Hobbs (1971) they occur in some 4 per cent of hospital patients and are likely to be the cause of symptoms in at least 2 per cent. In general, however, secondary immunological deficiencies are less severe in their effects than are primary.

Table 1.2 shows the incidence of secondary immunoglobulin deficiencies, with an indication of the typical serum immunoglobulin findings, as reported by Hobbs (1968).

OTHER CLASSIFICATIONS

Dysgammaglobulinaemias

Another system of classification is based on analysis of the γ-globulin fraction. In this way two groups are defined:

Table 1.2. Incidence of secondary immunological deficiency. (Reproduced from J. R. Hobbs, *Proc. Roy. Soc. Med.*, 1968, **61**, 883, by permission of The Royal Society of Medicine and Prof. Hobbs.)

	Total number studied	Number with subnormal serum concentration			Patients with IgG < 2 g/l
		IgG	IgA	IgM	
Physiological hypogammaglobulinaemia					
Prematurity	170	113			24
Delayed maturity	ca. 1000	37	3	3	13
Catabolic hypogammaglobulinaemia					
Nephrotic syndrome	69	61	11	2	14
Protein-losing enteropathy	18	10	5	3	2
Severe malnutrition	17	8	0	0	0
Dystrophia myotonica	7	4	0	2	2
Thoracic duct fistula	1	1	0	0	0
Hypogammaglobulinaemia with marrow disorders					
Marrow hypoplasia	35	18	3	2	4
Extensive bony metastases	ca. 200	22	5	18	2
Myelosclerosis	8	5	3	2	1
Paroxysmal nocturnal haemoglobinuria	21	4	2	1	0
Immunoglobulin deficiency probably due to toxic factors					
Prolonged uraemia	39	29	18	23	3
High levels of corticosteroids	ca. 100	3	0	1	0
Cytotoxic therapy	54	3	3	4	1
Diazoxide therapy	2	2	0	0	0
Gluten-sensitive enteropathy	79	4	2	32	0
Thyrotoxicosis	30	3	0	2	0
Diabetes mellitus without proteinuria	ca. 50	6	0	1	0
Following severe infection	ca. 100	3	0	0	0
Congenital heart disease (? rubella *in utero*)	ca. 100	7	7	3	3
Immunoglobulin deficiency with primary reticuloendothelial-neoplasia					
Reticulosarcoma	20	2	3	6	0
Myocosis fungoides	8	1	1	1	0
Hodgkin's disease	68	6	11	28	0

Table 1.2. *(Contd.)*

	Total number studied	Number with subnormal serum concentration			Patients with IgG < 2 g/l
		IgG	IgA	IgM	
Lymphosarcoma	44	15	24	28	1
Giant follicular lymphoma	13	5	8	8	3
Chronic lymphatic leukaemia	58	35	44	44	6
Thymoma	3	3	3	3	3
Myelomatosis-paraprotein type:					
IgG	150	120*	140	141	68%
IgA	70	56		59	28%
Bence Jones protein only	60	46	47	57	18%
IgD	9	7	6	9	11%
IgM	7	7	7		14%
No paraprotein detected	6	6	6	6	17%
Macroglobulinaemia:					
IgM	42	22	32		5%

*Estimated figure.

1. the hypogammaglobulinaemias, in which the deficiency of the γ-globulin can be diagnosed by simple electrophoretic analysis of the serum; and

2. the *dysgammaglobulinaemias*, in which the total quantity of γ-globulin appears on electrophoretic analysis to be normal, any defect being revealed only by measurement of the different immunoglobulins or by testing for specific antibodies.

One special type of dysgammaglobulinaemia (type VI), however, is characterized by a severe antibody deficiency in the presence of normal concentrations of serum immunoglobulins. Table 1.3 is based upon the classification of Hobbs (1969) (see also Hobbs, 1971). Unfortunately, other systems of numbering the dysgammaglobulinaemias are sometimes employed, and this can lead to confusion.

Strictly speaking, the term dysgammaglobulinaemia should be used only when a deficiency of antibody has been established by challenging the patient with a series of antigens. In practice, however, most patients with dysgammaglobulinaemia have a severe deficiency of one or more immunoglobulins, and for convenience the term may therefore be applied in the case of patients who appear to have a normal concentration of (total) γ-globulin and yet have such a deficiency as revealed by estimation of the individual immunoglobulins.

It should be noted that some disorders that are grouped together according to their plasma immunoglobulin concentrations may show variations in other features. For example, one condition classified as a type I dysgammaglobulin-

Table 1.3. Serum immunoglobulin concentrations in dysgammaglobulinaemia. (Reproduced from J. R. Hobbs, *Developmental Immunology* (Ed. M. Adinolfi), Spastics International Press, London, 1969, by permission of Spastics International Medical Publications and Prof. Hobbs.)

	Immunoglobulins*		
Type	IgG	IgA	IgM
I	40–100	**< 10**	**< 10**
II	**< 20**	**< 10**	70–2000
III	**< 40**	50–200	50–200
IV	50–300	**< 10**	50–800
V	50–200	50–200	**< 10**
VI	**50–170**	**50–170**	**50–170**
VII	**< 20**	200–400	**< 10**

*Concentrations are expressed as percentage of the mean adult normal value. The most constant findings are shown in bold type.

aemia has been found to be restricted almost entirely to boys (Barandun *et al.*, 1958), whereas another condition also classified as type I has entirely different characteristics and occurs in women (Gilbert and Hong, 1964). Again, patients with 'acquired idiopathic hypogammaglobulinaemia' sometimes have relatives with 'dysgammaglobulinaemias', the type varying from one relative to another. The classification in terms of immunoglobulins overlaps that of Seligmann and his colleagues (1968). Many patients showing dysgammaglobulinaemia fall into their fourth group (Table 1.1), i.e. non-sex-linked primary immunoglobulin aberrations. For a fuller discussion of the intricacies of these various systems of classification the reader is referred to the reviews of Rosen and Janeway (1966), Good *et al.* (1968), Soothill (1968), Franglen (1970), Hobbs (1969, 1971), and Fudenberg *et al.* (1971). The last-named paper includes a new WHO classification of primary immunodeficiency disorders differing somewhat from that proposed in the earlier WHO report (Allison *et al.*, 1968).

IgD AND IgE IN IMMUNODEFICIENCY DISEASES

Serum IgD and IgE concentrations in immunodeficiency diseases have been studied by a number of investigators, including Buckley and Fiscus (1974), who also reviewed previous findings. Although no clear patterns of susceptibility to infection associated with deficiency or excess of IgD and IgE production emerged from their observations, certain interesting trends were noted, such as a raised mean IgE concentration in a group of patients with selective IgA deficiency, and in patients with the Wiskott–Aldrich syndrome; concentrations of both immunoglobulins were generally, though not invariably, quite low in patients having marked deficiencies of all three major immunoglobulins.

IMMUNOLOGICAL DEFICIENCY IN CANCER

Although the relationship between cancer and the immune response is ill-defined, the idea of an immunological surveillance mechanism, which recognizes and destroys cells that have undergone neoplastic transformation, has been widely accepted. The hypothesis of immunological surveillance was presented by Thomas (1959) and developed by Burnet (1969, 1970). Modifications to the original hypothesis have been proposed, and certain of its assumptions questioned (Gleichmann *et al.*, 1972; Laroye, 1973, 1974; Gleichmann and Gleichmann, 1973a,b; MacGregor, 1973); indeed, the suggestion has been made that impairment of cell-mediated immunity may be a result rather than a cause of malignancy (Watkins, 1973). Whether a contributing cause of the disease, or its effect, deficiencies of cell-mediated immune response in patients with cancer have been demonstrated by the findings of prolonged survival of homografts (Kelly *et al.*, 1958; Southam, 1960), diminished delayed hypersensitivity responses to a purified protein derivative of tuberculin (Schier *et al.*, 1956), and an inhibition, by plasma from patients with cancer, of the normal response of lymphocytes to phytohaemagglutinin (Silk, 1967; Gatti *et al.*, 1970; Whittaker *et al.*, 1971). This response of lymphocytes to phytohaemagglutinin, and to certain other plant extracts, is regarded as a measure of cell-mediated immunity, reflecting the integrity of thymus-derived lymphocytes; and the finding of a diminished response suggested the presence of a humoral factor, in cancer, which would suppress lymphocyte activity and enable the tumour to grow without inhibition. Such a humoral factor, if present before the development of a tumour, might weaken the immunosurveillance mechanism and permit the growth and spread of neoplastic cells.

The presence of immunosuppressive factors in mammalian sera has been reported by a number of investigators (Kamrin, 1959; Mowbray, 1963; Cooperband *et al.*, 1968; Riggio *et al.*, 1969; Gatti, 1971; Hsu and LoGerfo, 1972; Veit and Michael, 1972, 1973). They appear to be associated with the α-globulin fraction of the plasma proteins; and α-globulin-rich fractions isolated from human plasma were shown to suppress phytohaemagglutinin- and antigen-induced proliferation of human lymphocytes *in vitro* (Cooperband *et al.*, 1968) and to prolong the survival of skin allografts in rabbits and mice (Mannick and Schmid, 1967). Further work has been in accord with these findings (Glasgow *et al.*, 1971a,b), and an immunosuppressive peptide fraction was isolated from normal human plasma (Occhino *et al.*, 1973) and shown to suppress T-lymphocyte-mediated immune responses and to prolong the survival of renal allografts in rats (Menzoian *et al.*, 1974a,b). An immunosuppressive peptide, closely resembling that previously isolated in trace amounts from large pools of normal human blood, was subsequently isolated from the serum of patients with cancer (Nimberg *et al.*, 1975); the same fractionation procedures failed, however, to recover any of this peptide from the serum of normal volunteers or patients without cancer.

It has been suggested that a high concentration of circulating immunosuppressive peptides contributes to the inability of some patients with cancer to mount an effective immune response against their tumours (Glasgow *et al.*, 1974). It is possible that there are a number of such immunosuppressive proteins or peptides in the α-globulin fraction; the glycoferroprotein α2H-globulin has an immunosuppressive effect on the response of lymphocytes to stimulation by phytohaemagglutinin (Buffe and Rimbaut, 1975), and this and similar *in vitro* methods of immunological assessment have demonstrated an immunosuppressive effect of pregnancy-associated α_2-macroglobulin (Stimson, 1972, 1975a,b; von Schoultz *et al.*, 1973; Than *et al.*, 1975a,b).

It should be noted that the above is a somewhat over-simplified account, since there have been reports indicating the absence of an inhibitory factor in the serum of cancer patients (Nelson, 1969; Golob *et al.*, 1969) and indeed one report that the phytohaemagglutinin response of lymphocytes from healthy persons was *enhanced* in the presence of plasma from patients with advanced intestinal cancer (McIllmurray *et al.*, 1973); again, some workers have found that any allogeneic serum causes a decrease in the lymphocyte response to phytohaemagglutinin and have concluded that the inhibition reported to occur in the presence of serum from patients with cancer is a non-specific manifestation of this effect (Al-Sarraf *et al.*, 1971). Whitehead and his colleagues (1974) attempted to clarify the situation by comparing the phytohaemagglutinin response of lymphocytes from patients with benign breast lesions, early breast cancer, and advanced breast cancer in the presence of five different types of serum, *viz.* autologous serum, AB serum from a healthy donor, pooled serum from patients with advanced cancer of the breast, pooled serum from patients with advanced cancer of the colon, and fetal bovine serum. From statistical analysis of their results they concluded that the inhibition produced was due to the 'non-self' serum rather than to a specific inhibitory factor, but that such a factor may be present in the serum of patients with advanced cancer of the colon.

The relationship of cancer to immunodeficiency is discussed by Good and his colleagues in a number of papers, the most recent being that by Kersey, Spector, and Good (1973). From a comprehensive review of the literature, Gatti and Good (1971) estimated that the incidence of malignancy in patients with primary immunodeficiencies is roughly 10,000 times that of the general age-matched population. It is consistent with these observations that immunosuppressive therapy after organ transplantation is associated with a significant risk of *de novo* malignancy (Starzl, 1968; Doak *et al.*, 1968; Penn *et al.*, 1969, 1971; Penn, 1970).

PROTEIN CHANGES IN INFECTIONS

The most important changes in the plasma proteins in infections involve the immunoglobulins, the complement system and that group of proteins known as 'acute-phase reactants'.

Immunoglobulins

As will be evident from Chapter 2, a high incidence of bacterial infections is found in patients with monoclonal gammopathies, presumably owing to the suppression of 'normal' immunoglobulins. Patients with IgG-type monoclonal gammopathy are particularly susceptible to gram-positive microorganisms, and patients with IgM-type to gram-negative microorganisms (Ritzmann *et al.*, 1970). *Polyclonal* gammopathy may accompany a wide range of clinical disorders, including chronic infections (tuberculosis, syphilis, deep fungal diseases, lymphogranuloma venereum, chronic bronchitis with bronchiectasis, etc.) (Ritzmann, 1975).

Numerous studies of the immune response in mammals have indicated that IgM antibodies are the first to appear, shortly after immunization, and that IgG antibodies are produced later, particularly in response to secondary stimulation (see Bandilla *et al.* (1969) for references). However, the analytical methods used in most of these studies have been criticized as magnifying the relative amount of IgM antibody present. Using a sensitive radioimmuno-precipitation method, Bandilla and his coworkers investigated the response of healthy volunteers to the injection of haemocyanin from the horseshoe crab (*Limulus polyphemus*). In the few individuals who made a measurable primary response to this antigen, characteristically the IgA and IgM antibodies appeared at an early stage (within 4 days), whereas measurable amounts of IgG antibody could not be found until 18 days after immunization; however, a second injection produced a rapid rise in IgG antibody, the concentrations of IgA and IgM antibodies also increasing but to a lesser degree.

Acute-phase reactants

In general, bacterial infections are associated with large increases in the concentration of C-reactive protein, α_1-acid glycoprotein, α_1-antitrypsin, and haptoglobin, to name but four of the so-called acute-phase reactants (see Chapter 8). Viral infections are usually characterized by relatively lower concentrations of C-reactive protein and α_1-acid glycoprotein, with moderately raised concentrations of α_1-antitrypsin and haptoglobin (Fischer and Gill, 1975). 'Acute-phase protein profiles' have been used to monitor the clinical course of patients with serious infections, and to guide therapy (Fischer and Gill, 1975).

As might be expected, the α-globulins are increased in concentration in acute febrile infections (Petermann, 1960). In chronic infections of many types the albumin concentration is lowered and there is a tendency for all the electrophoretic globulin fractions to become raised (Luetscher, 1947). Such diseases as tuberculosis, leprosy, and kala-azar are usually associated with pronounced hypergammaglobulinaemia (Gross *et al.*, 1959). Seibert and her colleagues have studied extensively the protein changes in tuberculosis (Seibert *et al.*, 1947).

Complement system

Total complement activity and the concentrations of various complement components may vary widely in infectious diseases. Decreased serum concentrations of complement have been reported in bacterial endocarditis complicated by glomerulonephritis (Williams and Kunkel, 1962). A similar combination of infection, glomerulonephritis, and hypocomplementaemia has been noted also in staphylococcal bacteraemia due to infected ventriculoatrial shunts (Stickler *et al.*, 1968), in ECHO virus type 9 infections (Yuceoglu *et al.*, 1966) and in quartan malaria (Ward and Kibukamusoke, 1969). Evidence of complement activation offers an important means of predicting the occurrence of glomerulonephritis in such conditions and monitoring its treatment.

In bacteraemia due to gram-negative organisms, low serum C3 concentrations were observed in patients with shock or who died of the infection, but not otherwise (McCabe, 1973). In acute viral hepatitis, total complement activity, and the serum concentrations of the components measured (C3, C4, and C1q), were found to vary widely; however, a correlation was observed between high titres of hepatitis-associated antigen and low concentrations of complement (particularly C4) in patients with joint and skin symptoms (Alpert *et al.*, 1971). It was suggested that complement-fixing immune complexes were present and that these had a rôle in the pathogenesis of these extrahepatic manifestations of viral hepatitis.

Abnormalities of complement have been observed also in meningococcal infection (Greenwood *et al.*, 1976). In the case of acute meningococcaemia, most patients with this condition were found to have low serum concentrations of C3, C4, C1q, factor B, and, especially, properdin. Such complement activation (presumably mediated by both the classical and the alternative pathways) can lead to the release of vasoactive amines (Bokisch *et al.*, 1969) and activation of the coagulation system (Zimmerman and Müller-Eberhard, 1971), and it was suggested that it might play an important part in initiating the circulatory collapse and intravascular coagulation that are prominent features of acute meningococcaemia (Greenwood *et al.*, 1976).

The complement system is also involved in measles (Charlesworth *et al.*, 1976) and bronchial asthma (Kay *et al.*, 1974).

Pre-existing deficiencies of specific components of the complement system which predispose to infection are discussed in the next section.

RÔLE OF THE COMPLEMENT SYSTEM IN IMMUNE DEFICIENCY

A number of rare and in some cases inadequately characterized syndromes are known in which the immune deficiency is apparently due to defects in the complement system. Failure of C3 activation, whether due to a deficiency of C3 itself, as in the two patients investigated by Alper and Ballow and their respective coworkers (Alper *et al.*, 1972; Ballow *et al.*, 1975), or to a deficiency of C3b inactivator, is associated with severe susceptibility to bacterial infection; in the patient with a deficiency of C3b inactivator investigated by Alper and his colleagues, plasma immunoglobulin concentrations were normal but C3 concentrations were very low (Alper *et al.*, 1970, 1972b; Alper and Rosen, 1971). In yet another patient, who showed increased susceptibility to infection with pyogenic bacteria, the concentration of C3 was markedly reduced; the patient's serum contained a circulating enzyme capable of cleaving C3 both *in vitro* and *in vivo* (Alper *et al.*, 1973).

The suggestion has been made that a physiological deficiency of the whole complement system or of one of its components, possibly C3, might be of importance in the epidemic type of *Pneumocystis* pneumonia in infants with no impairment of immunoglobulin synthesis (Brzosko *et al.*, 1971).

Low concentrations of C1q have been reported in hypogammaglobulinaemia, particularly of the Swiss type (O'Connell *et al.*, 1967; Gewurz *et al.*, 1968); the deficiency is likely to be due not to a defect in synthesis but rather to a redistribution of C1q between plasma and extracellular fluid and to increased catabolism (Kohler and Müller-Eberhard, 1972).

A family with C1r deficiency has been described (Day *et al.*, 1972), as well as a further patient (Pickering *et al.*, 1970). Three siblings in the affected family died in childhood, two probably from infection and one from a disease resembling systemic lupus erythematosus; and of the two remaining siblings one also had a disease resembling systemic lupus erythematosus, while the other suffered from arthralgia and recurrent infections.

A family with hereditary deficiency of C5 was studied by Rosenfeld and Leddy (1974); one member of the family, a young woman, had systemic lupus erythematosus and frequent bacterial infections, and C5 was absent; a healthy half-sister had barely measurable amounts of C5 in the serum.

A defect of humoral mediation of phagocytosis, attributed to a functional abnormality of C5 and associated with increased susceptibility to bacterial infections, has been described (Miller and Nilsson, 1970).

Absence of C6 in a child with repeated episodes of meningococcal meningitis has been reported (Lim *et al.*, 1976).

Finally, a single case of C8 deficiency in a woman who suffered from repeated disseminated gonococcal infection has been reported (Petersen *et al.*, 1976).

A number of other complement deficiencies, associated with conditions other than infections, have been described (see Lachmann, 1975, and Whicher, 1978).

LABORATORY INVESTIGATION OF PROTEINS IN IMMUNE DEFICIENCY STATES

The demonstration of a low γ-globulin fraction by simple electrophoresis of the serum proteins using cellulose acetate or agar gel may be supplemented by immunoelectrophoretic analysis to pin-point the abnormality. One or both of these procedures may, in the light of the clinical and other findings, be all that is required. It should be noted, however, that even gross deficiencies of certain immunoglobulins may remain undetected by electrophoresis, and that simple immunoelectrophoretic techniques are not quantitative and require experience for interpretation of the patterns. It follows that abnormalities cannot be excluded by either of these methods, but they are nevertheless useful for preliminary screening.

It will be clear from the preceding discussions and from Table 1.1, however, that the diagnosis of a primary immunological deficiency cannot be made on the basis of serum immunoglobulin findings alone; nor does the presence of normal concentrations of IgG, IgA, and IgM rule out the possibility of a deficiency of antibodies. Failure to respond to antigenic stimulation is sometimes seen in patients with normal or even high concentrations of all three immunoglobulins, as well as in patients with isolated immunoglobulin deficiencies (Fudenberg *et al.*, 1971). Nevertheless, it is important to determine the serum immunoglobulins quantitatively, and to examine the serum proteins electrophoretically. Combined immune deficiency is sometimes associated with a lymphoma, and it is therefore advisable to examine the concentrated urine for Bence Jones protein and the serum protein electrophoretic pattern for monoclonal immunoglobulin bands. The bands may be faint, and they may be obscured by the major protein fractions, even as far anodally as albumin in the case of certain serum Bence Jones proteins (Heremans and Masson, 1973). These examinations should, if possible, be done before any treatment with immunoglobulin is started. Other tests are necessary, however, if the presence of a primary immunological deficiency disease is to be firmly established. Seligmann and his colleagues (1968) have recommended that these should include an evaluation of humoral and cellular-type responses to standardized antigens; repeated lymphocyte counts; examination of the thymic region and, when necessary, rectal and regional lymph node biopsies (especially after antigenic stimulation); family studies; a careful check for prenatal infections or other influences; and chromosome analysis. Such exhaustive investigation may not be practicable in every case; indeed, these recommendations were made largely in the interest of future analysis and better classification of the primary immune deficiencies.

Serum immunoglobulins

Although there is no sharp threshold for the diagnosis of immunoglobulin deficiency, markedly subnormal concentrations of serum immunoglobulins may be taken as supporting such a diagnosis if associated with symptoms. As mentioned earlier, normal concentrations for children are very different from those for adults, and the age of the patient must always be taken into consideration when results are being interpreted.

Craig, J., D. Gitlin, and T. Jewett (1954), *Amer. J. Dis. Child.*, **88**, 626.
Day, N. K., H. Geiger, R. Stroud, M. deBracco, B. Mancado, D. Windhorst, and R. A. Good (1972), *J. Clin. Invest.*, **51**, 1102.
Di George, A. M. (1965), *J. Pediat.*, **67**, 907.
Dissing, J., and B. Knudsen (1972), *Lancet*, **ii**, 1316.
Doak, P. B., J. Z. Montgomerie, J. D. K. North, and F. Smith (1968), *Brit. Med. J.*, **ii**, 746.
Epstein, W. L., H. H. Fudenberg, W. B. Reed, E. Boder, and R. P. Sedgwick (1966), *Int. Arch. Allergy*, **30**, 15.
Faulk, W. P., W. S. Kiyasu, M. D. Cooper, and H. H. Fudenberg (1971), *Pediatrics*, **47**, 399.
Fischer, C. L., and C. W. Gill (1975), in *Serum Protein Abnormalities: Diagnostic and Clinical Aspects* (Eds. S. E. Ritzmann and J. C. Daniels), Little, Brown, Boston, p. 331.
Franglen, G. (1970), *Brit. J. Hosp. Med.*, **3**, 651.
Fudenberg, H. H., *et al.* (1967), in J. Killander (Ed.), *Gamma globulins*, Nobel Symposium III, Almqvist and Wiksells, Stockholm, p. 585. (Cited by Allison *et al.*, 1968.)
Fudenberg, H. H., R. A. Good, H. C. Goodman, W. Hitzig, H. G. Kunkel, I. M. Roitt, F. S. Rosen, D. S. Rowe, M. Seligmann, and J. R. Soothill (1971), *Bull. Wld. Hlth. Org.*, **45**, 125.
Fulginiti, V. A., W. E. Hathaway, D. S. Pearlman, W. R. Blackburn, C. W. Reiquam, J. H. Githens, H. N. Claman, and C. H. Kempe, (1966a), *Lancet*, **ii**, 5.
Fulginiti, V. A., O. F. Sieber, H. N. Claman, and D. Merrill (1966b), *J. Pediat.*, **68**, 723.
Gatti, R. A. (1971), *Lancet*, **i**, 1351.
Gatti, R. A., and R. A. Good (1971), *Cancer*, **28**, 89.
Gatti, R. A., N. Platt, H. H. Pomerance, R. Hong, L. O. Langer, H. E. M. Kay, and R. A. Good (1969), *J. Pediat.*, **75**, 675.
Gatti, R. A., D. B. Garrioch, and R. A. Good (1970), in *Proceedings of the Fifth Leukocyte Culture Conference* (Ed. J. E. Harris), Academic Press, New York, p. 339.
Gewurz, H., R. J. Pickering, C. L. Christian, R. Snyderman, S. E. Mergenhagen, and R. A. Good (1968), *Clin. Exp. Immunol.*, **3**, 437.
Giblett, E. R., J. E. Anderson, F. Cohen, B. Pollara, and H. J. Meuwissen (1972), *Lancet*, **ii**, 1067.
Giedion, A. von, and J. J. Scheidegger (1957), *Helv. paediat. Acta*, **12**, 241.
Gilbert, C., and R. Hong (1964), *Amer. J. Med.*, **37**, 602.
Gitlin, D., and J. M. Craig (1963), *Pediatrics*, **32**, 517.
Gitlin, D., C. A. Janeway, L. Apt, and J. M. Craig (1959), *Cellular and Humoral Aspects of the Hypersensitivity States*, Hoeber-Harper, New York, p. 375.
Glanzmann, E., and P. Riniker (1950), *Ann. Paediat.*, **175**, 1.
Glasgow, A. H., S. R. Cooperband, J. C. Occhino, K. Schmid, and J. A. Mannick (1971a), *Proc. Soc. Exp. Biol. Med.*, **138**, 753.
Glasgow, A. H., S. R. Cooperband, K. Schmid, J. T. Parker, J. C. Occhino, and J. A. Mannick (1971b), *Transplantation Proc.*, **3**, 835.
Glasgow, A. H., R. B. Nimberg, J. O. Menzoian, I. Saporoschetz, S. R. Cooperband, and K. Schmid (1974), *New Engl. J. Med.*, **291**, 1263.
Gleichmann, E., and H. Gleichmann (1973a), *Klin. Woch.*, **51**, 255, 260.
Gleichmann, H., and E. Gleichmann (1973b), *Lancet*, **i**, 883.
Gleichmann, E., H. Gleichmann, and R. S. Schwartz (1972), *J. Nat. Cancer Inst.*, **49**, 793.
Goldman, J. M., and J. R. Hobbs (1967), *Immunology*, **13**, 421.
Golob, E. K., T. Israsena, A. C. Quatrale, and K. L. Becker (1969), *Cancer*, **23**, 306.
Good, R. A. (1955), *J. Lab. Clin. Med.*, **46**, 167.
Good. R. A., and S. J. Zak (1956), *Pediatrics*, **18**, 109.
Good, R. A., W. D. Kelly, J. Rötstein, and R. L. Varco (1962), *Progr. Allergy*, **6**, 187.
Good, R. A., R. D. A. Peterson, D. Y. Perey, J. Finstad, and M. D. Cooper (1968), in

Immunologic Deficiency Diseases in Man: Birth Defects—Original Article Series, Vol. 4, No. 1 (Eds. D. Bergsma and R. A. Good), National Foundation, New York, p. 17.
Greenwood, B. M., I. I. Onyewotu, and H. C. Whittle (1976), *Brit. Med. J.*, **i**, 797.
Gross, P. A. M., D. Gitlin, and C. A. Janeway (1959), *New Engl. J. Med.*, **260**, 121.
Hay, F. C., M. G. R. Hull, and G. Torrigiani (1971), *Clin. Exp. Immunol.*, **9**, 355.
Heremans, J. F., and P. A. Crabbé (1968), in *Immunologic Deficiency Diseases in Man: Birth Defects—Original Article Series*, Vol. 4, No. 1 (Eds. D. Bergsma and R. A. Good), National Foundation, New York, p. 298.
Heremans, J. F., and P. L. Masson (1973), *Clin. Chem.*, **19**, 294.
Hitzig, W. H., and H. Willi (1961), *Schweiz. med. Wschr.*, **91**, 1625.
Hobbs, J. R. (1968), *Proc. Roy. Soc. Med.*, **61**, 883.
Hobbs, J. R. (1969), in *Developmental Immunology* (Ed. M. Adinolfi), Spastics International Press, London, p. 114.
Hobbs, J. R. (1971), *Adv. Clin. Chem.*, **14**, 219.
Hobbs, J. R., and J. A. Davis (1967), *Lancet*, **i**, 757.
Hobbs, J. R., R. D. G. Milner, and P. J. Watt (1967), *Brit. Med. J.*, **iv**, 583.
Hoyer, J. R., M. D. Cooper, A. E. Gabrielsen, and R. A. Good (1968), *Medicine (Baltimore)*, **47**, 201.
Hsu, C. C. S., and P. LoGerfo (1972), *Proc. Soc. Exp. Biol. Med.*, **139**, 575.
Janeway, C. A., and D. Gitlin (1957), *Adv. Pediat.*, **9**, 65.
Janeway, C. A., L. Apt, and D. Gitlin (1953), *Trans. Assoc. Amer. Phycns.*, **66**, 200.
Jeunet, F., and R. A. Good (1968), in *Immunological Deficiency Diseases in Man: Birth Defects—Original Article Series*, Vol. 4, No. 1 (Eds. R. A. Good and D. Bergsma), National Foundation, New York, p. 192.
Johansson, S. G. O., and T. Berg (1967), *Acta Paediat. Scand.*, **56**, 572.
Kadowaki, J.-I., R. I. Thompson, W. W. Zuelzer, P. V. Woolley, Jr., A. J. Brough, and D. Gruber (1965), *Lancet*, **ii**, 1152.
Kalff, M. W. (1970), *Clin. Chim. Acta*, **28**, 277.
Kamrin, B. B. (1959), *Proc. Soc. Exp. Biol. Med.*, **100**, 58.
Kay, A. B., G. D. Bacon, B. A. Mercer, H. Simpson, and J. W. Crofton (1974), *Lancet*, **ii**, 916.
Kelly, W. D., R. A. Good, and R. L. Varco (1958), *Surg. Gynec. Obstet.*, **107**, 565.
Kersey, J. H., B. D. Spector, and R. A. Good (1973), *Adv. Cancer Res.*, **18**, 211.
Kohler, P. F., and H. J. Müller-Eberhard (1972), *J. Clin. Invest.*, **51**, 868.
Koistinen, J. (1975), *Vox Sang.*, **29**, 192.
Lachmann, P. J. (1975), in *Clinical Aspects of Immunology* (Eds. P. G. H. Gell, R. R. A. Coombs, and P. J. Lachmann), 3rd edn., Blackwell, Oxford, p. 323.
Lancet (1975), Annotation, **ii**, 1291.
Lancet (1976), Annotation, **i**, 895.
Laroye, G. J. (1973), *Lancet*, **i**, 641.
Laroye, G. J. (1974), *Lancet*, **i**, 1097.
Lim, D., A. Gewurz, T. F. Lint, M. Ghaze, B. Sepheri, and H. Gewurz (1976), *J. Pediatrics*, **89**, 42.
Luetscher, J. A. (1947), *Physiol. Revs.*, **27**, 621.
Lux, S. E., R. B. Johnson, Jr., C. S. August, B. Say, V. B. Penchaszadeh, F. S. Rosen, and V. A. McKusick (1970), *New Engl. J. Med.*, **282**, 231.
MacGregor, G. A. (1973), *Lancet*, **i**, 1185.
Mancini, G., A. O. Carbonara, and J. F. Heremans (1965), *Immunochemistry*, **2**, 255.
Mannick, J. A., and K. Schmid (1967), *Transplantation*, **5**, 1231.
Masseyef, R., and J. Lamy (1966), *Clin. Chim. Acta*, **14**, 285.
McCabe, W. R. (1973), *New Engl. J. Med.*, **288**, 21.
McFarlane, H. (1966), *Lancet*, **ii**, 445.
McIllmurray, M. B., M. Gray, and M. J. S. Langman (1973), *Lancet*, **ii**, 452.
Menzoian, J. O., A. H. Glasgow, R. B. Nimberg, M. B. Constantian, R. L. Stevens, S. R. Cooperband, K. Schmid, and J. A. Mannick (1974a), *Transplantation*, **18**, 391.

Menzoian, J. O., A. H. Glasgow, R. D. Nimberg, S. R. Cooperband, K. Schmid, I. Saporoschetz, and J. A. Mannick (1974b), *J. Immunol.*, **113**, 266.

Meshaka, G., P. Burtin, F. Danon, B. Delpech, and M. Seligmann (1966), in *Protides of the Biological Fluids: Proceedings of 14th Colloquium, Bruges, 1965* (Ed. H. Peeters), Elsevier, Amsterdam, p. 715.

Meuwissen, H. J., B. Pollara, R. J. Pickering, and I. H. Porter (1975), Eds., *Combined Immunodeficiency Disease and Adenosine Deaminase Deficiency: A Molecular Defect*, Academic Press, New York.

Michaux, J. L. (1966), *Ann. Soc. belg. Méd. trop.*, **46**, Suppl. 5.

Miller, M. E., and U. R. Nilsson (1970), *New Engl. J. Med.*, **282**, 354.

Mohammed, I., A. M. Tomkins, and B. M. Greenwood (1973), *Lancet*, **i**, 481.

Moore, E. C., and H. J. Meuwissen (1975), in *Combined Immunodeficiency Disease and Adenosine Deaminase Deficiency: A Molecular Defect* (eds. H. J. Meuwissen, B. Pollara, R. J. Pickering, and I. H. Porter), Academic Press, New York, p. 219.

Morell, A., W. D. Terry, and Th. Waldmann (1970), *J. Clin. Invest.*, **49**, 673.

Morell, A., F. Skvaril, E. van Loghem, and M. Kleemola (1971), *Vox Sang.*, **21**, 481.

Morell, A., F. Skvaril, W. H. Hitzig, and S. Barandun (1972), *J. Pediat.*, **80**, 960.

Mowbray, J. F. (1963), *Transplantation*, **1**, 15.

Nelson, H. S. (1969), *J. Nat. Cancer Inst.*, **42**, 765.

Nezelof, C., M.-L. Jammet, P. Lortholary, B. Labrune, and M. Lamy (1964), *Arch. franç. Pédiat.*, **21**, 897.

Nimberg, R. B., A. H. Glasgow, J. D. Menzoian, M. B. Constantian, S. R. Cooperband, J. A. Mannick, and K. Schmid (1975), *Cancer Res.*, **35**, 1489.

Occhino, J. C., A. H. Glasgow, S. R. Cooperband, J. A. Mannick, and K. Schmid (1973), *J. Immunol.*, **110**, 685.

O'Connell, E. J., P. Enriquez, J. W. Linman, G. J. Gleich, and F. C. McDuffie (1967), *J. Lab. Clin. Med.*, **70**, 715.

Penn, I. (1970), *Recent Results in Cancer Research*, Vol. 35, Springer, Berlin.

Penn, I., W. Hammond, L. Brettschneider, and T. E. Starzl (1969), *Transplantation Proc.*, **1**, 106.

Penn, I., C. G. Halgrimson, and T. E. Starzl (1971), *Transplantation Proc.*, **3**, 773.

Petermann, M. L. (1960), in *The Plasma Proteins* (Ed. F. W. Putnam), Academic Press, New York, p. 309.

Petersen, B. H., J. A. Graham, and G. F. Brooks (1976), *J. Clin. Invest.*, **57**, 283.

Peterson, R. D. A., M. D. Cooper, and R. A. Good (1966), *Amer. J. Med.*, **41**, 342.

Pickering, R. J., G. B. Naff, R. M. Stroud, R. A. Good, and H. Gewurz (1970), *J. Exp. Med.*, **131**, 803.

Pollara, B., R. J. Pickering, and H. J. Meuwissen (1973), *Pediat. Res.*, **7**, 362.

Rhodes, K., A. Scott, R. L. Markham, and M. E. Monk-Jones (1969), *Ann. Rheum. Dis.*, **28**, 104.

Riggio, R. R., G. H. Schwartz, F. G. Bull, K. H. Stenzel, and A. L. Rubin (1969), *Transplantation*, **8**, 689.

Ritzmann, S. E. (1975), in *Serum Protein Abnormalities: Diagnostic and Clinical Aspects* (Eds. S. E. Ritzmann and J. C. Daniels), Little, Brown, Boston, p. 351.

Ritzmann, S. E., J. C. Daniels, and W. C. Levin (1970), in *Leukemia-Lymphoma*, Year Book, Chicago, p. 169. (Cited by Ritzmann, 1975.)

Rockey, J. H., L. A. Hanson, J. F. Heremans, and H. G. Kunkel (1964), *J. Lab. Clin. Med.*, **63**, 205.

Rosen, F. S., and C. A. Janeway (1966), *New Engl. J. Med.*, **275**, 709, 769.

Rosenfeld, S. I., and J. P. Leddy (1974), *J. Clin. Invest.*, **53**, 67a.

Ross, I. N., and R. A. Thompson (1976), *J. Clin. Path.*, **29**, 773.

Rowe, D. S. (1972), *Lancet*, **ii**, 1232.

Rowe, D. S., I. A. McGregor, S. J. Smith, P. Hall, and K. Williams (1968), *Clin. Exp. Immunol.*, **3**, 63.

Samuel, A. M., U. R. Deshpande, and B. Singh (1970), *Ind. J. Med. Res.*, **58**, 56.

Schier, W. W., A. Roth, G. Ostroff, and M. H. Shrift (1956), *Amer. J. Med.*, **20**, 94.
Sehgal, S., and B. K. Aikat (1970), *Ind. J. Med. Res.*, **58**, 289.
Seibert, F. B., M. V. Seibert, A. J. Atno, and H. W. Campbell (1947), *J. Clin. Invest.*, **26**, 90.
Seligmann, M., H. H. Fudenberg, and R. A. Good (1968), *Amer. J. Med.*, **45**, 817.
Silk, M. (1967), *Cancer*, **20**, 2088.
Soothill, J. F. (1968), *Proc. Roy. Soc. Med.*, **61**, 881.
Southam, C. M. (1960), *Cancer Res.*, **20**, 271.
Spiegelberg, H. L., B. G. Fishkin, and H. M. Grey (1968), *J. Clin. Invest.*, **47**, 2323.
Starzl, T. E. (1968), *Ann. Surg.*, **168**, 416.
Stickler, G. B., M. H. Shin, E. C. Burke, K. E. Holley, R. H. Miller, and W. E. Segar (1968), *New Engl. J. Med.*, **279**, 1077.
Stiehm, E. R., and H. H. Fudenberg (1966), *Pediatrics*, **37**, 715.
Stiehm, E. R., and R. M. McIntosh (1967), *Clin. Exp. Immunol.*, **2**, 179.
Stimson, W. H. (1972), *Lancet*, **i**, 684.
Stimson, W. H. (1975a), *Behring Inst. Mitt.*, **57**, 42.
Stimson, W. H. (1975b), *Lancet*, **ii**, 989.
Stoelinga, G. B. A., P. J. J. van Munster, and J. P. Slooff (1969), *Acta paediat. scand.*, **58**, 352.
Stoop, J. W., B. J. M. Zegers, P. C. Sander, and R. E. Ballieux (1969), *Clin. Exp. Immunol.*, **4**, 101.
Than, G. N., I. F. Csaba, N. J. Karg, D. G. Szabó, M. Ambrus, and G. Bajtai (1975a), *Lancet*, **ii**, 515.
Than, G. N., I. F. Csaba, D. G. Szabó, M. Paál, M. Ambrus, and G. Bajtai (1975b), *IRCS Med. Sci.*, **3**, 309.
Thomas, L. (1959), in *Cellular and Humoral Aspects of the Hypersensitive States* (Ed. H. S. Lawrence), Hoeber-Harper, New York, p. 529.
Tobler, R., and H. Cottier (1958), *Helv. paediat. Acta*, **13**, 313.
Turner, M. W., and A. Voller (1966), *J. Trop. Med. Hyg.*, **69**, 99.
Uffelman, J. A., W. E. Engelhard, and C. R. Jolliff (1970), *Clin. Chim. Acta*, **28**, 185.
Veit, B. C., and J. G. Michael (1972), *Nature New Biol.*, **235**, 238.
Veit, B., and J. G. Michael (1973), *J. Immunol.*, **111**, 341.
von Schoultz, B., T. Stigbrand, and A. Tärnvik (1973), *FEBS Lett.*, **38**, 23.
Waldmann, T. A., and K. R. McIntire (1972), *Lancet*, **ii**, 1112.
Wang, A. C., W. P. Faulk, M. A. Stuckey, and H. H. Fudenberg (1970), *Immunochemistry*, **7**, 703.
Ward, P. A., and J. W. Kibukamusoke (1969), *Lancet*, **i**, 283.
Watkins, S. M. (1973), *Lancet*, **i**, 1255.
West, C. D., R. Hong, and N. H. Holland (1962), *J. Clin. Invest.*, **41**, 2054.
Whicher, J. T. (1978), *Clin. Chem.*, **24**, 7.
Whitehead, R. H., P. M. Bolton, and R. G. Newcombe (1974), *Europ. J. Cancer*, **10**, 815.
Whittaker, M. G., K. Rees, and C. G. Clark (1971), *Lancet*, **i**, 892.
Williams, R. C., and H. G. Kunkel (1962), *J. Clin. Invest.*, **41**, 666.
Yeung, C. Y., and J. R. Hobbs (1968), *Lancet*, **i**, 1167.
Yuceoglu, A. M., S. Berkovich, and S. Minkowitz (1966), *J. Pediat.*, **69**, 603.
Zimmerman, T. S., and H. J. Müller-Eberhard (1971), *J. Exp. Med.*, **134**, 1601.

CHAPTER 2

Paraproteinaemias

Some diseases are associated with the production of a greatly increased amount of relatively homogeneous immunoglobulin—a so-called *paraprotein*—by a single proliferating clone of plasma cells. Conditions in which this happens are referred to as *monoclonal gammopathies*, in contrast to *polyclonal gammopathies*, in which plasma cells are producing, in response to antigenic stimulation, an immunoglobulin or mixture of immunoglobulins having greater diversity of electrophoretic mobility. An infection, for example, will generally present the body with many antigenic proteins, and elicit a broad spectrum of antibodies which contain most of the classes of heavy and light immunoglobulin chains. On electrophoresis of the patient's serum these antibodies will show a spread of electrophoretic mobilities ranging from the α_2- to the slowest γ-globulin region, and by the use of appropriate antisera they can be shown to be polyclonal in origin. By contrast, paraprotein molecules have an identical electrophoretic mobility and migrate as a single narrow band, which appears as a spike on scanning the electrophoretic strip (Figure 2.1). On testing with

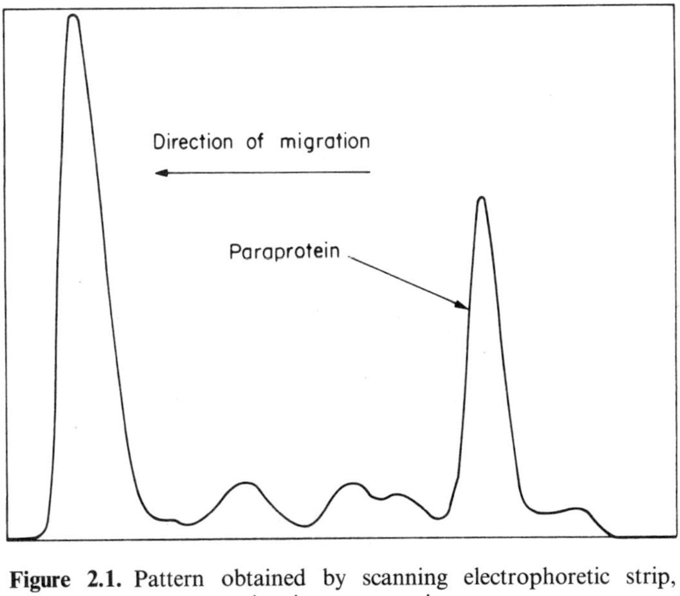

Figure 2.1. Pattern obtained by scanning electrophoretic strip, showing paraprotein

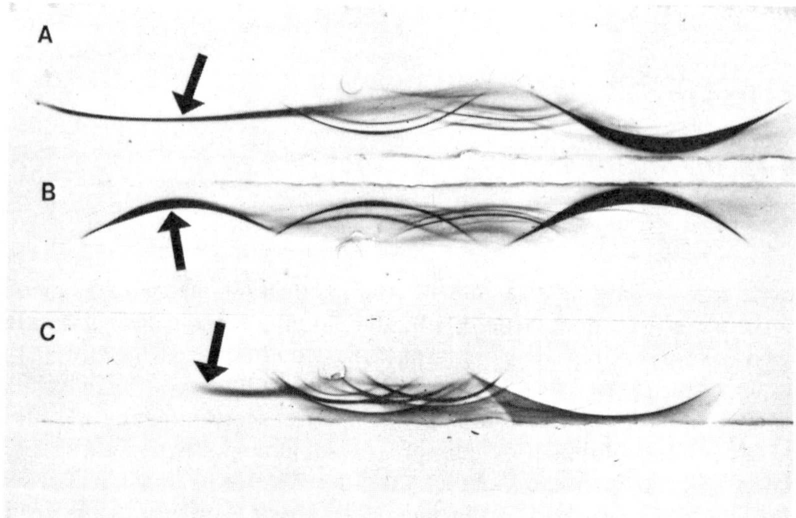

Figure 2.2. Typical immunoelectrophoretic patterns, showing albumin at right and IgG (indicated by arrow) at left. The anode was at the right-hand end of the plate and the serum sample was applied at the central spot: (A) normal serum; (B) serum from patient with multiple myelomatosis showing abnormal IgG; (C) serum from patient with immunoglobulin deficiency. (Reproduced, with permission, from J. W. Keyser, *Chem. Brit.*, 1972, **8**, 480.)

appropriate antisera paraproteins are found to contain immunoglobulin determinants of a single subclass of heavy chain and/or a single subclass of light chain. The relative homogeneity of the paraprotein under the conditions usually employed in immunoelectrophoresis leads to the formation of abnormally shaped precipitin arcs, as illustrated in Figure 2.2 in the case of an IgG myeloma. A polyclonal increase, on the other hand, would not alter the essential shape of the precipitin line.

The presence of a paraprotein in the blood or urine is generally evidence that a monoclone of cells is present—in other words, that the patient has an immunocytoma.

A few cases in which more than one monoclonal immunoglobulin appears in the same serum have been described (see Natvig and Kunkel, 1973).

ELECTROPHORESIS OF PARAPROTEINS IN STARCH GEL OR ACRYLAMIDE GEL

Reference has been made above to the relative homogeneity and restricted range of electrophoretic mobility of paraproteins under the conditions usually employed, *viz.* electrophoresis on cellulose acetate in barbitone buffer of pH 8.6 or thereabouts. A somewhat different picture is obtained if the electrophoretic separation is carried out in starch gel. Under these conditions many myeloma proteins are found to comprise a number of components (Owen

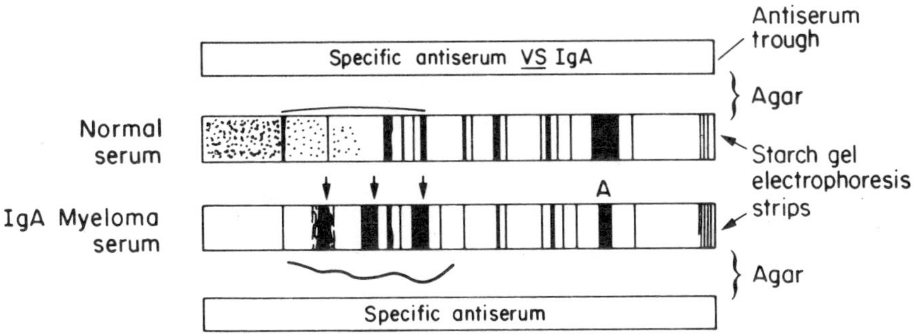

Figure 2.3. Starch gel immunoelectrophoresis of IgA myeloma serum, demonstrating that the anomalous bands in the serum are IgA. After electrophoretic separation half of the sliced gel was stained, while a strip containing the electrophoretically separated proteins was cut from the unstained half of the gel, placed on a glass plate, and surrounded with agar. When the agar had hardened, a trough was cut and specific antiserum against human IgA was added. After 48–168 hours the plates were photographed. The drawing was made by combining the findings from the stained half of the gel with the results of the immuno-starch-gel test. (After J. L. Fahey, *J. Clin. Invest.*, 1963, **42**, 111, by permission of the American Society for Clinical Investigation, Inc., and Dr. Fahey.)

et al., 1958; Flynn and Stow, 1958; Fine *et al.*, 1959; Laurell, 1961; Engle *et al.*, 1961). Fahey (1963) detected heterogeneity in 54 out of a total of 77 sera from patients with myeloma. As in an earlier study of myeloma globulins in mice (Fahey, 1961), the heterogeneity appeared to be of two types: electrophoretic, revealed by the presence of multiple, closely spaced components, apparently differing in net charge; and polymer-type heterogeneity, producing several widely spaced bands. The pattern of heterogeneity was found to be characteristic for each myeloma protein, no two patients having identical patterns. Electrophoretic heterogeneity was seen only with γ- (i.e. IgG-) myeloma proteins, and polymer-type heterogeneity only with β_{2A}- (i.e. IgA-) myeloma proteins. It is not known whether myeloma protein heterogeneity has any clinical or morphological significance. Figure 2.3 illustrates how the discrete bands in the starch gel may be characterized immunologically. Figure 2.4 shows a typical IgA myeloma pattern obtained by electrophoretic separation in acrylamide gel.

Many workers believe that much of the heterogeneity detected in starch or acrylamide gels could be due to post-synthetic alternations undergone by the protein.

CONDITIONS IN WHICH PARAPROTEINS OCCUR

By far the largest group of patients in whom paraproteins may be found are those with myelomatosis. Essentially a neoplastic disease of plasma cells, this is characterized by the presence of skeletal lesions and is commonly associated with anaemia, hypercalcaemia, impairment of renal function, coagulation defects, and an increased susceptibility to infection. Diagnosis is

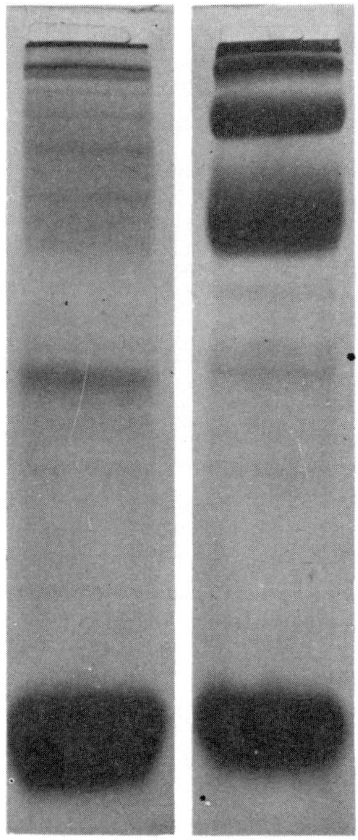

Figure 2.4. Acrylamide gel separation of plasma proteins. Left: normal serum; right: serum from a patient with IgA myeloma. (Reproduced from J. W. Keyser, *Analyt. Biochem.*, 1964, **9**, 249, by permission of Academic Press, Inc.)

based upon the demonstration of a monoclonal protein in the serum or urine, together with radiological evidence of osteolytic lesions (or, in a minority of cases, localized rarefaction or fractures) and the finding of increased numbers of plasma cells in the bone marrow. In about 50 per cent of cases of myelomatosis the paraprotein is IgG, and in about 25 per cent IgA; IgM and IgD myelomas are much less common, and IgE exceedingly rare. In about 20 per cent of cases the only monoclonal protein present is Bence Jones protein (Hobbs).

While about 0.5 per cent of patients with myelomatosis show the presence of an IgM paraprotein, this is more commonly found in macroglobulinaemia, a condition associated commonly with lymphadenopathy, splenic enlargement, and a bleeding tendency, but only rarely with osteolytic lesions. Syndromes with the clinical features of both myelomatosis and macroglobulinaemia also occur (Waldenström, 1962a,b). About 10–15 per cent of patients with macroglobulinaemia have Bence Jones proteinuria.

Urinary Bence Jones proteins are composed of immunoglobulin light chains (Edelman and Gally, 1962), present often in the form of dimers. They belong to either type kappa or type lambda and are relatively homogeneous on electrophoresis.

Heavy-chain diseases

A group of rare conditions is recognized in which heavy-chain fragments corresponding mostly to the Fc portion of the immunoglobulin molecule are excreted in the urine.

γ-Heavy-chain disease

This was the first heavy-chain disease to be described (Franklin *et al.*, 1963, 1964; Osserman and Takatsuki, 1964). The clinical features of the disorder are characteristic, despite some variation in its manifestations (Seligmann, 1972; Frangione and Franklin, 1973), and commonly include lymphadenopathy, anaemia, and fever, often accompanied by malaise, weakness, and hepato- or splenomegaly. The disease can progress rapidly, death occurring usually from infection or malignancy in a few months. In most cases the disease resembles a malignant lymphoma rather than myeloma; however, diagnosis must be based on careful immunochemical characterization of the serum and urine proteins, since other pathological features are variable and not specific (Franklin, 1975).

The γ-heavy-chain disease proteins are a heterogeneous group of molecules ranging from an intact heavy chain (Adlersberg *et al.*, 1975) to proteins having various types of internal deletions. Diagnosis is generally based on demonstration by immunoelectrophoresis of a protein in the serum or urine, or both, which migrates in the β-γ region and reacts with antisera to γ-chains but not with antisera to Fab fragments or light chains. In most cases the abnormal band was broad and heterogeneous and was accompanied by a reduction in the amount of the normal γ-globulins and by a depressed immune response. None of the patients so far (Franklin, 1975) studied had Bence Jones proteinuria.

α-Chain disease

α-Chain disease is the most frequent of the heavy-chain diseases and was first described by Seligmann and his coworkers (Seligmann *et al.*, 1968; Rambaud *et al.*, 1968). It is characterized by a diffuse plasma-cell proliferation which affects the IgA secretory system and results in the synthesis of an abnormal immunoglobulin molecule devoid of light chains and closely related to the Fc fragment of the IgA_1 molecule. Most of the recognized cases of this condition have suffered from severe malabsorption, the plasma-cell infiltrate being localized in the small intestine and mesenteric lymph nodes (Seligmann *et al.*, 1971); however, a respiratory form of the disease has been reported (Stoop *et al.*, 1971; Faux *et al.*, 1973; Florin-Christensen *et al.*, 1974). The pathogenesis of α-chain disease and its possible relationship to 'Mediterranean lymphoma' (Ramot *et al.*, 1965; Eidelman *et al.*, 1966; Seijffers *et al.*, 1968) have been reviewed by Rambaud and Matuchansky (1973).

The protein abnormality is not always readily detectable on routine serum protein electrophoresis, and in a case recently described it was found (Brouet *et al.*, 1977) that the α-chain disease protein, previously present in the patient's serum, had nearly disappeared at the time when lymphoma developed; when the protein is detectable it appears as an abnormal broad band, usually in the α_2- or β-globulin region. (The characteristic narrow band suggestive of a monoclonal immunoglobulin abnormality is always absent.) The serum concentrations of normal IgA, IgG, and IgM are usually decreased; and in most of the cases studied in which the abnormal protein was not noticeable, serum electrophoresis showed only a decrease in the albumin and a moderate to severe hypogammaglobulinaemia. Usually only traces of the abnormal protein occur in the urine. Bence Jones proteinuria is always absent.

μ-Heavy-chain disease

This is probably the least common of the recognized types of heavy-chain disease, only about 8 patients with the condition having been reported. Of these, 6 had chronic lymphocytic leukaemia. Most of the patients produced large amounts of Bence Jones protein. In the majority the only serum protein abnormality found on routine electrophoresis was marked hypogammaglobulinaemia, though in two cases a readily detectable abnormal band was seen. In the majority of cases the diagnosis was made by immunoelectrophoresis, which revealed a rapidly migrating component reacting with antisera to μ-chains but not antisera to light chains. This protein was not found in the urine of any of the patients.

The γ- and μ-heavy-chain diseases and related disorders have been reviewed by Franklin (1975).

Paraproteins in other conditions

Paraproteins are found in patients with a number of other malignant and also several benign immunocytomata. Table 2.1 shows the clinical diagnosis established in a series of nearly 700 patients in whom paraproteins had been detected (Hobbs, 1971a).

Although paraproteins have been reported to occur in patients with non-lymphoplasmocytic disorders such as autoimmune diseases, chronic liver diseases, chronic infections, and various neoplasms, it should be remembered that they are found in a proportion of apparently healthy subjects (Axelsson *et al.*, 1966). Nevertheless, the presence of a paraprotein in the blood or urine of a patient should initially be considered as indicating potential malignancy,

Table 2.1. Diagnosis in 691 patients with paraproteins. (Reproduced from J. R. Hobbs, *Adv. Clin. Chem.*, 1971, **14**, 219, by permission of Academic Press, Inc., and Prof. Hobbs.)

A. *Malignant immunocytomata*		74% of total
Myelomatosis (including 5 plasma cell leukaemia)	420	
Waldenström's macroglobulinaemia	32	
Soft-tissue plasmacytoma	20	
Lymphosarcoma	26	
Reticulosarcoma (including 5 atypical Hodgkin's)	6	
Chronic lymphatic leukaemia	5	
Atypical myelosclerosis	2	
Giant follicular lymphoma	1	
Arabian lymphoma of gut (α-chain)	3	
B. *Benign immunocytomata*		23% of total
(i) Followed up for at least 5 years	112	
(ii) Monoclonal antibody		
Primary cold agglutinins (8 others had lymphoma)	37	
Lichen myxoedematosis	4	
Transient paraproteins	5	
C. *Uncertain*	18	3% of total

and prolonged follow-up is necessary before the condition may be regarded as benign.

RELATIONSHIP OF PARAPROTEINS TO NORMAL IMMUNOGLOBULINS

It is clear that the myeloma proteins and Waldenström-type macroglobulins are closely related to the normal immunoglobulins. Early evidence of their close antigenic relationship (Kunkel *et al.*, 1951) has been fully confirmed, and there is little evidence that these proteins—with one clear exception—are in any way abnormal.

The exception alluded to above is found in the heavy-chain disease syndromes. In one case, studied in detail by Deutsch and his collaborators (Deutsch and Suzuki, 1971; Kunkel and Deutsch, 1971), the special protein, an IgG_1, was found to lack the Gm(f) marker in the Fab region of the immunoglobulin molecule, and detailed investigation of other markers as well as family studies showed that the protein was not a genetic variant but was rather an abnormal product of a specific clone of cells. In a second case, investigated by Osserman and Takatsuki (1963), the heavy-chain protein—again an IgG belonging to subclass 1—was also shown to be an abnormal product arising in one clone of cells and not the product of an altered gene. More recent structural studies have demonstrated large deletions in several of the heavy-chain disease proteins (Frangione and Milstein, 1969; Franklin and Frangione, 1971).

EFFECTS DUE TO PARAPROTEINS

The presence of a paraprotein in the blood can produce a number of effects, perhaps the best known of which is renal damage. In 'myeloma kidney', found in some 10% of patients with myelomatosis, the distal tubules become blocked by casts containing paraproteins (Bence Jones protein and IgA have been identified), with giant cell formation. Another complication is amyloidosis, which can lead to nephrosis and azotaemia. This and other types of renal involvement have been reviewed by Hobbs (1971a).

The interesting finding of a low plasma sodium concentration (e.g. 120 mmol/l) has been reported (Tarail *et al.*, 1962; Frick *et al.*, 1967; Hobbs, 1967) in some patients with IgG myelomatosis. The effect is apparently due to: (1) occupation of normal plasma water space by the large amounts of paraprotein; and (2) the high isoelectric point of the paraprotein, which allows it to act as a base at normal blood pH (Tarail *et al.*, 1962; Frick *et al.*, 1967). Dialysis of the plasma against sodium chloride containing 145 mmol/l fails to raise its sodium content to normal, and this clearly contraindicates any attempt to raise the patient's plasma sodium by administration of electrolytes.

The presence of cryoglobulins can cause symptoms as a result of aggregation on cooling. Raynaud's phenomenon is a common symptom and may be due to four kinds of cold aggregates: cryofibrinogen (see Zlotnick *et al.*, 1969); cold agglutinins; monoclonal cryoglobulins; and mixed cryoglobulins.

The term 'monoclonal cryoglobulin' is used when paraproteins complex with themselves so that the precipitate contains predominantly only the heavy- and light-chain classes of the paraprotein. Such monoclonal cryoglobulins may be IgG or IgM in class, and occur in some 2 per cent of all cases of myelomatosis. IgM cryoglobulins occur in about 6 per cent of all cases of macroglobulinaemia, and are apparently associated especially with lymphosarcoma.

In a few cases Bence Jones protein has been found to precipitate in the cold; however, this occurred below 20 °C and caused no symptoms in the patients.

Many patients with macroglobulinaemia, and a few with other types of paraprotein, exhibit a 'viscosity syndrome', which can be detected by viscosity measurements on whole blood, plasma, or serum. Usually, the viscosity of the blood in macroglobulinaemia is simply related to the serum concentration of IgM, the clinical syndrome presenting at concentrations above 30 g/l. In the case of IgG, IgA, or Bence Jones proteins the viscosity seems to depend on unusual forms of these proteins or on the formation of complexes or polymerization (see below).

Hobbs (1971a) lists the following symptoms and signs directly attributable to the viscosity of such paraproteins: severe lassitude, impaired phagocytosis, impaired platelet function, anaemia, distension of retinal veins (leading to perivenous haemorrhages and blindness), coma, renal failure, and simulation of congestive heart failure. Clearly, many symptoms or findings in patients with monoclonal proteins in the blood are directly referable to the physio-chemical properties of these proteins. For further information the reader is referred to the reviews of Cohen and Martin (1970) and Hobbs (1971a).

Immunological deficiency

One of the most important effects of the production of monoclonal immunoglobulins is a state of immunological deficiency characterized by reduced concentrations of normal immunoglobulins and a diminished capacity to form circulating antibodies. Consequently many patients with myelomatosis suffer from infection, and this is often the cause of death. The reduction in the concentration of normal immunoglobulins is readily demonstrated by electrophoresis on filter paper or cellulose acetate, as well as by immuno-electrophoresis or other methods.

PROGNOSIS OF IMMUNOCYTOMA

Four biochemical features are of great value in distinguishing between malignant and benign immunocytomata (Table 2.2). The presence of immuno-globulin fragments such as Bence Jones protein in the urine, the suppression of normal immunoglobulin synthesis, an elevated concentration of serum paraprotein, and, perhaps most strikingly, a progressive rise in the paraprotein concentration—all these are strongly associated with a poor prognosis.

Rate of growth of tumour

Repeated measurement of the concentration of the paraprotein can provide information on the rate of growth of the tumour clone (Hobbs, 1971b). In

Table 2.2. Biochemical features of value in the prognosis of immunocytomata. (Reproduced, with permission, from J. R. Hobbs, *Brit. Med. J.*, 1971, **i**, 67.)

Feature	Patients with immunocytomata: 517 malignant*	112 benign†
1. Immunoglobulin fragments (Bence Jones protein, etc.)	84%	0%
2. Suppression of normal immunoglobulins	98%	10%
3. Serum paraprotein more than 10 g/l	92%	15%
4. Progressive rise in paraprotein	(of those followed up untreated) 99%	1%

*Proven by biopsy.
†Followed for 5 years.

order to evaluate measurements of paraprotein concentration it is necessary to remember that the exchangeable pool of protein (P) and hence its concentration in the serum is determined by the ratio of its rate of biosynthesis (S)—and hence the number of cells synthesizing it—to its fractional rate of catabolism (K):

$$P = \frac{S}{K}$$

It has been shown that the fractional turnover rate of IgD is much higher than that for IgA or IgM, and that these in turn are much higher than that for IgG (see Waldmann and Strober, 1969). The turnover rate of IgE is even higher than that of IgD (Waldmann *et al.*, 1971). It follows that the tumour masses corresponding to a given concentration of these monoclonal proteins in the serum are much greater in the case of IgE and IgD myeloma than with myelomata associated with the production of IgA or IgM or especially IgG paraproteins. Figure 2.5 illustrates the relationships between the concentrations of IgE, IgA, IgM, and IgG in the serum and the rates of biosynthesis of these proteins. It should be noted that the fractional turnover rate of normal polyclonal IgG increases with increasing concentration of this protein in the plasma; this is reflected in the rapid upward curvature of the line relating rate of biosynthesis (and hence tumour mass) and serum concentration (Figure 2.5). Whether idiotypic IgG paraprotein behaves similarly is uncertain.

Hobbs (1971b) has calculated that to maintain a serum concentration in a 70-kg patient of 28 g IgA paraprotein per litre (i.e. the average concentration at clinical presentation) would require the daily production of about 15 g of the protein, corresponding to about 1 kg of immunocytoma. A comparable figure was obtained from a consideration of the number of myeloma cells in bone marrow biopsies. This mass of tumour would be equivalent to 4.6×10^{11} tumour cells, which, with little more than one further doubling, would become 10^{12} cells and death would ensue. These calculations are broadly in accord with the observations, made before the introduction of the drug melphalan, that less than half the patients with myeloma survived one year from presentation (Feinleib and MacMahon, 1960; Innes and Newall, 1961). Hobbs has also calculated that at the first chance of detecting IgG paraprotein in human serum there could only be about 20 g of immunocytoma, corresponding to some 9×10^9 cells, in a 70-kg patient, and that from such chance detection it would, on average, be 5 years before clinical evidence of myelomatosis emerged. By examining concentrated urine it is possible to detect Bence Jones protein at concentrations of 10 mg/l, corresponding to the excretion of about 14 mg/day, and this could represent as little as 3 g of immunocytoma.

Biochemical differentiation

The original idea that Bence Jones proteins are break-down products of myeloma proteins was disproved when Putnam and Miyake (1958) injected

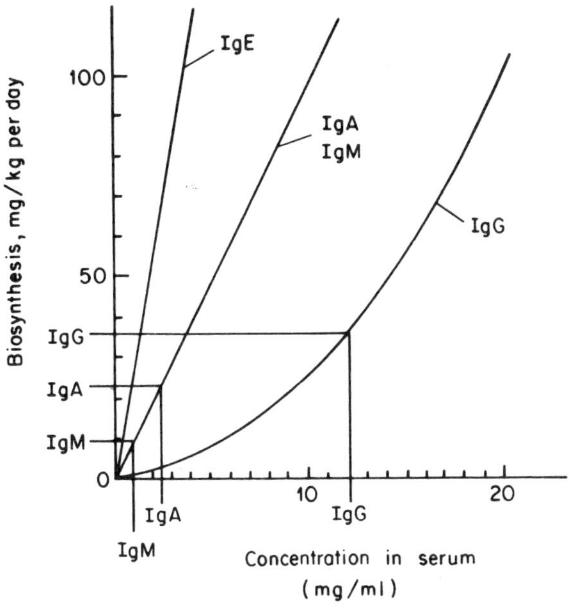

Figure 2.5. Relationships between the concentrations of IgE, IgA, IgM, and IgG in the serum and the rate of biosynthesis of these proteins. (Reproduced from J. F. Heremans and P. L. Masson, *Clin. Chem.*, 1973, **19**, 299, by permission of Dr. Masson and the American Association for Clinical Chemistry.)

labelled glutamate into a patient with myelomatosis and found much higher specific activity in the Bence Jones protein than in the myeloma protein. From the demonstration of *de novo* synthesis of Bence Jones protein Hobbs has developed a concept of 'biochemical dedifferentiation', according to which the malignant myeloma cell has acquired in imbalance in heavy- and light-chain synthesis, presumably by dedifferentiation, and often produces an excess of light-chain protein. In some 20 per cent of patients with myelomatosis this process of dedifferentiation has gone further and only light chains are synthesized and released: such Bence Jones myelomata grow faster, can present in younger persons, appear to be more invasive, and carry a worse prognosis (Hobbs, 1969). A few myelomata produce half light chains and/or only small amounts of Bence Jones proteins in relation to the mass of the tumour; and others, the so-called non-paraprotein myelomata, even fail to produce any recognizable heavy or light chain at all. According to Hobbs (1971b), 'more biochemical dedifferentiation parallels more malignant dedifferentiation'.

MOLECULAR SIZE OF PARAPROTEINS

A high production of monoclonal 19S IgM occurs in some lymphomata, in Waldenström's macroglobulinaemia, in IgM myelomatosis, and in primary cold agglutinin disease. It may also be associated with chronic lymphatic leukaemia and rheumatoid arthritis, and sometimes occurs in benign conditions. The presence of 7S IgM as well as 19S IgM in the serum of some patients has also been reported. Solomon and Kunkel (1967) found 7S IgM in a patient with a neoplastic lesion of the plasma-cell/lymphatic system, and Bush and his coworkers (1969) and Hansson and Laurell (1969) in patients with macroglobulin diseases. The last-named workers separated the 7S subunits from the 19S IgM by means of crossed immunoelectrophoresis, and the other two groups did so by sucrose density-gradient ultracentrifugation.

Using a simple thin-layer 'Sephadex' technique, Carter and Hobbs (1971) investigated sera from 117 patients with diseases associated with a high production of monoclonal IgM. They found that 2 out of 3 patients with IgM myelomatosis, 15 of 33 with lymphoma, and 5 of 25 with Waldenström's macroglobulinaemia had 7S IgM in the serum, but that this was absent from the serum of 9 patients with benign monoclonal macroglobulinaemia. Although the significance of its presence in the serum of adults is unknown, these observations suggest that the finding of 7S IgM in the serum of patients producing monoclonal IgM may be of prognostic significance. 7S IgM has been found in cord serum from the newborn child (Perchalski *et al.*, 1968).

CRYOGLOBULINS

In 1933 Wintrobe and Buell described a case of multiple myeloma in which a precipitate formed in the serum at reduced temperature, to redissolve on heating; and in 1947 Lerner and Watson applied the term *cryoglobulin* to a protein with similar properties from the serum of a patient with glomerulonephritis, urticaria, and purpura. Since then cryoglobulins, i.e. reversibly cold-precipitable globulins, have been found in a variety of clinical conditions. Since cryoglobulins are found in the serum of some patients with myelomatosis it has been suggested that the phenomenon of precipitation in the cold may simply reflect the physicochemical characteristics, such as reduced solubility at low temperatures, of certain homogeneous proteins (Abrams *et al.*, 1949). There is evidence that many cryoglobulins consist of immune complexes, i.e. antigen–antibody complexes; it is suggested that the IgG components of the complex may represent autoantigens, while the IgM or IgA—and in some cases part of the IgG itself—may represent the antibodies; and these mixtures of antigens and antibodies, plus in certain cases co-factors such as complement, may precipitate at reduced temperatures. There is also evidence that in certain infectious diseases the cryoglobulins consist of a complex containing deoxyribonucleic acid, ribonucleic acid, or viruses, with the antibodies to these heteroantigens, together with the co-factors (Andres, 1969). These relationships are summarized in Table 2.3.

Four types of cryoglobulins or *cold aggregates* are recognized.

Table 2.3. Classification of cryoglobulins. (After R. M. Nakamura and E. S. Tucker, *Serum Protein Abnormalities: Diagnostic and Clinical Aspects* (Eds. S. E. Ritzmann and J. C. Daniels), Little, Brown, Boston, 1975, p. 301, by permission of Little, Brown & Co. and Drs. Nakamura and Tucker.)

Type	Immunoglobulins*	Diseases†
Pure monoclonal	IgG, IgM, IgA, or Bence Jones proteins	Myeloma, Waldenström's macroglobulinaemia, lymphoma, other malignancy, cold-agglutinin disease
Mixed monoclonal‡	IgM + IgG, IgA + IgG, IgG + IgG — In each case one component is monoclonal	Primary or secondary Waldenström's macroglobulinaemia, myeloma, lymphoma
Polyclonal	One or more polyclonal immunoglobulins	Rheumatoid arthritis, systemic lupus erythematosus, bacterial or viral infections

*Any of the immunoglobulins may or may not have rheumatoid factor activity.
†In some cases a cryoglobulin is not associated with a specific disease and is called *essential* or *idiopathic*.
‡Many of these contain also specific antigens, antibodies, and complement.

Mixed cryoglobulins

These are the immune complexes referred to above. By lodging in the walls of vessels, where they fix fibrinogen and complement, they cause a vasculitis (which is evident as skin nodules), as well as synovitis, serositis, and glomerulonephritis. Such complexes are found in systemic lumpus erythematosus, rheumatoid arthritis, Sjögren's syndrome, sarcoidosis, leprosy, syphilis, certain viral infections (cytomegalovirus, Epstein–Barr), and post-streptococcal glomerulonephritis. The majority of mixed cryoglobulins contain IgG and IgM. Some, as indicated above, contain deoxyribonucleic acid, and the possible rôle of this in the development of nephritis and vasculitis is discussed in later chapters.

Monoclonal cryoglobulins

Sometimes immunocytomata produce immunoglobulins that polymerize at reduced temperatures, and the term *monoclonal cryoglobulinaemia* is applied to conditions in which this occurs, the cryoprecipitate containing predominantly only the heavy and light chains of the paraprotein. Such cryoglobulins may be IgG or IgM in class, a majority of the IgG cryoglobulins belonging to subclasses IgG_3 and IgG_2 (Virella and Hobbs, 1971). Patients have a tendency to the hyperviscosity syndrome. There are associated skin lesions, which are flat, often with central necrosis, due to occlusion of peripheral vessels.

Cryofibrinogen

This results either from an abnormality affecting the synthesis of fibrinogen, or from some change in the protein occurring after synthesis. Skin lesions, similar to those produced in monoclonal cryoglobulinaemia, can occur, as can thrombophlebitis migrans.

Cold agglutinins

Strictly speaking these are not cryoproteins, since they do not themselves precipitate on cooling; however, they do agglutinate red cells reversibly in the cold, and hence can be considered under the general heading 'cold aggregates'. The presenting clinical features are Raynaud's phenomenon and haemolytic anaemia. Primary cold agglutinins are monoclonal, with one particular subclass of IgM (Cooper *et al.*, 1970) and nearly always kappa-type light chains; those secondary to infections with mycoplasma, rickettsia, listeria, or infectious mononucleosis are transient and polyclonal, with both kappa and lambda light chains (Costea *et al.*, 1966).

Clinical symptoms

Some of the effects of cryoglobulins have been indicated above. Raynaud's phenomenon may be the presenting feature with any of the four types of cold aggregate. Indeed, in monoclonal cryoglobulinaemia the symptoms brought about by cold may be obvious long before the discovery, on follow up, of an invasive immunocytoma. However, if a cryoglobulin does not precipitate above 21°C (i.e. the lowest skin temperature encountered under natural conditions), exposure to cold is unlikely to cause symptoms in the patient.

For further information on cryoglobulins the reader is referred to the review by Hobbs (1971a) (see also Barnett *et al.* (1970), and a study of cryoglobulinaemia in renal diseases by Druet and his colleagues (1973)).

LABORATORY INVESTIGATION OF PARAPROTEINS

Both serum and urine should be examined.

Serum

Since paraproteins are sometimes cryoglobulins (i.e. globulins that precipitate on cooling), the serum should be separated from the cells at 37°C in order to avoid possible loss of the abnormal protein. (The investigation of cryoglobulins is discussed in Appendix 16.) A paraprotein is evident on cellulose acetate or agar gel electrophoresis as a narrow band, usually superimposed on a diffuse background of either normal or diminished immunoglobulins. Occasionally, however, a faint monoclonal band may be found much nearer the anodal part of the pattern, indeed as far anodally as albumin in the case of certain serum Bence Jones proteins (Heremans and Masson, 1973). Electrophoresis on filter paper is far less satisfactory, since small amounts of paraproteins may be completely missed by this method.

A number of proteins can give narrow bands on electrophoresis and may be mistaken for paraproteins. A faint false 'monoclonal' band in the mid-gamma region may be given by C-reactive protein, which is likely to be present in patients with acute inflammatory conditions as well as after various kinds of trauma; haemoglobin produces a band in the β-region; old or uraemic sera produce misleading bands, and so do fibrinogen and its break-down products. The fibrinogen band may obscure the immunoglobulin pattern, especially in the β_2-globulin region, and for this reason serum is to be preferred to plasma for the analysis.

Heremans and Masson (1973) have drawn attention to a source of error which is found in the imbalance that may occur in polyclonal hypergammaglobulinaemia; in extreme cases discrete antibody bands may be misinterpreted as monoclonal bands. The most striking instance is that in which an apparently monoclonal band appears in serum lacking in immunoglobulins, during reconstitutive therapy (marrow graft) of combined immune deficiency, the band subsequently fading and being replaced by a more diffuse zone (Rádl *et al.*, 1972). This is presumably because at the onset of reconstitutive therapy perhaps only one or at most a few immunocyte clones are able to respond to the antigenic stimulation. An analogous mechanism is possibly responsible for the pattern of restricted heterogeneity and predominant IgM concentration commonly found in the fetus or the newborn child with a viral, toxoplasmal, or bacterial infection (Stiehm *et al.*, 1966). Table 2.4 lists the various factors which are responsible for restricted heterogeneity of the immune response and which may consequently pose a problem of differential diagnosis with monoclonal immunoglobulin disorders. Sometimes it is very difficult to distinguish between genuine products of the tumour and homogeneous antibodies, and a decision must often be made on clinical grounds.

Immunoelectrophoretic analysis of the serum will establish the type of heavy and/or light chain present in the paraprotein.

Light-chain typing of paraproteins is a useful though generally not an essential investigation. Kohn (1973) recommends immunoelectrophoresis of serum diluted 1:10 or 1:20 (depending on the amount of paraprotein present); in this way the amount of normal 'background' immunoglobulins is reduced and their interference with the light-chain typing is minimized.

The abnormal component having been characterized as a paraprotein, its concentration in the serum should be measured. This is most easily done by cellulose acetate electrophoresis (see Appendix 5). The use of immunodiffusion methods for this purpose is unsatisfactory unless a specimen of the pure paraprotein is available as a standard.

A progressive rise in the concentration of paraprotein indicates a poor prognosis.

Table 2.4. Factors responsible for restricted heterogeneity of the immune response. (Reproduced from J. F. Heremans and P. L. Masson, *Clin. Chem.*, 1973, **19**, 294, with the permission of the American Association for Clinical Chemistry and Dr. Masson.)

Factors	Examples
1. Factors involving the antigen	Antibodies to blood groups A_1 (Rochant *et al.*, 1972) or I (Feizi, 1967; de Boissezon *et al.*, 1970)
Nature of the antigen (few antigenic determinants or special steric requirements for fitting of antibody)	Restricted heterogeneity Ig patterns in acute viral diseases?
2. Factors involving the host (immunological immaturity: few clones available)	Restricted heterogeneity (pseudomonoclonal) patterns in immune deficiency, especially after marrow graft (Rádl *et al.*, 1972)
	Restricted heterogeneity and IgM predominance in infections of fetus or newborn
3. Factors involving host–antigen interaction	
(a) Mucosal portal of entry (favouring IgA response)	Rise of serum IgA during urinary infections
(b) Restriction of the antigen to a site poor in immuno-competent cells (clonal selection between few competitors)	Pronounced banding in cerebrospinal fluid immunoglobulins in chronic infectious or autoimmune diseases of the brain (see Chapter 10)
(c) Prolonged low-grade stimulation due to persistence of antigen (exhaustive clonal selection)	Restricted heterogeneity on dense background in autoimmune disorders and chronic parasitic diseases of the blood (filariasis) (Michaux, 1966)

Serum immunoglobulins of classes other than that of the paraprotein (e.g. IgA and IgM in the case of an IgG myeloma) should be measured. Malignant monoclonal proliferations are usually associated with diminished production of all the immunoglobulin classes, including the polyclonal part of that class to which the paraprotein itself belongs, whereas this phenomenon is not seen in benign conditions.

Molecular size of paraproteins

This may be of some prognostic significance (see above) and can be investigated by the simple technique described in Appendix 15.

Urine

The urine, cleared of bacteria by passage through an ultrafilter with a pore size of 0.2 μm, is concentrated 300-fold and subjected to electrophoresis in parallel with the patient's serum. Failure to remove bacteria may result in extensive loss of Bence Jones protein during the concentration process. In addition, immunoelectrophoresis should be performed and the paraprotein typed with anti-kappa and anti-lambda sera.

Light chains occur normally in the urine in small concentrations, and increased concentrations of these normal B-chains are found in a number of other conditions besides myeloma. They may be distinguished from Bence Jones protein by their more diffuse electrophoretic mobility and by their containing both kappa and lambda classes of light chain.

Investigation of cryoglobulins

For the detection of cryoglobulins the plasma or serum must be separated at 37 °C. The specimen is then kept at 4 °C and examined at intervals as described in Appendix 16; any cold aggregate is then redissolved and its temperature of precipitation ascertained by careful cooling. Most cryoproteins causing symptoms on exposure to cold precipitate above 28 °C (Hobbs, 1971a).

It is important to differentiate monoclonal from mixed cryoglobulins. The latter are distinguished from other types of cold aggregate by their content of usually more than one class of heavy chain and both types of light chain. According to Hobbs (1971a) careful measurement of immunoglobulins both in serum kept at 37 °C (with the addition of azide to inhibit bacterial action) and in the supernatant obtained after keeping the serum at 4 °C can indicate how much IgM, IgG, or IgA has been removed in the precipitate. Alternatively the immunoglobulin content of the cryoprecipitate itself may be measured (Barnett *et al.*, 1970). The best assessment would appear to be based on gel filtration with 'Sephadex' G-200 (Barnett *et al.*, 1970).

REFERENCES

Abrams, A., P. P. Cohen, and O. O. Meyer (1949), *J. Biol. Chem.*, **181**, 237.

Adlersberg, J. B., E. C. Franklin, and B. Frangione (1975), *Proc. Nat. Acad. Sci.*, **72**, 723.

Andres, G. A. (1969), *Vox Sang.*, **16**, 345.

Axelsson, U., R. Bachmann, and J. Hallen (1966), *Acta. Med. Scand.*, **179**, 235.

Barnett, E. V., R. Bluestone, A. Cracchiolo, III, L. S. Goldberg, G. L. Kantor, and R. M. McIntosh (1970), *Ann. Int. Med.*, **73**, 95.

Brouet, J. C., D. Y. Mason, F. Danon, J. L. Preud'homme, M. Seligmann, F. Reyes, F. Navab, A. Galian, E. Rene, and J. C. Rambaud (1977), *Lancet*, **i**, 861.

Bush, S. T., H. A. Swedlund, and G. J. Gleich (1969), *J. Lab. Clin. Med.*, **73**, 194.

Carter, P. M., and J. R. Hobbs (1971), *Brit. Med. J.*, **ii**, 260.

Cohen, S., and N. H. Martin (1970), in *Biochemical Disorders in Human Disease*, 3rd ed. (Eds. R. H. S. Thompson and I. D. P. Wootton), Churchill, London, p. 523.

Cooper, A. G., S. I. Chavin, and E. C. Franklin (1970), *Immunochem.*, **7**, 479.

Costea, N., V. Yakulis, and P. Heller (1966), *Science*, **152**, 1520.

de Boissezon, J. F., Y. Marty, R. Bierme, and J. Ducos (1970), *Ann. Inst. Pasteur, Paris*, **119**, 141.

Deutsch, H. F., and T. Suzuki (1971), *J. Immunol.*, **107**, 929.

Druet, P., P. Letonturier, A. Contet, and C. Mandet (1973), *Clin. Exp. Immunol.*, **15**, 483.
Edelman, G. M., and J. A. Gally (1962), *J. Exp. Med.*, **116**, 207.
Eidelman, S., R. A. Parkins, and C. Rubin (1966), *Medicine (Baltimore)*, **45**, 111.
Engle, R. L., Jr., K. R. Woods, G. B. Castillo, and J. H. Pert (1961), *J. Lab. Clin. Med.*, **58**, 1.
Fahey, J. L. (1961), *J. Exp. Med.*, **114**, 399.
Fahey, J. L. (1963), *J. Clin. Invest.*, **42**, 111.
Faux, J. A., J. D. Crain, F. S. Rosen, and E. Merler (1973), *Clin. Immunol. Immunopath.*, **1**, 282.
Feinleib, M., and B. MacMahon (1960), *J. Nat. Cancer Inst.*, **24**, 1259.
Feizi, T. (1967), *Nature*, **215**, 540.
Fine, J. M., R. Creyssel, and P. Morel (1959), *Rev. Hémat.*, **14**, 75.
Florin-Christensen, A., D. Doniach, and P. B. Newcomb (1974), *Brit. Med. J.*, **ii**, 413.
Flynn, F. V., and E. A. Stow (1958), *J. Clin. Path.*, **11**, 338.
Frangione, B., and E. C. Franklin (1973), *Semin. Hémat.*, **10**, 53.
Frangione, B., and C. Milstein (1969), *Nature*, **223**, 807.
Franklin, E. C. (1975), *J. Clin. Path.*, **27**, Suppl. (Assoc. Clin. Path.) 6, 65.
Franklin, E. C., and B. Frangione (1971), *J. Immunol.*, **107**, 1527.
Franklin, E. C., M. Meltzer, F. Guggenheim, and J. Lowenstein (1963), *Fed. Proc.*, **22**, 264.
Franklin, E. C., J. Lowenstein, B. Bigelow, and M. Meltzer (1964), *Amer. J. Med.*, **37**, 332.
Frick, P. G., J. R. Schmid, H. J. Kistler, and W. H. Hitzig (1967), *Helv. Med. Acta.*, **33**, 317.
Hansson, U.-B., and C.-B. Laurell (1969), *Scand, J. Clin. Lab. Invest.*, **24**, 199.
Heremans, J. F., and P. L. Masson (1973), *Clin. Chem.*, **19**, 294.
Hobbs, J. R. (1967), *Medical News*, Nov., 10.
Hobbs, J. R. (1969), *Brit. J. Haematol.*, **16**, 607.
Hobbs, J. R. (1971a), *Adv. Clin. Chem.*, **14**, 219.
Hobbs, J. R. (1971b), *Brit. Med. J.*, **i**, 67.
Innes, J., and J. Newall (1961), *Lancet*, **i**, 239.
Keyser, J. W. (1964), *Analyt Biochem.*, **9**, 249.
Kohn, J. (1973), in *Recent Advances in Clinical Pathology*, Series 6 (Ed. S. C. Dyke), Churchill Livingstone, Edinburgh and London, p. 363.
Kunkel, H. G., and H. F. Deutsch (1971), *J. Immunol.*, **107**, 930.
Kunkel, H. G., R. J. Slater, and R. A. Good (1951), *Proc. Soc. Exp. Biol. Med.*, **76**, 190.
Laurell, C.-B. (1961), *Acta. Med. Scand.*, Suppl. 367, 17.
Lerner, A. B., and C. J. Watson (1947), *Amer. J. Med. Sci.*, **214**, 410.
Michaux, J. L. (1966), *Ann. Soc. Belge Méd. Trop.*, **46**, 483.
Natvig, J. B., and H. G. Kunkel (1973), *Adv. Immunol.*, **16**, 1.
Osserman, E. F., and K. Takatsuki (1963), *Medicine (Baltimore)*, **42**, 357.
Osserman, E. F., and K. Takatsuki (1964), *Amer. J. Med.*, **37**, 351.
Owen, J. A., C. Got, and H. J. Silberman (1958), *Clin. Chim. Acta*, **3**, 605.
Perchalski, J. E., L. W. Clem, and J. A. Small, Jr. (1968), *Amer. J. Med. Sci.*, **256**, 107.
Putnam, F. W., and A. Miyake (1958), *J. Biol. Chem.*, **231**, 671.
Rádl, J., L. F. Dooren, V. P. Eijsvoogel, J. J. Van Went, and W. Hijmans (1972), *Clin. Exp. Immunol.*, **10**, 367.
Rambaud, J. C., and C. Matuchansky (1973), *Lancet*, **i**, 1430.
Rambaud, J. C., C. Bognel, A. Prost, J. J. Bernier, Y. Le Quintrec, A. Lambling, F. Danon, D. Hurez, and M. Seligmann (1968), *Digestion*, **1**, 321.
Ramot, B., N. Shanin, and J. J. Bubis (1965), *Israel J. Med. Sci.*, **1**, 221.
Rochant, H., H. Tonthat, M. F. Etievant, L. Intrator, R. Sylvestre, and B. Dreyfus (1972), *Vox. Sang.*, **22**, 45.
Seijffers, M. J., M. Levy, and G. Hermann (1968), *Gastroenterology*, **55**, 118.
Seligmann, M. (1972), *Rev. Europ. Etud. Clin. Biol.*, **17**, 349.

Seligmann, M., F. Danon, D. Hurez, E. Mihaesco, and J. L. Preud'homme (1968), *Science*, **162**, 1396.
Seligmann, M., E. Mihaesco, and B. Frangione (1971), *Ann. N. Y. Acad. Sci.*, **190**, 487.
Solomon, A., and H. G. Kunkel (1967), *Amer. J. Med.*, **42**, 1334.
Stiehm, E. R., R. J. Ammann, and J. D. Cherry (1966), *New Engl. J. Med.*, **275**, 971.
Stoop, J. W., R. E. Ballieux, W. Hijmans, and B. J. M. Zegers (1971), *Clin. Exp. Immunol.*, **9**, 625.
Tarail, R., K. W. Buchwald, J. F. Holland, and O. S. Selawry (1962), *Proc. Soc. Exp. Biol. Med.*, **110**, 145.
Virella, G., and J. R. Hobbs (1971), *Clin. Exp. Immunol.*, **9**, 973.
Waldenström, J. (1962a), *Progr. Allergy*, **6**, 320.
Waldenström, J. (1962b), *Progr. Haematol.*, **3**, 266.
Waldmann, T. A., and W. Strober (1969), *Progr. Allergy*, **13**, 1.
Waldmann, T. A., W. Strober, and R. M. Blaese (1971), *Progr. Immunol.*, Academic Press, New York, p. 891.
Wintrobe, M. M., and M. V. Buell (1933), *Bull. Johns Hopkins Hosp.*, **52**, 156.
Zlotnick, A., W. Shahin, and E. A. Rachmilewitz (1969), *Acta Haematol.*, **42**, 8.

CHAPTER 3

Liver diseases

The rôle of the liver in synthesizing most of the plasma proteins, with the exception of the immunoglobulins, is well established; and it is not surprising, therefore, that diseases of the liver often result in substantial changes in the concentrations of various plasma proteins. These changes are slow to develop, however, and do not immediately reflect acute liver damage. It has been calculated, for example, that complete cessation of albumin synthesis—were this to occur—would result in only a 25 per cent decrease in the serum concentration after about 8 days. Consequently patients with severe viral hepatitis may initially be found to have normal serum albumin concentrations. In chronic liver disease the characteristic findings are lowered serum albumin and raised globulin concentrations, and the combined effect of these changes may be a total protein concentration with normal limits. Possible reasons for the rise in the concentration of serum globulin are discussed below.

The investigation of serum proteins in diseases of the liver and biliary tract has involved several types of procedures: serum albumin estimation, turbidity and flocculation tests, estimations of enzyme activity, seromucoid estimation, electrophoresis, and, more recently, specific immunochemical determinations of various globulins. These immunochemical determinations have enabled many of the older electrophoretic observations to be reinterpreted in terms of specific changes in the globulins.

It will be convenient to dispose briefly of the flocculation tests and seromucoid estimation and then to consider the electrophoretic and specific protein changes and changes in enzyme activity found in various types of liver disease.

TURBIDITY AND FLOCCULATION TESTS

It is often necessary to distinguish between hepatocellular disease and extrahepatic obstruction as a cause of jaundice, and these tests, often loosely called flocculation tests, have played an important part in aiding differential diagnosis. Results are usually positive in hepatocellular disease and negative in cholestatic jaundice; however, positive results are also found in such primarily non-hepatic diseases as malaria, infectious mononucleosis, kala-azar, myelomatosis, and the collagen diseases.

Tests of this type include the cephalin–cholesterol flocculation (Hanger, 1939), thymol turbidity (Maclagan, 1944), and zinc sulphate (Kunkel, 1947) tests. These and a number of other flocculation tests appear to depend on an increase in the γ-globulin concentration, especially if the albumin concentration is reduced (Maclagan, 1948). In the thymol turbidity test, phospholipid is necessary for the production of turbidity (Maclagan and Bunn, 1947). Maclagan and Bunn (1947) furthermore demonstrated not only that albumin inhibits this reaction but also that in hepatitis it is a less effective inhibitor than is normal albumin. The mechanism and interrelationships of the various flocculation tests were reviewed by Maclagan and his associates (1952) and by Reinhold (1955).

SEROMUCOID

Seromucoid is the name given to the mixture of proteins—mainly α_1-acid glycoprotein—soluble in 0.6 M perchloric acid (Winzler *et al.*, 1948). Greenspan and his colleagues (Greenspan *et al.*, 1951, 1952; Greenspan and Dreiling, 1953; Greenspan, 1954) reported that many patients with hepatocellular disease had low serum concentrations of seromucoid whereas in obstructive biliary disease and in hepatomegaly due to metastatic carcinoma high values were frequent. Estimation of the seromucoid concentration was accordingly proposed as an aid to the differential diagnosis of jaundice. Mandel and his coworkers (1955) confirmed the presence of subnormal concentrations in patients with benign and malignant biliary obstruction. However, since complications likely to raise the seromucoid concentration were present in most of their patients with 'primary' hepatic disease, only a minority of these had a subnormal concentration; and even after exclusion of patients with extrahepatic complications the incidence of diagnostic, subnormal seromucoid concentrations was far below that expected from earlier reports. They concluded that although the finding of such a subnormal concentration in a jaundiced patient is strongly indicative of parenchymal disease of the liver, this diagnosis cannot be excluded by a normal or increased concentration; furthermore, the finding of normal or increased concentrations of seromucoid is of very limited value, since these may be due to a variety of causes. More recent observations have supported the finding of Mandel and his colleagues of a lowered seromucoid concentration in only a minority of patients with hepatocellular disease, while confirming the existence of elevations in most patients with obstructive jaundice and especially in patients with obstruction due to carcinoma or with secondary deposits in the liver (Keyser *et al.*, 1962).

Shields and his colleagues (1963), who made a similar study, concluded that the estimation of seromucoid was of great value in distinguishing hepatic from post-hepatic jaundice.

The estimation of seromucoid would appear to have a place in the differential diagnosis of hepatobiliary disease, provided the results are interpreted cautiously, with due regard to the many factors that can influence the concentration of this fraction. Because of this limitation it is not to be expected that the estimation will help decisively in more than a minority of cases.

Other applications of seromucoid estimations have been reviewed (Keyser, 1964).

ELECTROPHORESIS

In the 1940s and 1950s many investigators studied the electrophoretic changes found in various disorders of the liver and biliary tract. Although most of their observations were made with filter paper as the supporting medium, their conclusions appear to be essentially in accord with more recent findings based on the use of cellulose acetate. The main findings may be summarized briefly as follows.

In chronic liver disease there is a lowering of the serum albumin concentration and an increase in γ-globulin. As mentioned above, this change forms the basis of the flocculation tests. The fall in serum albumin concentration is only slight in mild or early infective hepatitis, but in severe cases it is more pronounced. Particularly low values are found in diffuse hepatic fibrosis.

A striking increase in the concentration of γ-globulin is found in hepatic cirrhosis. This seems to be due to an increased production of γ-globulins and not to delayed removal from the blood (Havens *et al.*, 1954). It has been suggested that the liver may normally play an important rôle in regulating the immune response to exogenous antigens through its ability to sequester them and possibly render them non-immunogenic (Franzl, 1962), and that hyperglobulinaemia in chronic liver disease may be due to failure of the diseased liver to perform this function (Triger and Wright, 1973). Whatever the mechanism, the electrophoretic pattern of the serum proteins in hepatic cirrhosis is rather characteristic: in addition to the decrease in albumin, the appearance of fast-moving γ-globulins leads to poor resolution between the β- and γ-globulin bands, with the appearance of a β–γ 'veil' or 'bridge'. This β–γ fusion is largely the result of an increase in the concentration of IgA, which mainly has γ_1-globulin mobility. A further feature of the cirrhotic pattern is a normal α_2-globulin concentration; and in some cases the finding of an increased γ-globulin together with a normal α_2-globulin concentration may help in differentiating diffuse hepatic fibrosis from a secondary hepatic neoplasm, in the presence of which there tends to be a normal γ-globulin with an increased α_2-globulin fraction (Seibert *et al.*, 1947; Rafsky *et al.*, 1950; Kay, 1954): The absence of an increase in the α_2-globulin in chronic hepatic disease is attributed to impairment of liver function, since a rise in this fraction, due largely to an increased production of haptoglobins and α_2-macroglobulin, is found in most diseases, as well as after trauma (see Chapter 8).

In infective hepatitis the γ-globulin fraction tends to rise with increasing hepatocellular damage (Ricketts and Sterling, 1949; Hartmann and Steinebach, 1950; Viollier, 1951; Church and Blackburn, 1954), and an increased γ-globulin concentration appears to be a most unfavourable finding (Owen and Robertson, 1956).

In obstructive jaundice there is an increase in the α_1- and β-globulins, and this is correlated with the concentration of serum lipids. This pattern may be useful in distinguishing biliary obstruction from non-biliary cirrhosis: a high concentration of lipoproteins strongly supports a biliary aetiology, especially if there is little lowering of the albumin concentration (Sherlock, 1971). In this connexion it is important to note that, unless specific lipoprotein staining is employed, paper or cellulose acetate electrophoresis does not record the increase in the β-globulin fraction due to lipoprotein that was found by means of the classical Tiselius method in the jaundice of extrahepatic biliary obstruction and the 'obstructive' phase of infective hepatitis.

The classical electrophoretic pattern of chronic liver disease contrasts with that of chronic aggressive hepatitis (formerly called 'juvenile cirrhosis'), in which the serum albumin concentration can be maintained, the α_2-globulin is initially raised and the γ-globulin usually shows a large increase from the onset of the disease. An additional important feature of the electrophoretic pattern is, in many cases, an absence of β–γ fusion, and this serves to distinguish 'juvenile cirrhosis' from other types of cirrhosis (excluding biliary) (Hobbs, 1967). This absence of β–γ fusion is apparently due to the fact that the increase in the γ-globulin fraction is largely in the slow IgG, there being no increase in IgA and a reduction in β_{1C}-globulin (Hobbs, 1966). Chronic aggressive hepatitis, as well as certain other liver diseases, has been suspected of having an autoimmune origin; however, destruction of liver cells as a response to an autoimmune process does not appear to have been demonstrated.

There is evidence, however, that some diseases of the liver are accompanied by processes closely associated with autoimmune phenomena (Doniach *et al.*, 1966; Doniach and Walker, 1969). Among the hepatic diseases fulfilling the criteria of primary autoimmune disorders are, according to Read (1971): active chronic hepatitis, primary biliary cirrhosis, the liver disease accompanying certain collagen diseases, and possibly cryptogenic cirrhosis. Immunological aspects of liver disease have been reviewed by Wright (1975) and by Sherlock (1977).

The serum electrophoretic pattern in haemolytic jaundice may show an increase in γ-globulin, again without β–γ fusion; the albumin concentration is normal, while the α_1-globulin is raised and the α_2-globulin lowered. This latter feature is of some diagnostic importance, and is a result of the binding of haemoglobin with haptoglobin and the rapid removal of the complex. If the α_2-globulin is found to be increased the presence of haemolytic jaundice is unlikely.

It should be noted that a normal serum electrophoretic pattern in the presence of jaundice can be very informative in largely excluding a pre-existing cirrhosis, provided the patient has not had a massive transfusion of blood (Hobbs, 1967).

An increase in the concentration of γ-globulin found one or two weeks after the onset of jaundice is an indication of an infective aetiology. It is not diagnostic of viral hepatitis, being found also in glandular fever, infective cholangitis, and serum sickness.

Figure 3.1 summarizes many of the points mentioned above and illustrates six types of serum electrophoretic pattern which can be helpful in the differential diagnosis of jaundice.

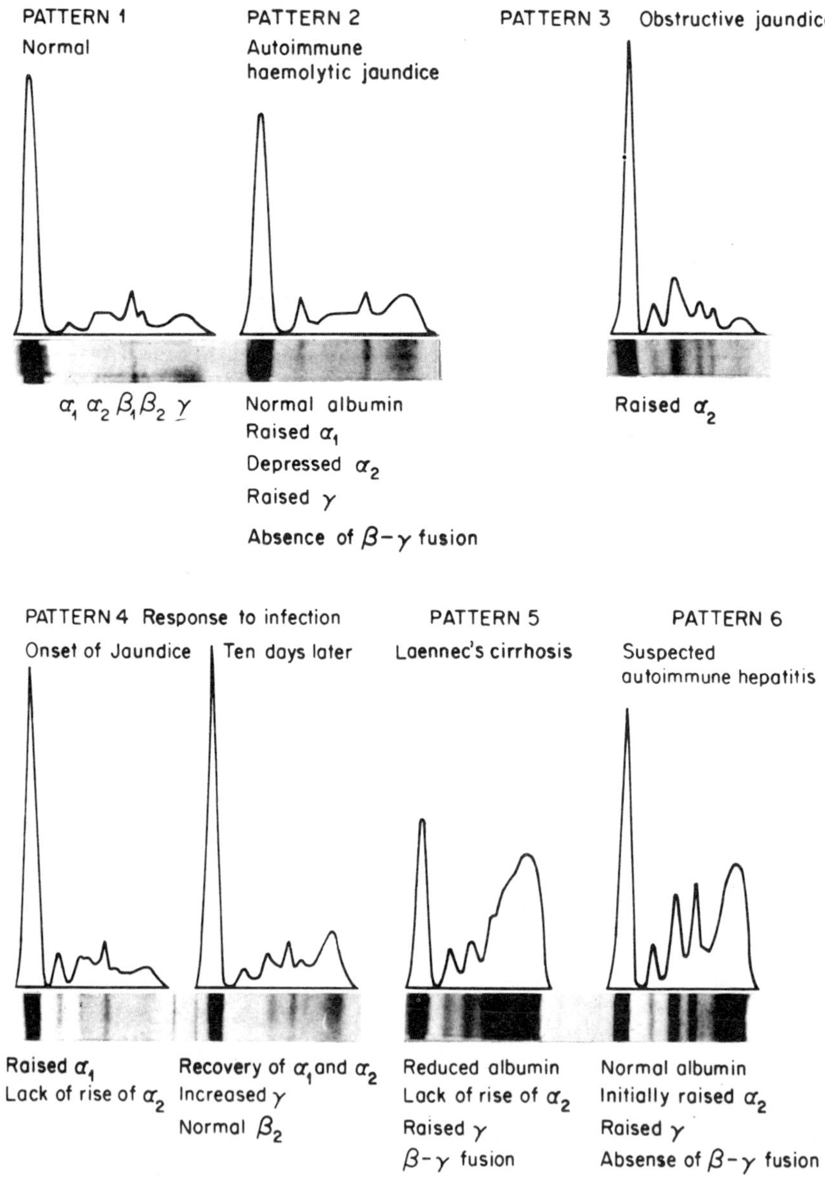

Figure 3.1. Six patterns of serum electrophoresis on cellulose acetate which can be helpful in the differential diagnosis of jaundice. (Reproduced from J. R. Hobbs, *Proc. Roy. Soc. Med.*, 1967, **60**, 1250, by permission of The Royal Society of Medicine and Professor Hobbs.)

SPECIFIC PROTEIN CHANGES IN LIVER DISEASE

Immunoglobulins

A large number of investigators have studied immunoglobulin concentrations in patients with liver disease. The following brief outline of the main findings is based on the summary of Hobbs (1967), who gives references to some twenty publications.

A dominant increase in IgM occurs in primary biliary cirrhosis, though in some cases the disease overlaps with chronic aggressive hepatitis and then both IgG and IgM may be raised. Both of these patterns are distinct from that seen in secondary biliary cirrhosis (Hobbs, 1966), when IgG, IgA, and IgM are all, typically, increased to about twice the mean normal concentrations. A dominant increase in IgM can also be found in the early stages of acute hepatitis; later a less striking increase in IgG may follow.

A dominant increase in IgG occurs in macronodular chronic aggressive hepatitis. In this condition the IgG concentration correlates well with the clinical condition of the patient, falling with improvement on treatment with prednisone.

A dominant increase in IgA is found in the micronodular Laennec type of cirrhosis, which may result from damage by alcohol or iron and occurs in Wilson's disease.

A raised IgA concentration may be associated with heavy drinking, in the absence of overt liver disease, as well as in alcoholism (Varsamis *et al.*, 1974).

Figures 3.2–3.5 show the serum immunoglobulin patterns characteristic of a variety of diseases. Although none of the patterns is absolutely specific for a particular liver disease, measurement of the serum immunoglobulins can, according to Hobbs (1967), be very helpful in the differential diagnosis of liver diseases. It must be noted, however, that overlapping does occur among the various diagnostic groups, and in a proportion of cases the immunoglobulin measurements may prove to be of little value; thus, markedly raised concentrations of IgG, IgA, and IgM were found by Feizi (1968) among patients in almost all the diagnostic groups that he studied.

α-Fetoprotein and primary carcinoma of the liver

The appearance of fetal antigens in the blood of patients with neoplastic diseases is well recognized. One of these antigens, α-fetoprotein, is a normal constituent of the plasma in the human fetus, where it reaches its maximum concentration between the twelfth and sixteenth weeks of fetal life (Gitlin and Boesman, 1966; Foli *et al.*, 1969). The concentration falls rapidly after birth and the protein is virtually absent from the serum of healthy children and adults, though sensitive radioimmunoassay techniques have demonstrated that extremely small amounts persist and that these are increased in pregnancy. The protein reappears in patients with primary carcinoma of the

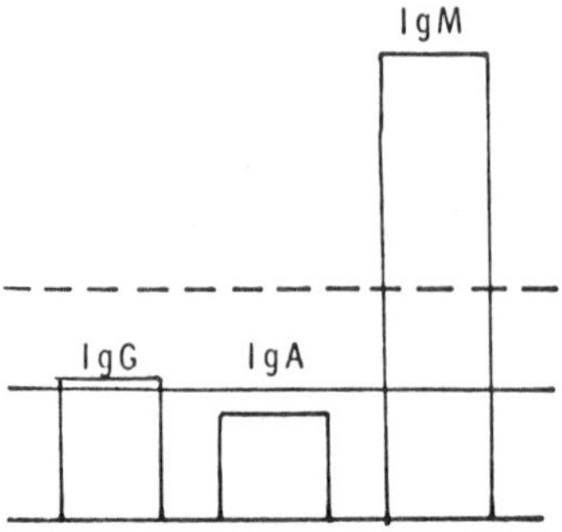

Figure 3.2 Serum immunoglobulin pattern typical of primary biliary cirrhosis. The solid line represents the 100% mean normal adult concentration, the broken line the 2SD upper limit of normal. In over half the patients the serum IgM concentration is above that shown and in 95% it exceeds the upper limit of normal. This pattern also occurs with trypanosomiasis, toxoplasmosis, syphilis, rubella, bartonellosis, Q fever, tropical splenomegaly, New Guinea amyloidosis, and some patients with fibrosing alveolitis. (Reproduced from J. R. Hobbs, *Brit. J. Hosp. Med.*, 1970, **3**, 669, by permission of Hospital Medical Publications Ltd. and Prof. Hobbs.)

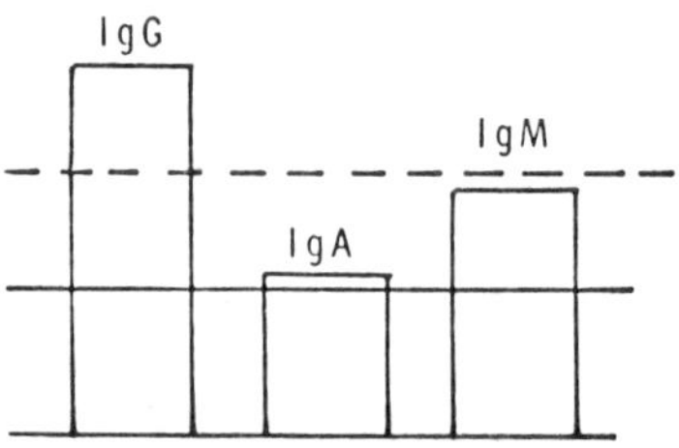

Figure 3.3. Serum immunoglobulin pattern typical of chronic aggressive hepatitis. Lines as in Figure 3.2. 98% of patients have an IgG above the upper normal limit. This pattern is also seen in systematic lupus erythematosus, leprosy, and some patients with scleroderma or malaria. (Reproduced from J. R. Hobbs, *Brit. J. Hosp. Med.*, 1970, **3**, 669, by permission of Hospital Medical Publications Ltd. and Prof. Hobbs.)

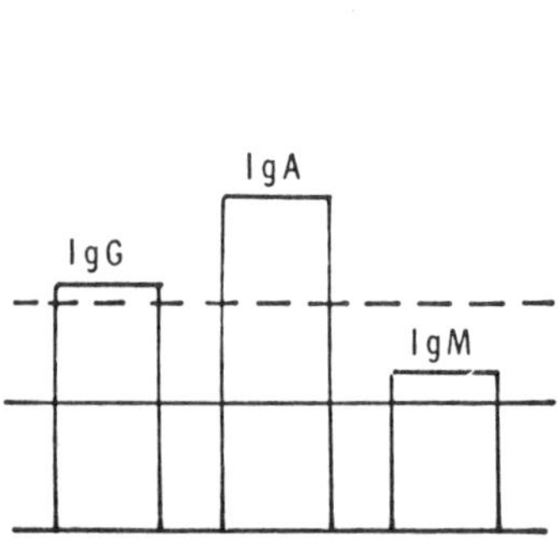

Figure 3.4. Serum immunoglobulin pattern typical of Laennec's micronodular cirrhosis. Lines as in Figure 3.2. 95% of patients have an IgA above the upper normal limit. This pattern is also seen in rheumatic fever, Sjögren's syndrome, infantile malabsorption, and some cases of acute nephritis and fibrosing alveolitis; while IgA elevation is seen in a whole range of gut, chest, and skin diseases, these do not so often have an associated elevation of IgG. (Reproduced from J. R. Hobbs, *Brit. J. Hosp. Med.*, 1970, **3**, 669, by permission of Hospital Medical Publications Ltd. and Prof. Hobbs.)

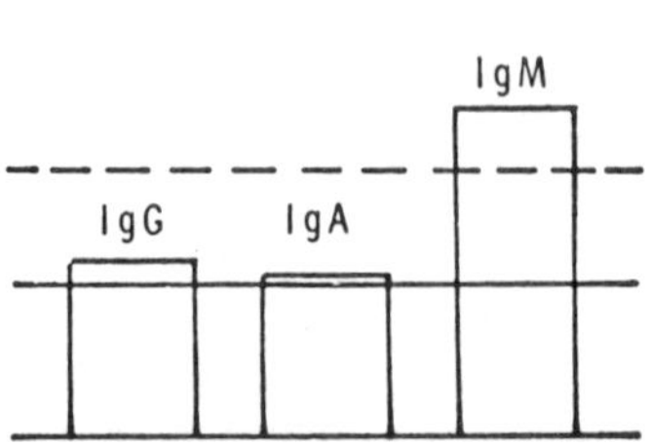

Figure 3.5. Serum immunoglobulin pattern typical of acute hepatitis. Lines as in Figure 3.2. 86% of patients have an IgM above the upper limit of normal. This pattern is also seen in malaria, filariasis, pneumocystis, brucellosis, listeriosis, mycoplasma, Q fever, typhus, and other viral infections. (Reproduced from J. R. Hobbs, *Brit. J. Hosp. Med.*, 1970, **3**, 669, by permission of Hospital Medical Publications Ltd. and Prof. Hobbs.)

liver (Tatarinov, 1965; Abelev, 1968), and its presence, in amounts often detectable by simple immunodiffusion tests, is strong evidence for the diagnosis (Uriel *et al.*, 1967; Alpert *et al.*, 1968). However, increased amounts are also found in a proportion of patients with embryonal tumours of the ovary and testis (Masopust *et al.*, 1968; Bourgeaux *et al.*, 1971) and transiently in patients with acute viral hepatitis associated with the presence of Australia antigen (p. 54) (Smith, 1971). Since the aetiology of primary carcinoma of the liver is unknown, it is of interest that, of 5 patients with cirrhosis complicated by this condition and showing positive tests for Australia (hepatitis-associated) antigen, 2 were also found to have raised α-fetoprotein concentrations (Sherlock *et al.*, 1970). This suggests that viral hepatitis, and the cirrhosis which in rare cases follows it, might represent a pre-cancerous condition (Sherlock *et al.*, 1970).

Ruoslahti, Salaspuro, and their colleagues (1974) found raised serum α-fetoprotein concentrations in some 10 per cent of patients with liver diseases other than primary liver cancer, and suggested that such raised concentrations might reflect the extent of regeneration.

Although, as mentioned above, greatly increased serum concentrations of α-fetoprotein are mostly indicative of primary carcinoma of the liver, there have been reports of positive tests in gastric and pancreatic carcinoma (Bourreille *et al.*, 1970; Alpert *et al.*, 1971b; Andrieu *et al.*, 1971; Bernades *et al.*, 1971., Kozower *et al.*, 1971; Mehlman *et al.*, 1971); most of the patients were found to have liver metastases. Serum α-fetoprotein is also sometimes increased in infants with hepatitis (Masopust *et al.*, 1968; Kang *et al.*, 1972) and occasionally in adults with cirrhosis or hepatitis (O'Conor *et al.*, 1970; Kresno *et al.*, 1970). The findings in Indian childhood cirrhosis are conflicting (Nayak *et al.*, 1972; Agarwal *et al.*, 1974).

Estimation of the serum α-fetoprotein concentration was found to be helpful in differentiating between neonatal hepatitis and biliary atresia, hepatitis being associated with high concentrations (Zeltzer *et al.*, 1974). It was suggested that in neonatal hepatitis the proliferating hepatocytes may have an increased capacity to revert to a fetal state, with a renewal of α-fetoprotein synthesis, whereas in biliary atresia there is proliferation of bile-duct endothelium, which is incapable of synthesizing α-fetoprotein. Kattamis and his colleagues (1974) suggested that differentiation is aided by testing for Australia antigen (see below) at the same time. They also found that failure to detect α-fetoprotein by counter-electrophoresis suggests a poor prognosis.

Serial measurement of serum α-fetoprotein concentrations may be helpful in assessing the results of liver transplantation in patients with hepatoma (Alpert *et al.*, 1971c).

The use of α-fetoprotein estimations as a screening test for detecting fetal neural-tube abnormalities is discussed in Chapter 11.

Carcinoembryonic antigen (CEA) in liver diseases

Carcinoembryonic antigen (CEA) is a tumour-associated protein which is

Table 3.1. Hepatobiliary diseases in which raised plasma CEA concentrations have been reported

Disease	References
Metastases to liver	Dhar *et al.*, 1972; Meeker *et al.*, 1973; Chu and Nemoto, 1973
Hepatoma	Lo Gerfo *et al.*, 1971; Laurence *et al.*, 1972; Dykes and King, 1972; Booth *et al.*, 1973; Khoo and Mackay, 1973
Carcinoma of gall-bladder, bile ducts	Lo Gerfo *et al.*, 1971; Dykes and King, 1972; Booth *et al.*, 1973
Cirrhosis (mostly alcoholic)	Lo Gerfo *et al.*, 1971; Dykes and King, 1972; Moore *et al.*, 1972; Booth *et al.*, 1973; Khoo and Mackay, 1973
Viral hepatitis	Booth *et al.*, 1973
Active chronic hepatitis	Booth *et al.*, 1973; Khoo and Mackay, 1973
Cholecystitis	Lo Gerfo *et al.*, 1971; Meeker *et al.*, 1973; Booth *et al.*, 1973; Hansen *et al.*, 1974
Cholelithiasis	Hansen *et al.*, 1974
Benign extrahepatic biliary tract obstruction and inflammation	Lurie *et al.*, 1975

discussed more fully in Chapter 9. Raised concentrations of CEA in the blood have been reported in a number of malignant and benign hepatobiliary diseases (Table 3.1). It is evident that patients with jaundice and raised plasma CEA concentrations do not necessarily have cancer. In addition to the diseases listed in Table 3.1, raised CEA concentrations are often found in carcinoma of the pancreas (Ona *et al.*, 1973; Zamchek, 1974) and in pancreatitis (Khoo and Mackay, 1973; Delwiche *et al.*, 1973). The suggestion has been made that raised CEA concentrations in patients with cancer of the head of the pancreas may be due partly to biliary tract obstruction; in patients in whom there is such obstruction a sharp temporary fall in circulating CEA concentrations has been observed immediately after relief of the obstruction (Lurie *et al.*, 1975).

Hepatitis-associated antigen (Australia antigen)

In 1965 Blumberg and his colleagues discovered that the serum of two haemophiliac patients who had received multiple blood transfusions contained an antibody that reacted with an antigen contained in a single serum in their panel; this serum came from an Australian Aborigine (Blumberg *et al.*, 1967). The antibody, an IgG, was detected in many patients who had received multiple blood transfusions, and the antigen was later found to be present in some 20 per cent of patients with viral hepatitis. Of the two known types of viral hepatitis, serum hepatitis or homologous serum jaundice is almost always associated with the presence of hepatitis-associated antigen (HAA) in the serum, though whether HAA is identical with the virus causing the infection is unknown. In a group of 12 recipients of HAA-positive blood only 9 developed hepatitis, while 4 out of 69 controls receiving HAA-negative blood developed the disease (Gocke *et al.*, 1969). Again, although the antigen is apparently demonstrable in the serum of practically all patients with serum hepatitis, it is only rarely that the homologous antibody has been found in these sera during or after illness (Shulman and Barker, 1969; Almeida and Waterson, 1969). Many findings of this sort can be better understood if it is postulated that the antigen particles do not represent the integral virus itself but are simply a part of the virus molecule or a by-product of its synthesis (Almeida and Waterson, 1970).

HAA is a globulin with alpha mobility (Alter and Blumberg, 1966). A variety of techniques are available for its detection in serum, including immunodiffusion, crossed immunoelectrophoresis, radioimmunoassay, and electron microscopy.

Caeruloplasmin and hepatolenticular degeneration

Patients with Wilson's disease (hepatolenticular degeneration) have low serum concentrations of caeruloplasmin (Scheinberg and Gitlin, 1952), and it has been suggested that this is the most typical single biochemical abnormality associated with the condition (Bearn and Kunkel, 1954). Wilson's disease may present in childhood as cirrhosis or subacute hepatitis (Walshe, 1957; Chalmers *et al.*, 1957; Scheinberg and Sternlieb, 1959), and in such cases the diagnosis often depends upon the biochemical findings. The report of low concentrations of caeruloplasmin and copper in the blood serum of patients with severe hepatitis, but without Wilson's disease, shows that additional criteria must be employed before Wilson's disease is diagnosed (Walshe and Briggs, 1962). The low serum concentration of caeruloplasmin in these patients was presumably due to failure of the synthetic functions of the liver (cf. Sternlieb and Scheinberg, 1961).

The recent report of reduced copper oxidase activity of caeruloplasmin in two families with Wilson's disease (Gollan *et al.*, 1977) suggests the desirability of carrying out both measurements in parallel during the investigation of suspected Wilson's disease, especially when measurement of caeruloplasmin by the immunochemical method gives results within the normal range.

Serum concentrations of caeruloplasmin are also decreased in the nephrotic syndrome, kwashiorkor, sprue, and scleroderma of the small bowel. Most, if not all, oestrogen-containing drugs cause increases in serum caeruloplasmin concentration, as do pregnancy, leukaemia, infectious diseases, myocardial infarction, and trauma generally.

Complement in liver disease

Low serum concentrations of total haemolytic complement have been reported in a number of liver diseases, including active chronic hepatitis

(Pagaltsos *et al.*, 1971). In another study, in which C3, C4, and C1q were measured as well as total haemolytic complement, it was found that low concentrations of C3 and C4 were most common in active chronic hepatitis and cryptogenic cirrhosis, whereas the concentration of C1q was normal (Finlayson *et al.*, 1972). No correlation could be found between the low concentrations of C3 and C4 and the activity of the disease, or the presence of autoantibodies or hepatitis B antigen; they were, however, correlated with low serum albumin concentrations and a prolonged prothrombin time, suggesting that defective synthesis by the liver, rather than utilization in immune complex formation, was the cause of the lowering.

It is possible, nevertheless, that complement, together with hepatitis B antigen, may play a part in the pathogenesis of certain extrahepatic lesions. Both have been demonstrated in blood-vessel walls in a patient with polyarteritis nodosa (Gocke *et al.*, 1970) and in the glomerular basement membrane of a patient who had a persistence of the antigen in his serum after post-transfusion hepatitis and who developed membranous glomerulonephritis (Combes *et al.*, 1971). Another line of evidence is found in the low serum level of complement at the time of development of arthritis preceding the onset of hepatitis (Alpert *et al.*, 1971a, Onion *et al.*, 1971).

α_1-Antitrypsin deficiency and liver disease

The glycoprotein α_1-antitrypsin, which forms about 90 per cent of the α_1-globulin band seen on electrophoresis of the plasma proteins, exists as a number of allelomorphs, identifiable by their electrophoretic mobility in starch gel. More than 25 alleles have been described, and six or more of the phenotypes (SS, SZ, ZZ, S^-, Z^-, and the homozygous null) are associated with severe lowering of the serum concentration of α_1-antitrypsin (i.e. to less than 0.6 g/l). Combination of S and Z with other alleles results in heterozygotes having serum concentrations between 0.3 and 1.8 g/l. In normal individuals concentrations in the region of 2.0–3.0 g/1 are found.

The protein inhibits trypsin and other enzymes with trypsin-like activity, and for this reason the genotypes are referred to as the Pi (i.e. protease inhibitor) genotypes (Fagerhol and Laurell, 1967). It is one of the acute-phase proteins (Chapter 8), and raised concentrations are found in the plasma after trauma and in infections or conditions associated with inflammation of any kind.

Clinically, the homozygous state is associated with a severe emphysematous type of chronic pulmonary disease in adults and with a predisposition to hepatic cirrhosis in children.

Pulmonary disease

The absence of an α_1-band on paper electrophoresis led Laurell and Eriksson (1963) to identify 5 patients with α_1-antitrypsin deficiency out of a total of some

1500 patients over a period of 6 months, and of these 5 patients 3 were found to have severe pulmonary disease. Subsequently Eriksson (1965) examined relatives of the α_1-antitrypsin-deficient patients and was able to demonstrate that three different levels of the protein occur in antitrypsin-deficient families, corresponding to normal, intermediate, and low. These findings corroborated the hypothesis (Eriksson, 1964) that α_1-antitrypsin deficiency is transmitted by a recessive gene, the homozygotes having low concentrations and the heterozygotes intermediate concentrations of the protein in the serum. Numerous studies have confirmed and extended this concept (Hunter *et al.*, 1968; Talamo *et al.*, 1968; Tarkoff *et al.*, 1968; Townley *et al.*, 1970).

The clinical consequences of homozygous α_1-antitrypsin deficiency in adults include, most prominently, a severe, degenerative, emphysematous type of chronic obstructive pulmonary disease (Guenter *et al.*, 1968; Meiers *et al.*, 1968; Stein *et al.*, 1971; Stevens *et al.*, 1971). It has been thought to occur possibly as a result of autodigestion of lung tissue by the proteolytic activity of proteases released from leukocytes during inflammatory episodes (Eriksson, 1965; Kueppers and Bearn, 1966; Sharp, 1971), though whether trypsin, elastase, or another enzyme is responsible for the tissue damage does not appear to have been established.

Hepatic cirrhosis

A more recently recognized clinical feature of α_1-antitrypsin deficiency is a predisposition to hepatic cirrhosis in homozygous α_1-antitrypsin-deficient children (Sharp *et al.*, 1969). It seems that the protein is synthesized normally within the hepatocytes but is not released, and intracellular accumulation of α_1-antitrypsin occurs (Gordon *et al.*, 1972; Lieberman *et al.*, 1972). The condition can lead to childhood cirrhosis. However, the rarity of liver disease in individuals with homozygous α_1-antitrypsin deficiency suggests that infantile cirrhosis does not result directly from the abnormal intrahepatic accumulation of the protein (Gordon *et al.*, 1972; Lieberman *et al.*, 1972).

Cirrhosis accompanied by accumulation of α_1-antitrypsin in the liver has been found in an adult with homozygous α_1-antitrypsin deficiency (Cohen *et al.*, 1973) and one with heterozygous deficiency (Campra *et al.*, 1973).

In liver disease accompanying α_1-antitrypsin deficiency, prominent, magenta-coloured, diastase-resistant, periodic acid-Schiff-positive globules are found in periportal hepatocytes. These appear to correspond to the amorphous material which is seen on electron microscopy to distend the endoplasmic reticulum and which fluoresces with specific fluorescent-labelled antibody to α_1-antitrypsin (Sharp, 1971). However, these globules occur in α_1-antitrypsin-deficient individuals whether liver disease is present or not; moreover, the incidence of liver disease is greater in some families than in others. It has therefore been suggested that a second, associated genetic factor may be necessary for liver disease to occur. Such a factor might have a part in controlling protease/antiprotease balance in tissues, though this appears to be speculative at present.

Polymorphism of α_1-antitrypsin

The genetically determined polymorphism of α_1-antitrypsin has been the subject of a number of studies and more than 20 variants have been described. Bell and Carrell (1973), and independently Cox (1973), have produced evidence that the abnormal serum protein occurring in the homozygous deficiency state (ZZ) results from partial loss of sialic acid from the molecule. This is compatible with the electrophoretic behaviour of α_1-antitrypsin and explains its defective release from the liver cells and hence the low plasma concentrations in the deficiency state. It was also proposed that most of the other variants are explicable in terms of single amino acid substitution; in the case of the S variant, 'peptide maps' prepared from normal and S-variant homozygous phenotypes showed a single substitution of valine for glutamic acid in the latter, which is compatible with a single point mutation in the genetic code and explains the slow electrophoretic mobility of the S variant (Owen and Carrell, 1976).

Other serum protein changes in liver disease

A number of investigators have studied groups of serum proteins in various liver diseases. Hällén and Laurell (1972) determined the plasma concentrations of 21 specific proteins in patients with liver cirrhosis in a quiescent state. Concentrations of haptoglobin and orosomucoid (α_1-acid glycoprotein) were normal or decreased, while α_1-antitrypsin, fibrinogen, and C-reactive protein were slightly increased or normal. Prealbumin, prothrombin, and β_2-glycoprotein I concentrations were most frequently decreased. Of the proteins studied, prealbumin seemed to be the most sensitive indicator of impaired liver function.

In a more recent study carried out by Skrede and his collaborators (1975), certain proteins—prealbumin, retinol-binding protein, albumin, α-lipoprotein, and the group of clotting factors measured by the 'Normotest' (Nyegaard & Co., Oslo, Norway)—were found to be usually highly intercorrelated, the frequency of lowered concentrations being, with some exceptions, similar for a particular liver disease. Decreased protein synthesis by the liver was presumably the cause of the lowered concentrations of this group of proteins. The concentrations of haptoglobin and the C3 component of complement, and the total iron-binding capacity of the serum, respectively, were also lowered in some liver diseases. That of α_1-antitrypsin was often increased in liver diseases, especially in patients with hepatic tumours. Retention of bile was often accompanied by relatively high concentrations of caeruloplasmin, the C3 component of complement, and α-lipoprotein and by high 'Normotest' values.

PLASMA ENZYME CHANGE IN LIVER DISEASE

The literature dealing with enzyme changes in diseases of the liver and hepatobiliary tract is voluminous, and only the briefest outline is possible here.

For fuller information on these changes and on the clinical applications of enzyme tests in liver disease the reader is referred to specialized reviews, such as those by Rosalki (1976), Batsakis and Briere (1967), and Wilkinson (1970, 1976).

Alkaline phosphatase

This appears to have been the first enzyme to have been measured for the investigation of patients with hepatic disease (Roberts, 1930, 1933). The chief value of this measurement lies in the help that it gives in differentiating between obstructive and parenchymal jaundice; the former is associated generally with high levels of activity (usually over 30 King-Armstrong or 10 Bodansky units), whereas in jaundice due to hepatocellular disease marginal or only slightly increased values are found. The cause of the raised level of alkaline phosphatase activity in hepatitis is not known with certainty, but may be an increased synthesis of the enzyme (Sebesta *et al.*, 1964; Kaplan and Righetti, 1969), some of which finds its way into the circulation.

In intracanalicular stasis due to chlorpromazine, elevation of serum alkaline phosphatase activity may be one of the first biochemical abnormalities to appear (Dickes *et al.*, 1957).

Toxic hepatitis, non-infectious hepatitis and infectious mononucleosis are associated with higher serum alkaline phosphatase levels than infective hepatitis. In infectious mononucleosis the incidence of raised serum alkaline phosphatase activity is greater than that of jaundice (Gall, 1947; Barondess and Erle, 1960).

In portal cirrhosis the serum alkaline phosphatase is normal or only slightly raised (West and Zimmerman, 1959).

Patients with 'space-occupying' lesions of the liver, such as occur for example in sarcoidosis and in metastatic carcinoma of the liver, have raised serum alkaline phosphatase activity; the estimation of this enzyme is of value for the early detection of metastases in the liver (Mendelsohn and Bodansky, 1952; Shay and Siplet, 1954). As might be expected, elevations occur also in many if not most patients with primary hepatoma (Galluzzi *et al.*, 1953).

Some patients with cardiac failure or long-standing chronic passive congestion of the liver have raised serum alkaline phosphatase (Felder *et al.*, 1950; Zimmerman and West, 1963).

Isoenzymes of alkaline phosphatase have been studied with a view to differentiating between liver and bone as the source of raised serum activity of the enzyme. Occasionally, electrophoretic separation gives a definite indication of the source of the enzyme; however, the principal liver enzyme is only slightly more negatively charged than the bone enzyme and the two bands often overlap. For this reason reliance is often placed on indirect tests, such as the estimation of serum *5′-nucleotidase* activity, which is increased in liver disease, or on the urinary excretion of hydroxyproline, which is increased in bone diseases.

The intestinal and placental isoenzymes, however, are readily distinguished from the liver and bone enzymes by their sensitivity to inhibition by L-phenylalanine (Fishman *et al.*, 1963; Ghosh and Fishman, 1967).

Aspartate transaminase and alanine transaminase

The activities of these transaminases in the serum are both markedly raised in acute hepatitis—up to 20 or 30 times the normal level, or even higher. According to Batsakis and Briere (1967), the finding of such high values, with the alanine transaminase higher than the aspartate transaminase activity and in the absence of exposure to hepatotoxins, is almost diagnostic of acute hepatitis.

Serum transaminase estimations are especially useful in the early diagnosis of viral hepatitis (Sherlock, 1971); measurements must be made at an early stage because normal values may be found within a week of the onset. In spite of falling values, the patient may develop fatal acute hepatic necrosis.

Almost 50 per cent of patients with hepatic metastases have somewhat raised serum transaminase activity (Korn *et al.*, 1962). Higher levels of activity are seen when the hepatic parenchyma is more extensively replaced. The increase in aspartate transaminase may not be accompanied by a corresponding increase in alanine transaminase activity.

There is no consistent pattern of transaminase activity in cirrhosis; results are particularly high in active chronic hepatitis (juvenile cirrhosis) (Sherlock, 1971).

Finally, the assay of aspartate and alanine transaminases if often of value in determining the aetiology of jaundice in the newborn (Kove *et al.*, 1957, 1960). Since adult concentrations of γ-globulin are not present in the serum of even normal, healthy infants, the turbidity tests mentioned above are useless in the diagnosis of neonatal hepatitis; and since reduction of bilirubin to urobilinogen occurs only when the gut has been colonized by bacteria, misleading results may be obtained in the routine urine tests. For these reasons, increased reliance is placed on serum enzyme tests.

Aspartate transaminase is present in large amounts in heart, liver, skeletal muscle, and kidney, and the serum activity of the enzyme increases whenever these tissues are acutely damaged. Very high serum values are found in patients with hepatocellular necrosis or with myocardial infarction.

Alanine transaminase is also present in the liver, though in smaller amounts than aspartate transaminase. Since, however, it constitutes in the liver a greater proportion of the transaminases than in heart and skeletal muscle, an increase in serum alanine transaminase is rather more specific for liver damage than is an increase in serum aspartate transaminase activity.

Lactate dehydrogenase

Although estimation of serum lactate dehydrogenase activity is much less useful for the detection of hepatic disease than estimation of the transaminases,

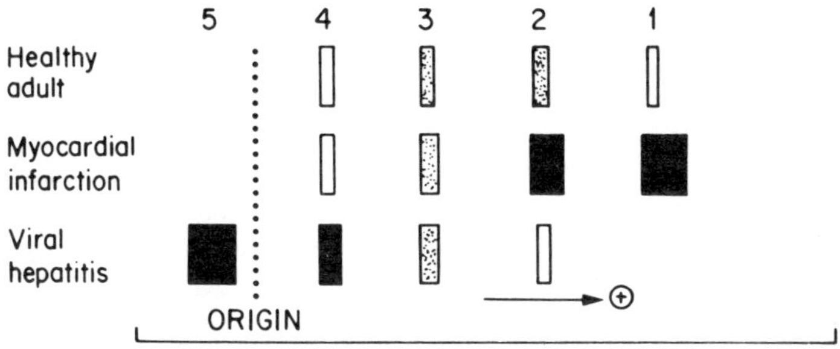

Figure 3.6. Diagram showing the serum lactate dehydrogenase isoenzyme pattern found in health, together with that seen 2 or 3 days after the onset of myocardial infarction or viral hepatitis. The patterns are those seen after staining the starch gel specifically for the enzyme by a tetrazolium technique. The density of shading reflects the relative concentrations of the isoenzymes, which are numbered at the top of the diagram. (Reproduced from F.V. Flynn, *Chromatographic and Electrophoretic Techniques, Vol. 2—Zone Electrophoresis*, 2nd edn., (Ed. I. Smith), Heinemann, London, 1968, by permission of Wm. Heinemann Medical Books Ltd. and Prof. Flynn.)

the investigation of its isoenzyme pattern has proved to be of value clinically. The lactate dehydrogenase isoenzyme patterns of normal serum and of serum from patients with myocardial infarction or liver disease are illustrated in Figure 3.6. In normal serum little if any of the slowest moving fraction, LD_5, can be demonstrated; hence even a slight increase in this fraction (which may be insufficient to increase the total lactate dehydrogenase activity significantly) can be of clinical importance. Such increases in the LD_5 fraction, with a total serum lactate dehydrogenase within normal limits, have been found in chronic liver diseases (Elliott and Wilkinson, 1963).

A study of the lactate dehydrogenase isoenzymes is of value in the differential diagnosis of jaundice, the LD_5 band being generally much more pronounced in hepatocellular disease than in biliary obstruction; this difference can be recognized more easily in the earlier stages of the disease, i.e. within a day or two of the onset of jaundice, than at a later stage (Wilkinson, 1970).

In acute hepatitis an increase in LD_4 and LD_5 often precedes the onset of jaundice by several days, and this observation has proved to be of value in the investigation of patients suspected of being in the incubation phase of the disease (Batsakis and Briere, 1967). Once jaundice is established, the concentration of LD_5 returns to normal; this does not mean that the disease is subsiding, but, according to Batsakis and Briere (1967), indicates rather that the tissue reservoir of LD_5 has been depleted. The same authors point out that a persistent prominence of LD_5, or a secondary increase after normalization, is strongly suggestive of the development of chronic hepatitis.

In various types of chronic liver disease, especially cirrhosis, rises in the LD_5 fraction are associated with exacerbation of necrosis; however, in uncomplicated cirrhosis the serum isoenzyme pattern is normal (Batsakis and Briere, 1967).

Isoenzyme fractionation is considered by some to be one of the most sensitive and specific indicators of active hepatocellular disarrangement or necrosis.

It should be noted that although electrophoresis is probably the technique most widely used for the separation of the isoenzymes of lactate dehydrogenase, a number of non-electrophoretic methods are available. One of these is based on the differential heat stability of the isoenzymes, LD_5 activity being destroyed by heating the serum for 30 minutes at 65 °C.

γ-Glutamyl transferase (γ-glutamyl transpeptidase)

The serum activity of this enzyme is raised in various types of liver disease. Its estimation is of little value in the differential diagnosis of jaundice, but appears to offer a highly sensitive test for disease of the liver and biliary tract (Kokot *et al.*, 1963; Mayr, 1972; Keane *et al.*, 1973; Adjarov and Iwanow, 1973; Kokot and Sledzinski, 1974). However, the high sensitivity of the test is not accompanied by organ specificity or selectivity; for example, diseases of the pancreas, the small and large intestine, the duodenum, and the kidneys may be associated with raised activity (Mayr, 1974).

Other enzymes

Although estimations of serum alkaline phosphatase and transaminase activity are the mainstay of enzyme investigations in liver disease, a number of other enzyme estimations have been suggested from time to time as being of clinical value: some of these are listed in Table 3.2. There can be little doubt that estimation of certain of these enzymes—for example, sorbitol dehydrogenase—would be applied more widely to the diagnosis of hepatic disease if other enzyme estimations had not already received general acceptance.

Table 3.2. Some other serum enzymes that have been estimated for the detection of liver damage

Enzyme	Significance of elevations	References
Isocitrate dehydrogenase	Indicator of hepatocellular damage, but ineffective in differentiating between types of jaundice	Cohen *et al.*, 1961; Batsakis *et al.*, 1964; Cohn *et al.*, 1965; Baron and Bell, 1959; Bell *et al.*, 1962
Sorbitol dehydrogenase	Indicator of hepatocellular damage	Gerlach, 1959; Asada and Galambos, 1963; Pitkänen and Servo, 1971
Leucine aminopeptidase	Indicator of hepatobiliary and pancreatic disease	See Chapter 9
Orthinine carbamoyl transferase	Indicator of hepatocellular damage	Reichard, 1961, 1962

LABORATORY INVESTIGATION OF PROTEINS IN LIVER DISEASE

In practice, the investigation of serum proteins (including enzymes) usually forms part of a group of tests which may include measurement of the serum concentration of bilirubin and an assessment of the ability of the liver to excrete various dyes. The choice of tests will depend upon the purpose of the investigation: this may be to provide an early warning of liver damage, for example in patients being treated with certain drugs, or else to arrive at an accurate diagnosis and to assess the extent of the damage in persons known to have a hepatic disorder. Taken together with the clinical findings, a suitable combination of these tests can be helpful in the diagnosis and follow-up of liver disease.

In assessing the results of specific protein estimations, the possible effects of other conditions must always be considered. For example, in the investigation of suspected α_1-antitrypsin deficiency it must be remembered that raised concentrations of this protein—up to two or three times the normal—are associated with inflammation, malignancy, or trauma; measurement of the protein is of little or no clinical value in such a situation. Various conditions other than Wilson's disease influencing the serum concentration of caeruloplasmin are mentioned on page 55.

REFERENCES

Abelev, G. I. (1968), *Cancer Res.*, **28**, 1344.

Adjarov, D., and E. D. Iwanow (1973), *Acta Hepato-Gastroenterol.*, **20**, 315.

Agarwal, S. S., S. K. Mehta, and P. C. Bajpai (1974), *Lancet*, **ii**, 175.

Almeida, J. D., and A. P. Waterson (1969), *Lancet*, **ii**, 983.

Almeida, J. D., and A. P. Waterson (1970), *Der Internist*, **2**, 73.

Alpert, M. E., J. Uriel, and B. de Nechaud (1968), *New Engl. J. Med.*, **278**, 984.

Alpert, E., K. J. Isselbacher, and P. H. Schur (1971a), *New Engl. J. Med.*, **285**, 185.

Alpert, E., W. V. Pinn, and K. J. Isselbacher (1971b), *New Engl. J. Med.*, **285**, 1058.

Alpert, E., T. E. Starzl, P. H. Schur, and K. J. Isselbacher (1971c), *Gastroenterology*, **61**, 144.

Alter, H. J., and B. S. Blumberg (1966), *Blood*, **27**, 297.

Andrieu, J., G. Breart, B. Rodier, and P. E. Robert (1971), *Presse Méd.*, **79**, 1595.

Asada, M., and J. T. Galambos (1963), *Gastroenterology*, **44**, 578.

Baron, D. N., and J. L. Bell (1959), *J. Clin. Path.*, **12**, 385.

Barondess, J. A., and H. Erle (1960), *Amer. J. Med.*, **29**, 43.

Batsakis, J. G., and R. O. Briere (1967), *Interpretive Enzymology*, Thomas, Illinois.

Batsakis, J. G., R. O. Briere, and J. A. Preston (1964), *Univ. Mich. Med. Center J.*, **30**, 278.

Bearn, A. G., and H. G. Kunkel (1954), *J. Clin. Invest.*, **33**, 400.

Bell, J. L., S. Shaldon, and D. N. Baron (1962), *Clin. Sci.*, **23**, 57.

Bell, O. F., and R. W. Carrell (1973), *Nature*, **243**, 410.

Bernades, P., M. Smadja, B. Rueff, A. Bonnefond, T. Tursz, E. Martin, C. Bognel, J. Barge, and J. Uriel (1971), *Presse Méd.*, **79**, 1585.

Blumberg, B. S., B. J. S. Gerstley, D. A. Hungerford, W. T. London, and A. I. Sutnick (1967), *Ann. Int. Med.*, **66**, 924.

Booth, S. N., J. P. G. King, J. C. Leonard, and P. W. Dykes (1973), *Gut*, **14**, 794.

Bourgeaux, Cl., F. Martin, F. Cabanne, P. Aupecle, and J. Guerrin (1971), *Presse Méd.*, **79**, 1589.
Bourreille, J., P. Metayer, F. Sauger, F. Matray, and A. Fondimare (1970), *Presse Méd.*, **78**, 1277.
Campra, J. L., J. R. Craig, R. L. Peters, and T. B. Reynolds (1973), *Ann. Int. Med.*, **78**, 233.
Chalmers, T. C., F. L. Iber, and L. L. Uzman (1957), *New Engl. J. Med.*, **256**, 235.
Chu, T. M., and T. Nemoto (1973), *J. Nat. Cancer Inst.*, **51**, 1119.
Church, D., and C. R. B. Blackburn (1954), *Aust. Ann. Med.*, **3**, 279 (cited by Owen and Robertson, 1956).
Cohen, N. N., H. P. Potter, and G. N. Bowers (1961), *Ann. Int. Med.*, **55**, 604.
Cohen, K. L., P. E. Rubin, R. E. Echevarria, H. L. Sharp, and P. O. Teague (1973), *Ann. Int. Med.*, **78**, 227.
Cohn, E. M., S. Winsten, and E. B. Abramson (1965), *Amer. J. Gastroenterol*, **44**, 45.
Combes, B., P. Stastny, J. Shorey, E. H. Eigenbrodt, A. Barrera, A. R. Hull, and N. W. Carter (1971), *Lancet*, **ii**, **234**.
Cox, D. W. (1973), *Lancet*, **ii**, 844.
Delwiche, R., N. Zamcheck, and N. Marcon (1973), *Cancer*, **31**, 328.
Dhar, P., T. Moore, N. Zamcheck, and H. Z. Kupchik (1972), *J. Amer. Med. Assoc.*, **221**, 31.
Dickes, R., V. Schenker, and L. Deutsch (1957), *New Engl. J. Med.*, **256**, 1.
Doniach, D., and J. G. Walker (1969), *Lancet*, **i**, 813.
Doniach, D., I. M. Roitt, J. G. Walker, and S. Sherlock (1966), *Clin. Exp. Immunol.*, **1**, 237.
Dykes, P. W., and J. King (1972), *Gut*, **13**, 1000.
Elliott, B. A., and J. H. Wilkinson (1963), *Clin. Sci.*, **24**, 343.
Eriksson, S. (1964), *Acta Med. Scand.*, **175**, 197.
Eriksson, S. (1965), *Acta Med. Scand.*, **177**, Suppl. 432.
Fagerhol, M. K., and C.-B. Laurell (1967), *Clin. Chim. Acta*, **16**, 199.
Feizi, T. (1968), *Gut*, **9**, 193.
Felder, L., A. Mund, and J. G. Parker (1950), *Circulation*, **2**, 286.
Finlayson, N. D. C., K. Krohn, M. H. Fauconnet, and K. E. Anderson (1972), *Gastroenterology*, **63**, 653.
Fishman, W. H., S. Green, and N. I. Inglis (1963), *Nature*, **198**, 685.
Foli, A. K., S. Sherlock, and M. Adinolfi (1969), *Lancet*, **ii**, 1267.
Franzl, R. E. (1962), *Nature*, **195**, 457.
Gall, E. A. (1947), *Amer. J. Clin. Path.*, **17**, 529.
Galluzzi, N. J., W. Weingarten, F. D. Regan, and A. A. Doerner (1953), *J. Amer. Med. Assoc.*, **152**, 15.
Gerlach, U. (1959), *Klin. Woch.*, **37**, 93.
Ghosh, N. K., and W. H. Fishman (1967), *Fed. Proc.*, **26**, 558.
Gitlin, D., and M. Boesman (1966), *J. Clin. Invest.*, **45**, 1826.
Gocke, D. J., H. B. Greenberg, and N. B. Kavey (1969), *Lancet*, **ii**, 248.
Gocke, D. J., K. Hsu, C. Morgan, S. Bombardieri, M. Lockshin, and C. L. Christian (1970), *Lancet*, **ii**, 1149.
Gollan, J. L., J. Stocks, T. L. Dormandy, and S. Sherlock (1977), *J. Clin. Path.*, **30**, 81.
Gordon, H. W., J. Dixon, J. C. Rogers, C. Mittman, and J. Lieberman (1972), *Human Path.*, **3**, 361.
Greenspan, E. M. (1954), *Arch. Int. Med.*, **93**, 863.
Greenspan, E. M., and D. A. Dreiling (1953), *Arch. Int. Med.*, **91**, 474.
Greenspan, E. M., I. Lehman, M. M. Graff, and E. B. Schoenbach (1951), *Cancer*, **4**, 972.
Greenspan, E. M., B. Tepper, L. L. Terry, and E. B. Schoenbach (1952), *J. Lab. Clin. Med.*, **39**, 44.
Guenter, C. A., M. H. Welch, T. R. Russell, R. M. Hyde, and J. F. Hammarsten (1968), *Arch. Int. Med.*, **122**, 254.

Hällén, J., and C.-B. Laurell (1972), *Scand. J. Clin. Lab. Invest.*, **29**, Suppl. 124, 97.
Hanger, F. M. (1939), *J. Clin. Invest.*, **18**, 261.
Hansen, H. J., J. J. Snyder, E. Miller, J. P. Vandevoorde, O. N. Miller, L. R. Hines, and J. J. Burns (1974), *Human Path.*, **5**, 139.
Hartmann, F., and K. Steinebach (1950), *Deut. Arch. klin. Med.*, **197**, 568.
Havens, W. P., Jr., J. Dickensheets, J. N. Bierly, and T. P. Eberhard (1954), *J. Immunol.*, **73**, 256.
Hobbs, J. R. (1966), in *Scientific Basis of Medicine, Ann. Revs.*, University of London—The Athlone Press, London, p. 106.
Hobbs, J. R. (1967), *Proc. Roy. Soc. Med.*, **60**, 1250.
Hunter, C. C., J. A. Pierce, and J. B. LaBorde (1968), *J. Amer. Med. Assoc.*, **205**, 93.
Kang, K.-Y., K. Higashino, Y. Takahashi, M. Hashinotsume, and Y. Yamamura (1972), *Clin. Chim. Acta*, **42**, 175.
Kaplan, M. M., and A. Righetti (1969), *Biochim. Biophys. Acta*, **184**, 667.
Kattamis, C. A., S. Laskari, and N. S. Matsaniotis (1974), *Lancet*, **ii**, 650.
Kay, H. E. M. (1954), *Brit. Med. J.*, **ii**, 1025.
Keane, P. M., L. Garcia, R. N. Gupta, and W. H. C. Walker (1973), *Clin. Biochem.*, **6**, 41.
Keyser, J. W. (1964), *Postgrad. Med. J.*, **40**, 184.
Keyser, J. W., R. B. Payne, and B. T. Stephens (1962), *Clin. Chem.*, **8**, 270.
Khoo, S. K., and I. R. Mackay (1973), *J. Clin. Path.*, **26**, 470.
Kokot, F., and Z. Sledzinski (1974), *Z. Klin. Chem. Klin. Biochem.*, **12**, 374.
Kokot, F., J. Kuska, and J. Maraszek (1963), *Z. inn. Med.*, **18**, 851.
Korn, R. J., M. West, D. P. Davis, and M. I. Gibbel (1962), *Surg. Clin. N. Amer.*, **42**, 249.
Kove, S., S. Goldstein, and F. Wróblewski (1957), *Pediatrics*, **20**, 590.
Kove, S., R. Perry, and F. Wróblewski (1960), *Amer. J. Dis. Child.*, **100**, 47.
Kozower, M., K. A. Fawaz, H. M. Miller, and M. M. Kaplan (1971), *New Engl. J. Med.*, **285**, 1059.
Kresno, S. B., R. Gandasoebrata, and P. Rümke (1970), *Lancet*, **i**, 1178.
Kueppers, F., and A. G. Bearn (1966), *Proc. Soc. Exp. Biol. Med.*, **121**, 1207.
Kunkel, H. G. (1947), *Proc. Soc. Exp. Biol. Med.*, **66**, 217.
Laurell, C.-B. and S. Eriksson (1963), *Scand. J. Clin. Lab. Invest.*, **15**, 132.
Laurence, D. J. R., U. Stevens, R. Bettelheim, D. Darcy, C. Leese, C. Turberville, P. Alexander, E. W. Johns, and A. M. Neville (1972), *Brit. Med. J.*, **iii**, 605.
Lieberman, J., C. Mittman, and H. W. Gordon (1972), *Science*, **175**, 63.
Lo Gerfo, P., J. Krupey, and H. J. Hansen (1971), *New Engl. J. Med.*, **285**, 138.
Lurie, B. B., M. S. Loewenstein, and N. Zamcheck (1975), *J. Amer. Med. Assoc.*, **233**, 326.
Maclagan, N. F. (1944), *Brit. J. Exp. Path.*, **25**, 234.
Maclagan, N. F. (1948), *Brit. Med. J.*, **ii**, 892.
Maclagan, N. F., and D. Bunn (1947), *Biochem. J.*, **41**, 580.
Maclagan, N. F., N. H. Martin, and J. B. Lunnon (1952), *J. Clin. Path.*, **5**, 1.
Mandel, E. E., T. L. Gorsuch, and G. E. Cooper (1955), *Clin. Chem.*, **1**, 221.
Masopust, J., K. Kithier, J. Rádl, J. Koutecký, and L. Kotál (1968), *Int. J. Cancer*, **3**, 364.
Mayr, K. (1972), *Wien. med. Woch.*, **122**, 393.
Mayr, K. (1974), *Ärzt. Lab.*, **20**, 325.
Meeker, W. R., R. Kashmiri, L. Hunter, W. Clapp, and W. O. Griffen, Jr. (1973), *Arch. Surg.*, **107**, 266.
Mehlman, D. J., B. H. Bulkley, and P. H. Wiernik (1971), *New Engl. J. Med.*, **285**, 1060.
Meiers, H. G., D. Beisenherz, H. Brüster, D. Strassburger, and H. Greuel (1968), *Deut. med. Woch.*, **93**, 1633.
Mendelsohn, M. L., and O. Bodansky (1952), *Cancer*, **5**, 1.
Moore, T., P. Dhar, N. Zamcheck, A. Keeley, L. Gottlieb, and H. Z., Kupchik (1972), *Gastroenterology*, **63**, 88.

Nayak, N. C., A. N. Maliviya, V. Chawla, and R. K. Chandra (1972), *Lancet*, **i**, 68.
O'Conor, G. T., Y. S. Tatarinov, G. I. Abelev, and J. Uriel (1970), *Cancer*, **25**, 1091.
Ona, F. V., N. Zamcheck, P. Dhar, T. Moore, and H. Z. Kupchik (1973), *Cancer*, **31**, 324.
Onion, D. K., C. S. Crumpacker, and B. C. Gilliland (1971), *Ann. Int. Med.*, **75**, 29.
Owen, J. A., and R. F. Robertson (1956), *Lancet*, **ii**, 1125.
Owen, M. C., and R. W. Carrell (1976), *Brit. Med. J.*, **i**, 130.
Pagaltsos, A. P., M. G. M. Smith, A. L. W. F. Eddleston, and R. Williams (1971), in *Immunology of the Liver* (Eds. M. Smith and R. Williams), Heinemann, London, p. 93.
Pitkänen, E., and C. Servo (1971), *Clin. Chim. Acta*, **33**, 273.
Rafsky, H. A., M. Weingarten, C. I. Krieger, K. G. Stern, and B. Newman (1950), *Gastroenterology*, **14**, 29.
Read, A. E. (1971), in *Immunology of the Liver* (Eds. M. Smith and R. Williams), Heinemann, London, p. 1.
Reichard, H. (1961), *J. Lab. Clin. Med.*, **57**, 78.
Reichard, H. (1962), *Acta Med. Scand.*, **172**, Suppl. 390.
Reinhold, J. G. (1955), *Clin. Chem.*, **1**, 351.
Ricketts, W. E., and K. Sterling (1949), *Clin. Invest.*, **28**, 1477.
Roberts, W. M. (1930), *Brit. J. Exp. Path.*, **11**, 90.
Roberts, W. M. (1933), *Brit. Med. J.*, **i**, 734.
Rosalki, S. B. (1976), in *The Principles and Practice of Diagnostic Enzymology* (Ed. J. H. Wilkinson), Arnold, London, p. 303.
Ruoslahti, E., M. Salaspuro, H. Pihko, L. Andersson, and M. Seppälä (1974), *Brit. Med. J.*, **i**, 527.
Scheinberg, I. H., and D. Gitlin (1952), *Science*, **116**, 484.
Scheinberg, I. H., and I. Sternlieb (1959), *Gastroenterology*, **37**, 550.
Sebesta, D. G., F. J. Bradshaw, and D. J. Prockop (1964), *Gastroenterology*, **47**, 166.
Seibert, F. B., M. V. Seibert, A. J. Atno, and H. W. Campbell (1947), *J. Clin. Invest.*, **26**, 90.
Sharp, H. L. (1971), *Hosp. Practice*, 83.
Sharp, H. L., R. A. Bridges, W. Krivit, and E. F. Freier (1969), *J. Lab. Clin. Med.*, **73**, 934.
Shay, H., and H. Siplet (1954), *J. Lab. Clin. Med.*, **43**, 741.
Sherlock, S. (1971), *Diseases of the Liver and Biliary System*, 4th edn. Blackwell, Oxford, p. 38.
Sherlock, S. (1977), *Proc. Roy. Soc. Med.*, **70**, 851.
Sherlock, S., R. A. Fox, S. P. Niazi, and P. J. Scheuer (1970), *Lancet*, **i**, 1243.
Shields, R., R. A. McAllister, and W. Burnett (1963), *Scot. Med. J.*, **8**, 185.
Shulman, N. R., and L. F. Barker (1969), *Science*, **165**, 304.
Skrede, S., J. P. Blomhoff, K. Elgjo, and E. Gjone (1975), *Scand. J. Clin. Lab. Invest.*, **35**, 399.
Smith, J. B. (1971), *Int. J. Cancer*, **8**, 421.
Stein, P. D., J. D. Leu, M. H. Welch, and C. A. Guenter (1971), *Circulation*, **43**, 227.
Sternlieb, I., and I. H. Scheinberg (1961), *Ann. N. Y. Acad. Sci.*, **94**, 71.
Stevens, P. M., V. S. Hnilica, P. C. Johnson, and R. L. Bell (1971), *Ann. Int. Med.*, **74**, 672.
Talamo, R. C., J. D. Allen, M. G. Kahan, and K. F. Austen (1968), *New Engl. J. Med.*, **278**, 345.
Tarkoff, M. P., F. Kueppers, and W. F. Miller (1968), *Amer., J. Med.*, **45**, 220.
Tatarinov, Yu. S. (1965), *Vopros. Med. Khim.*, **11**, 20; see *Fed. Proc.*, **25**, 344 (1966) (translation supplement).
Townley, R. G., F. Ryning, H. Lynch, and A. W. Brody (1970), *J. Amer. Med. Assoc.*, **214**, 325.
Triger, D. R., and R. Wright (1973), *Lancet*, **i**, 1494.
Uriel, J., B. de Nechaud, M. Stanislawski-Birencwajg, R. Masseyeff, L. Leblanc, C. Quenum, F. Loisillier, and P. Grabar (1967), *Compt. rend. Acad. Sci.*, **265**, 75.
Varsamis, J., F. Paraskevas, P. Averback, and J. D. Adamson (1974), *Lancet*, **i**, 1291.

Viollier, G. (1951), in *Liver Disease* (Eds. S. Sherlock and G. E. W. Wolstenholme), Churchill, London, p. 185.
Walshe, J. M. (1957), *Brit. Med. Bull.*, **13**, 132.
Walshe, J. M., and J. Briggs (1962), *Lancet*, **ii**, 263.
West, M., and H. J. Zimmerman (1959), *Med. Clin. N. Amer.*, **43**, 371.
Wilkinson, J. H. (1970), *Isoenzymes*, 2nd edn., Chapman and Hall, London, p. 178.
Wilkinson, J. H. (1976), *The Principles and Practice of Diagnostic Enzymology*, Arnold, London.
Winzler, R. J., A. W. Devor, J. W. Mehl, and I. M. Smyth (1948), *J. Clin. Invest.* **27**, 609.
Wright, R. (1975), in *Clinical Aspects of Immunology*, 3rd ed. (Eds. P. G. H. Gell, R. R. A. Coombs, and P. J. Lachmann), Blackwell, Oxford, p. 1269.
Zamcheck, N. (1974), *Adv. Int. Med.*, **19**, 413.
Zeltzer, P. M., R. C. Neerhout, E. W. Fonkalsrud, and E. R. Stiehm (1974), *Lancet*, **i,** 373.
Zimmerman, H. J., and M. West (1963), *Amer. J. Gastroenterol.*, **40**, 387.

CHAPTER 4

Renal diseases

PROTEINS OF NORMAL URINE

It is generally accepted that normal, healthy persons excrete small but significant amounts of protein in the urine. Estimates vary, no doubt largely on account of the variety of analytical methods employed, but are generally in the region of 40–80 mg of protein per day. Apart from *uromucoid*, which appears to originate in the renal tubular epithelium and perhaps other parts of the excretory system, and apart also from certain formed elements of urine found in disease (e.g. certain types of casts), the urinary proteins are substantially derived from the plasma by a process of filtration through the glomeruli, as has been demonstrated by clearance experiments with intravenously injected ^{131}I-labelled proteins and, indirectly, by observations on the intensity of proteinuria in relation to plasma protein concentrations (Schultze and Heremans, 1966). A detailed consideration of the mechanisms that have been proposed is beyond the scope of this book, but in general the glomerulus may be regarded as a molecular sieve which tends to retain molecules above a certain size. Modern theories emphasize the importance of diffusion as a mechanism for the transfer of proteins across the glomeruli. In accordance with the diffusion theory is the observation that there is no sharp limit to the size of protein molecules that can pass through the glomeruli, but rather that the glomerular clearance diminishes with increasing molecular size, tending asymptotically towards zero. One of the most recent proposals is that of Misra (1964, 1971), according to which the filtration function of the glomerular basement membrane depends largely on the dimensions of the spaces between and within randomly coiled macromolecules of glycoproteins; thus, the membrane may be analogous to the highly cross-linked gel of 'Sephadex' or to a wad of cotton wool. In the nephrotic syndrome, reorientation or rearrangement of the constituents of the membrane occurs, and this may alter the size of the interspaces and hence the ability of the membrane to restrict the passage of protein. For a fuller discussion of the mechanisms involved in glomerular filtration the reader is referred to the publications of Misra (1964, 1971, 1972) (see also Schultze and Heremans, 1966).

A great deal of evidence indicates that reabsorption of proteins by the renal tubules takes place, and that certain types of proteinuria are the result of an absolute or relative decrease in this tubular reabsorption (see Schultze and Heremans, 1966).

The *electrophoretic pattern* of the proteins of normal urine differs from that of serum mainly in the smaller amount of protein migrating with the velocity of albumin, and in the relatively poor resolution of the globulins. In addition, urinary albumin has a greater mobility than serum albumin. It is noteworthy that the urinary electrophoretic 'albumin' area includes also a number of non-albumin components, mainly acid polysaccharides (Heremans *et al.*, 1959, 1960). For a comprehensive account of the urinary proteins the reader is referred to Schultze and Heremans (1966) and Berggård (1970). Table 4.1 shows the plasma proteins and plasma protein subunits that have been identified in normal human urine.

Table 4.1. Plasma proteins and protein subunits identified in normal human urine. (After I. Berggård, *Proteins in Normal and Pathological Urine* (Eds. Y. Manuel, J. P. Revillard, and H. Betuel), Karger, Basel, 1970, by permission of S. Karger AG, Basel, and the authors.)

Protein	Reference
IgM	Peterson (see Berggård, 1970)
α_2-Macroglobulin	Berggård 1961; Revillard, 1964
Fibrinogen (or products of fibrinogenolysis)	Berggård, 1961
β_{1E}-Globulin (C4)	Berggård *et al.*, 1964
α_1-Lipoprotein	Berggård, 1961
Caeruloplasmin	Berggård, 1961; Rowe and Soothill, 1961
IgA	Patte *et al.*, 1958; Berggård, 1961
IgG	Franklin, 1959
β-$_{1A}$-Globulin	Berggård, 1961
Haptoglobin	Patte *et al.*, 1958; Berggård, 1961
Transferrin	Patte *et al.*, 1958
Haemopexin	Berggård *et al.*, 1964
Albumin	McGarry *et al.*, 1955; Grant, 1957
Prealbumin	Patte *et al.*, 1958
Gc-Globulin	Berggård *et al.*, 1964
$\alpha_{2\,HS}$-Glycoprotein	Berggård *et al.*, 1964
Fc fragment of IgG	Berggård and Bennich, 1967; Vaughan *et al.*, 1967
Ig light chains, dimers	Berggård and Peterson, 1967
α_1-Antitrypsin ('α_1-principale')	Patte *et al.*, 1958
α_1-Acid glycoprotein	Patte *et al.*, 1958; Biserte *et al.*, 1959
Zn-α_2-Glycoprotein	Berggård *et al.*, 1964
β_2-Glycoprotein	Poortmans, 1967
β-Trace protein	Hochwald and Thorbecke, 1962; Walravens *et al.*, 1968
α_2bT-Protein	Walravens *et al.*, 1968
α_2cT-Protein	Walravens *et al.*, 1968
3Sγ_1-Globulin	Poortmans *et al.*, 1967
Fc′-fragment of IgG	Turner and Rowe, 1966
Ig light chains, monomers	Berggård and Edelman, 1963
α_2-Microglobulin	Peterson (see Berggård, 1970)
β_2-Microglobulin	Berggård, 1965; Berggård and Bearn, 1968
Post-γ protein (γ trace protein)	Hochwald and Thorbecke, 1962

TYPES OF PROTEINURIA

Four major types of proteinuria are recognized (Hardwicke, 1974). These are:

1. Proteinuria associated with increased glomerular permeability.
2. Overflow proteinuria.
3. Proteinuria associated with renal tubular disease.
4. 'Nephrogenic' proteinuria.

A fifth type—proteinuria of undetermined mechanism—may also be distinguished.

Glomerular proteinuria

This is characterized by the loss, into the urine, of plasma proteins of the molecular size of albumin or greater, those proteins with a molecular radius greater than that of albumin having a relatively lower clearance (p. 71). The degree of selectivity of protein excretion varies from one patient to another, and is correlated with responsiveness to therapy. In the most selective proteinurias the clearance of IgG is less than 10 per cent of that of albumin.

Massive proteinuria of this type is found in the *nephrotic syndrome*, in which the amounts of protein lost in the urine range from 5 to 20 g or even more per day. A detailed consideration of the various conditions that may cause the nephrotic lesion is beyond the scope of this book. They all appear to involve a degree of damage to the glomerular capillary membranes, sometimes so slight as to be undetectable by optical microscopy but in other cases readily demonstrable. As well as in these conditions, in which the glomerular capillary membranes are damaged, a moderate to slight proteinuria of the same type may be associated with renal damage of almost any kind. In shock and in congestive heart failure it appears that the hypoxia and increased diffusion time in the glomerular capillaries, as well as the increased venous pressure in the case of congestive heart failure, are responsible for the increased glomerular permeability and slight proteinuria that result.

Urinary protein pattern

The predominant protein is albumin, which is responsible for a positive result with the usual clinical laboratory tests for albuminuria. Three other major protein constituents are transferrin, α_1-acid glycoprotein, and α_1-antitrypsin. All these proteins are of low molecular weight, and even in massive proteinuria the molecular-sieve effect of the glomeruli is to a large extent retained.

That this molecular-sieve effect is essentially intact in damaged glomeruli is evident in the way that the kidney deals with proteins of different molecular weights. For example, although large amounts of the smaller molecular forms of haptoglobin may be excreted in nephrotic urine (Jayle *et al.*, 1953; Jayle and Boussier, 1954), homozygous patients with haptoglobin 2–2 have no haptoglobin in their urine (Marnay, 1961); and most authors agree that the largest molecules, such as β_1- (α_2-) lipoproteins, IgM, α_2-macroglobulin, and fibrinogen are virtually absent from the majority of nephrotic urines or are present at most in traces. The molecular-sieve effect has been modelled in the experiments of Rowe (1956, 1957), who, by forcing normal serum or serum from patients with the nephrotic syndrome through nitrocellulose membranes of suitable pore size, obtained ultrafiltrates that were electrophoretically and immunoelectrophoretically similar to nephrotic urines.

In patients with the nephrotic syndrome the onset of renal insufficiency is often preceded by a progressive increase in the various globulin fractions in the urine (see Schultze and Heremans, 1966, for references). This phenomenon had already been observed before the introduction of electrophoresis, when the ratio of 'albumin' and 'globulin' was estimated by methods based on salting-out. Using data obtained by such methods, Bing (1936) calculated a 'renal factor'—

$$\frac{\text{relative albumin percentage in urine}}{\text{relative albumin percentage in blood}}.$$

The greater this ratio, the lower must be the permeability of the glomerulus to the large molecular weight globulins. More recently, electrophoretic values have been used in place of those obtained by salt fractionation, with very similar results. The introduction of specific immunological methods for the estimation of individual proteins provided a powerful tool in the search for better measures of selectivity, and made possible the clearance studies of Blainey and his coworkers (1960). These investigators applied the principle of the renal clearance method, in which the rate of urinary excretion of a substance is related to its concentration in the plasma:

$$\text{clearance} = \frac{UV}{P},$$

where U and P are the concentrations of the substance in urine and plasma respectively and V is the urinary flow rate. Figure 4.1 illustrates the relationship between the renal clearances of six different plasma proteins to their molecular weights in two patients with the nephrotic syndrome. Clearly, the patient for whom the steeper line was obtained had the higher selectivity of protein excretion. This selectivity may be expressed in terms of the angle, θ, subtended by the lines A and B to the abscissa.

In patients with heavy proteinuria (2 g or more per day) the selectivity is reported to correlate broadly with the different histological types of glomerulonephritis in both adults and children (Blainey *et al.*, 1960; Cameron and White, 1965; Hitzig *et al.*, 1965) and also with the clinical outcome and the response to steroids (Joachim *et al.*, 1964; Cameron, 1966). Joachim and his coworkers (1964) classified their patients into four groups according to the selectivity of protein excretion as indicated by the slope of the line (see Figure 4.1), *viz*: (a) highly selective (slope $> 67°$); intermediate ($63.1°$–$67°$); average ($54°$–$63°$);

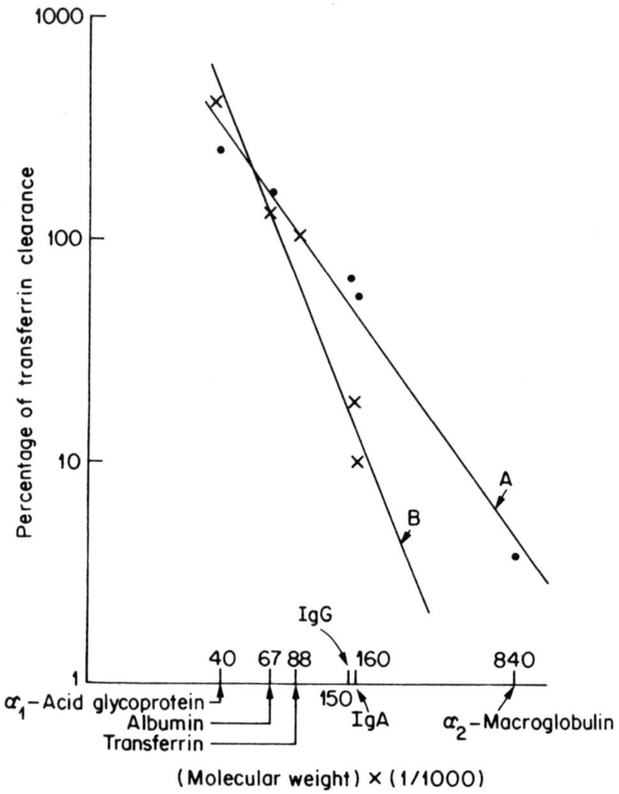

Figure 4.1. Pattern of selective protein excretion in two patients with the nephrotic syndrome. Line A represents the lower limit of average selectivity, line B the lower limit of high selectivity. (After G. R. Joachim *et al.*, *J. Clin. Invest.*, 1964, **43**, 2332, by permission of the American Society for Clinical Investigation.)

and poorly selective ($< 54°$). Those patients with primary renal disease who displayed high selectivity of protein excretion usually responded favourably to treatment with steroids. The nephrotic syndrome associated with chronic renal disease was characterized by average or low selectivity. However, Joachim and his colleagues did not confirm the correlation, referred to above, between selectivity and histological findings.

The degree of selectivity bears no relationship to the amount of protein excreted per day; thus a patient with a pure nephrotic syndrome who excreted 10 g of protein per litre of urine displayed a highly selective pattern of excretion, whereas another patient, with congestive heart failure and only slight proteinuria (0.15 g/l), had a much less selective pattern (Schultze and Heremans, 1966).

Assessment of the selectivity of proteinuria by methods that involve estimating the urinary clearances of from five to seven proteins by an immunochemical method, or by gel filtration (Hardwicke, 1965; Vere and Walduck, 1966), are time consuming and inconvenient for routine use. Simpler methods, requiring the measurement of only two proteins, have been described. Cameron and Blandford (1966) measured transferrin and IgG, expressing the clearance of IgG as a proportion of that of transferrin. They found that response to steroids was very unlikely unless this proportion or ratio was less than 0.20 and preferably as low as 0.10. MacLean and Robson (1967) reported, however, that indices of selectivity using these two proteins were unreliable and they recommended the measurement of albumin (or transferrin) and α_2-macroglobulin rather than IgG. For practical reasons Hardwicke and his coworkers (1970) recommended measurement of albumin and IgG and suggested that the administration of steroids is probably justified only in those patients having a clearance ratio of less than about 0.2 or 0.15.

Beetham and his coworkers (1974) made a careful study of various aspects of the immunochemical determination of the selectivity of proteinuria. They determined the selectivity from the relative clearances of α_1-acid glycoprotein, albumin, transferrin, and IgG in 190 children and adolescents, and found that the effectiveness of selectivity in predicting the response to steroids in the nephrotic syndrome was slightly superior when all four proteins were measured ('θ_4') than when transferrin and IgG alone were measured. If α_2-macroglobulin was included, so as to give a selectivity determination based on five proteins ('θ_5'), significantly different values were often obtained. The IgG–transferrin index of Cameron and Blandford was found to be a valid alternative to θ_4, and the α_2-macroglobulin–transferrin index a valid alternative to θ_5, but the two indices were not interchangeable. The former index provided sufficient information on which to predict the response to steroids.

Discrepancies have been found in a few cases. Hardwicke and his colleagues (1970) noted that in some patients the IgG clearance appeared to be anomalously high or low: high clearances were associated with amyloid disease and a malarial nephrotic syndrome, while a low clearance could be found in proliferative glomerulonephritis. Mills and his coworkers (1973) found that in a number of children with proteinuria (five with focal glomerulosclerosis, one membranoproliferative glomerulonephritis, and one Alport's syndrome), a progressive fall in selectivity occurred over a period of years when the assessment was based on four proteins—orosomucoid (α_1-acid glycoprotein), albumin, transferrin, and IgG—and further investigation suggested that this was due to an apparent increase in the clearance of IgG with the passage of time. Hardwicke and his colleagues (1974) have attributed anomalously high IgG clearances in such patients to the presence in their plasma of an IgG molecule having an abnormally low molecular size. Such a derivative would be preferentially filtered through the glomeruli. The origin and nature of this protein remain to be determined.

Other anomalies have been noted. Thus, in the clearance studies of Blainey and his colleagues (1960) it was found that although a plot of clearance against molecular weight gave a reasonably straight line with some patients, with others a curve was obtained. Possible reasons for this are discussed in a detailed review of clearance studies to which the reader is referred for further information (Hardwicke *et al.*, 1970). Pesce and his associates (1970) have emphasized that the relative clearances of some proteins are strikingly inconsistent with their relative molecular weights, and have suggested that the handling and passage from blood to urine of these proteins is different. It is possible that in certain cases such anomalies might be due to protein–protein interactions in the plasma or to the presence of break-down products in the urine.

Overflow proteinuria

As is to be expected, proteins having a molecular size less than that of albumin will pass through the glomerular filter more easily than albumin itself. The amounts filtered will depend both on their concentration in the plasma and on their molecular size, and if the concentration achieved in the glomerular filtrate is sufficient to exceed the reabsorptive capacity of the renal tubules these proteins will be excreted in the urine. This type of proteinuria is sometimes termed pre-renal, to emphasize that it is not caused by a renal defect. If this mechanism is operating, albumin may be detected in the urine but its clearance will not exceed the normal value of 0.02 per cent of the glomerular filtration rate, larger losses of albumin implying the presence of concurrent glomerular damage (Hardwicke, 1974).

Examples of proteins excreted by this overflow mechanism are Bence Jones protein (Harrison *et al.*, 1966); myoglobin and haemoglobin; and certain glycoproteins in the case of patients with high plasma concentrations associated with carcinoma, trauma, acute infections, and so on (Heremans, 1958a,b; de Vaux Saint-Cyr *et al.*, 1963). In these conditions the plasma concentrations of α_1- and α_2-globulins are increased. Among these are α_1-acid glycoprotein and α_1-antitrypsin, two proteins of low molecular weight (44,100 and 45,000 respectively) which are rapidly excreted in the urine. The large amount of α_1-acid glycoprotein in the urine is revealed by the intense staining of the α_1-globulin band on treatment with periodic acid and Schiff's reagent after electrophoresis at pH 8.6, and by the well-marked 'M_1-zone' obtained on electrophoresis at pH 4.5 or 4.7. Sometimes an 'inflammatory syndrome' is accompanied by increased glomerular permeability, as in congestive heart failure in patients with myocardial infarction, and in such cases the urine will contain large amounts of albumin as well as α_1-globulin (Heremans, 1958a,b).

Proteinuria associated with renal tubular disorders

Lesions of the renal tubules may be due to a variety of causes, including poisoning by cadmium, phenacetin, or vitamin D, chronic hypokalaemia, Bence Jones proteinuria, and a number of hereditary disorders such as Wilson's disease, galactosaemia, and the Fanconi syndrome. Sometimes, as in endemic Balkan nephropathy, the aetiology is unknown. The bulk of the urinary proteins in tubular proteinuria have low molecular weights, in the range 20,000 to 30,000, and this accounts for the fact that this type of proteinuria cannot be demonstrated by the classical heat-coagulation test, though certain other tests do detect it, positive reactions being obtained with trichloroacetic acid (4 per cent) and sulphosalicylic acid. Indeed, the electrophoretic mobilities, low molecular weights, and high carbohydrate contents of the urinary proteins found in tubular proteinuria are essentially similar to those of the proteins found, in much smaller amounts, in normal urine—as might be expected if the proteinuria is due to a failure to reabsorb proteins that are normal constituents of the glomerular filtrate.

Electrophoretic analysis of the urinary proteins at the usual alkaline pH generally shows strikingly raised α_2- and sometimes β-globulin peaks (Friberg, 1950; Butler and Flynn, 1958, 1961; Piscator, 1962; and others), but the albumin peak is proportionately much smaller than in glomerular proteinuria. In some patients a post-γ-globulin may be present, as can be demonstrated by starch gel electrophoresis (Butler and Flynn, 1961); however, although this post-γ-globulin is associated most frequently with conditions displaying gross renal tubular dysfunction, it is not restricted to such conditions, since some patients with proteinuria of glomerular origin were found to show a similar band. From the work of Osserman and Lawlor (1966) it would seem that this post γ fraction consists largely of lysozyme (see below). Butler and Flynn's study also suggested that the α_2-globulin fraction separated by paper electrophoresis in tubular proteinuria corresponded to various proteins migrating between the β-globulin and prealbumin in starch gel. Subsequent work (Butler *et al.*, 1962) using a combination of electrophoresis on filter paper and then in starch gel demonstrated the existence of a type of urine protein pattern particularly associated with diseases involving non-specific renal tubular dysfunction. Two protein zones appeared to be especially prominent: an α_2 'tubular' protein having a mobility slightly greater than that of serum albumin in starch gel, and, secondly, a β_2 'tubular' protein which had the mobility of β_2-globulin on paper electrophoresis and occurred approximately midway between albumin and transferrin in starch gel. Albumin and transferrin zones were also present but were much less prominent than in 'glomerular' patterns. Other features often seen were a post-γ protein, as mentioned above, and three or more bands within the γ-globulin zone. Serum from patients with renal tubular disorders was studied in the same way and showed no obvious abnormalities: there were no zones corresponding to the α_2 and β_2 'tubular' proteins, even when up to ten times the usual quantity of serum was applied.

More recently, electrophoretic separation of urinary proteins in polyacrylamide gel in the presence of sodium dodecyl sulphate (Shapiro *et al.*, 1967) has been found to be a valuable technique (Pesce *et al.*, 1972; Waldmann *et al.*, 1972; Virella and Pires, 1974; Pesce *et al.*, 1976). Since separation under these conditions depends mainly on molecular size (Dunker and Rueckert, 1969; Weber and Osborn, 1969), the type of pattern obtained can often establish the glomerular or tubular origin of the proteinuria. The results obtained by this

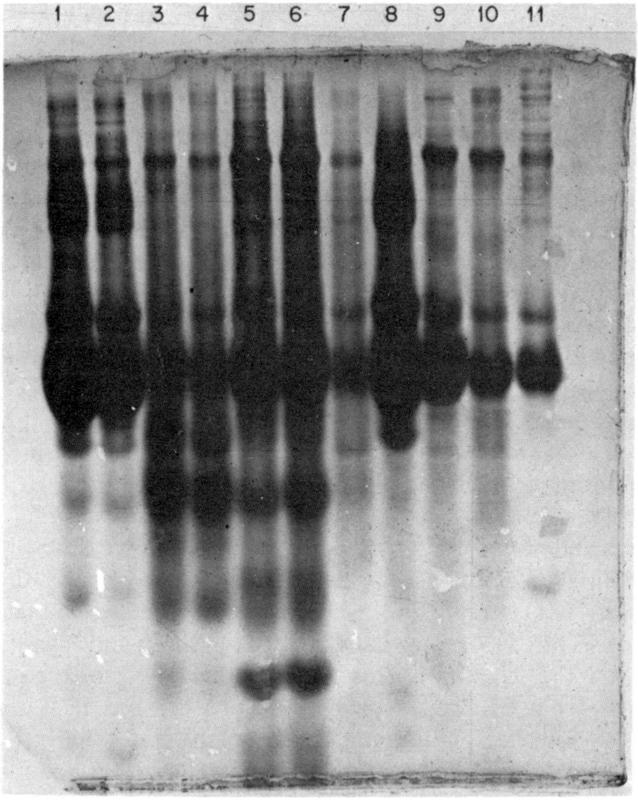

Figure 4.2. Differentiation of glomerular and tubular proteinuria by electrophoresis of urine in acrylamide gel after treatment with sodium dodecyl sulphate. Anode at lower end. Nos. 1–10, urine. No. 11, serum. Note large amount of low molecular weight proteins in Nos. 3–6 (tubular proteinuria). (Kindly supplied by Dr. M. Davies.)

method are essentially similar to those obtained by 'Sephadex'-gel filtration, but the electrophoretic method is rather more sensitive and much more suitable for dealing with large numbers of samples. The method has been used to characterize the proteinuria of patients with monoclonal gammopathies, and the results suggest that glomerular involvement is a common feature of multiple myelomatosis and macroglobulinaemia (Virella and Pires, 1974; Virella *et al.*, 1974).

Low molecular weight proteins

As mentioned above, low molecular weight proteins are presumed to be filtered at the glomerulus and reabsorbed by the proximal tubules. The evidence for this is mainly the excretion of considerable amounts of these proteins by patients with proximal tubular damage but not by healthy persons.

One protein that has been extensively studied is *β_2-microglobulin*, a low molecular weight protein (mol. wt. 11,600) of unknown function (Berggård and Bearn, 1968). It is normally present in the serum in trace amounts (up to about 3 mg/l) and the daily urinary excretion is about 100 μg (Bernier and Post, 1973). It is excreted in increased amounts, sometimes exceeding 50 mg/l, in proximal tubular disorders (Peterson *et al.*, 1969). The latter authors found that although most patients with tubular dysfunction excreted large amounts of β_2-microglobulin in the urine, they excreted normal or only slightly increased amounts of albumin; consequently the ratio urinary albumin/urinary β_2-microglobulin was high in glomerular proteinuria (falling within the range 1100–14,200), intermediate in normal proteinuria (33–163), and low in tubular proteinuria (1.0–13.3).

Irrespective of the kind of renal disease, patients with a low glomerular filtration rate usually have a large amount of β_2-microglobulin in their urine (Johansson and Ravnskov, 1972). There are, however, several exceptions to this generalization (Ravnskov and Johansson, 1974):

1. during early, acute rejection crises after renal transplantation the excretion of β_2-microglobulin decreased, in spite of the reduction in the glomerular filtration rate;
2. during the initial stages of severe, acute renal failure β_2-microglobulin was not detectable in the urine, in spite of a high serum concentration of the protein and in contrast to a pronounced excretion of albumin and low molecular weight proteins other than β_2-microglobulin; and
3. in a few patients with terminal, chronic renal failure β_2-microglobulin was not detectable in the urine.

It was concluded that factors other than proximal tubular function may influence the urinary excretion of this protein.

Studies of the urinary and serum concentrations of β_2-microglobulin in patients with various degrees of renal dysfunction suggest that there is a threshold, in the region of 4.5 mg/l, for the tubular reabsorption of this protein (Wibell and Evrin, 1974). In patients with a sufficiently large reduction in the glomerular filtration rate, β_2-microglobulin will contribute to a tubular proteinuria pattern, though in qualitative investigations this may sometimes be obscured by the simultaneous presence of glomerular proteinuria. It was also concluded that at serum concentrations below the threshold the urinary concentration of β_2-microglobulin probably provides a good assessment of the capacity of the renal tubules to reabsorb this protein, and may possibly reflect the capacity of the tubules to reabsorb low molecular weight proteins in general.

A study of the development of tubular proteinuria in endemic Balkan nephropathy (Hall and Vasiljević, 1974) showed that the first abnormality to appear in the urine proteins was an increase in β_2-microglobulin excretion. Later a 3s γ-globulin appeared, and later still there was an increase in retinol-binding protein (p. 79) and lysozyme (p. 78). These increases, which were confirmed by immunoelectrophoresis and the use of specific antisera, produced well-marked changes in the protein pattern on cellulose acetate electrophoresis. This sequence of changes occurs before azotaemia develops and before there is any detectable increase in the excretion of proteins with molecular weights above 30,000, the latter proteins being found in the urine in increased amounts only when glomerular function is diminished (Hall and Vasiljević, 1974).

The excretion of β_2-microglobulin after renal transplantation has also been studied by Bernier and Post (1973). After renal homotransplantation in patients with renal failure, the previously raised serum concentrations of β_2-microglobulin declined towards normal, apparently as a result of both urinary excretion and catabolism in the transplanted kidney, and it was suggested that measurement of serum and urine concentrations of this protein might ultimately provide a sensitive index of homograft viability.

Lysozyme (muramidase)

Lysozyme (muramidase), which has been referred to above, is a low molecular weight enzyme (mol. wt. 14,000–15,000) which brings about lysis of certain bacteria by enzymic cleavage of a specific polysaccharide of the bacterial cell wall. It is widely distributed, occurring in tears, nasal secretions, saliva, and extracts of various organs, especially the kidney, as well as in the white of the hen's egg (Fleming, 1922; Fleming and Allison, 1922). Many of the early biochemical and physicochemical investigations of lysozyme were concerned with hen's egg white, but in 1966 Osserman and Lawlor reported that large amounts of the enzyme are excreted in the urine of patients with monocytic and monomyelocytic leukaemia and showed that this material is identical with that normally occurring in tears, external secretions, white blood cells, and so on. Investigations of the renal handling of lysozyme (summarized by Osserman, 1970) appear to show that the enzyme reaching the kidney via the blood, plus that which is probably synthesized by cells within the kidney itself, must either be catabolized *in situ* or else be reabsorbed and returned to the blood by the proximal tubules. It has also been shown, both in man and in experimental animals, that proximal renal tubular damage results in lysozymuria. Rejection of a renal homograft has been shown to result in lysozymuria, in both man and experimental animals (Noble *et al.*, 1965), and this also appears to be related primarily to damage to the proximal convoluted tubules. According to Noble and his colleagues, lysozymuria is an accurate and sensitive index of rejection, apparently reflecting both the degree of macrophage-histiocyte activity and the extent of tubular damage in the grafted kidney. Subsequent studies have confirmed the value of urinary lysozyme estimations as an index of the state of kidney transplants (Shehadeh *et al.*, 1968; Osserman, 1970).

Harrison and his coworkers (1968) compared the renal clearances of lysozyme and ribonuclease with those of two other urinary proteins of lower molecular weight than albumin. They concluded that the urine concentrations and renal clearances of the two enzymes give useful indications of impaired renal tubular

Table 4.2 Probable mechanisms and extent of lysozymuria in renal and nonrenal diseases. (After E. F. Osserman, *Proteins in Normal and Pathological Urine* (Eds. Y. Manuel, J. P. Revillard, and H. Betuel), Karger, Basel, 1970, by permission of S. Karger AG, Basel, and the authors.)

Disease	Local synthesis	Proximal tubular damage	Raised serum concentration	Urine lysozyme (μg/ml)*
Pyelonephritis, genitourinary infections	×	×		5–50
Renal homograft rejection	×	×		10–200
Heavy-metal poisoning (especially cadmium)		×		10–200
Nephrotoxic syndrome		×		5–50
Chronic infections (especially tuberculosis)	×	×	×	5–50
Sarcoidosis	×	×	×	10–100
Monocytic and monomyelocytic leukaemia		×	××	10–1500

*Approximate range, based on a human lysozyme standard.

function. Other workers have also suggested that lysozymuria may be a relatively specific indication of renal tubular damage (Prockop and Davidson, 1964), though the absence of enzyme activity in the urine does not exclude tubular damage (Hayslett *et al.*, 1968).

Marked increases in serum and urine concentrations of the enzyme are found in monocytic and monomyelocytic leukaemia, apparently as a result of over-production by proliferating monocytic leukaemic cells (Osserman and Lawlor, 1966).

Table 4.2 summarizes the conditions in which lysozymuria has been reported.

Another protein characteristic of tubular proteinuria is the *retinol-binding protein* (mol. wt. 21,000), which was isolated from plasma by Kanai *et al.* (1968) and independently from urine and plasma by Peterson and his colleagues (Peterson, 1969; Peterson and Berggård, 1971). The average serum concentration was found to be 46 mg/l, and the average urinary excretion 0.11 mg/24 hours, in a small number of healthy persons. Urine from patients with tubular proteinuria, however, contained up to 150 mg/24 hours, and was found to be a good source for the isolation and purification of the protein. The structure and function of the retinol-binding protein have been reviewed by Rask and Peterson (1973). In normal serum, prealbumin and retinol-binding protein form a complex by which vitamin A (retinol) is transported.

The metabolism of lambda *light chains* and lysozyme has also been studied, together with that of β_2-microglobulin, by Bernier and his associates (1974). (Free lambda light chain was studied in preference to kappa because of the tendency of the former to exist as stable dimers and of the latter to exist in monomer–dimer equilibrium.) Serum concentrations of lambda chains,

β_2-microglobulin and lysozyme were found to be raised in patients with renal failure. After successful renal transplantation and the resumption of urine flow the concentrations returned to near normal.

Nephrogenic proteinuria

A number of ways in which this kind of proteinuria can occur are recognized. In the first place, certain proteins, for example IgA (Bienenstock and Tomasi, 1968), IgM (Goddard and Hobbs, 1968), and IgE (Barratt *et al.*, 1971) have been found in the urine in amounts greater than would be expected from the usual mechanisms of filtration, and it would appear that in such cases selective secretion into the urine is taking place. Occasionally chyluria, with loss of intestinal lymph in the urine, may be seen (p. 81). This appears to be related to the taking of food, or to other causes of an increased flow of lymph, rather than to the glomerular filtration rate (Hardwicke, 1974).

Another type of nephrogenic proteinuria consists in the loss of certain specifically renal proteins. These may be normal constituents, such as the Tamm–Horsfall mucoprotein (McQueen, 1962; Grant *et al.*, 1973), or abnormal constituents such as components of renal tubular cells and proteins similar immunologically to components of the glomerular basement membrane (see below). The experiments of McQueen (1962) appear to show that hyaline casts are not, as was generally thought, composed mainly of plasma proteins, but consist largely of the mucoprotein described by Tamm and Horsfall (1950, 1952), though small amounts of serum albumin were also found to be present.

PROTEINURIA OF UNDETERMINED MECHANISM

A few people, mostly adolescents, may excrete protein in the urine in more or less normal amounts when they are recumbent but show proteinuria when in the erect (orthostatic) and lordotic postures, without displaying any evidence of active renal disease. (The term *lordosis* refers to a posture in which there is an exaggeration of the forward lumbar curve of the spinal column.) The significance of this *postural proteinuria*, in which as much as 30 mg of protein may be excreted each minute, is still a matter of dispute; some individuals develop renal insufficiency after many years (King, 1959) while others may continue to show no evidence of renal disease. The urinary immunoelectrophoretic protein pattern reveals that albumin, transferrin, and low molecular weight α-globulins are the predominant components and that the γ-globulin fraction consists mainly of IgG and produces a single precipitin line (McKay and Slater, 1962). When the subject is recumbent there is a tendency for the urinary protein electrophoretic pattern to revert to normal.

Postural proteinuria may be inconstantly present from day to day ('transient'), or demonstrable consistently ('fixed'). Histological examination of renal biopsy specimens from persons with 'fixed' postural proteinuria has revealed changes in glomerular structure in many cases, while in others the structure was apparently normal (Robinson *et al.*, 1961a,b). The few histological observations that have been made on persons with 'transient' postural proteinuria do not allow of any definite conclusions.

The subject of postural proteinuria has been reviewed by Robinson (1970).

A somewhat different type of proteinuria, known as *exercise proteinuria*, appears in a proportion of individuals after strenuous exercise. It was first noted by Von Leube in 1878. Differences have been found between the immunoelectrophoretic patterns of protein excretion in exercise proteinuria and in postural proteinuria. In contrast to the single precipitin line developed by the IgG in postural proteinuria (and by the IgG of normal serum), double lines are found in exercise proteinuria and with certain nephrotic urines, and triple lines with normal urinary IgG (McKay and Slater, 1962). These findings have led to the suggestion that exercise proteinuria may result from an accentuation of the process responsible for the normal excretion of protein in the urine (McKay and Slater, 1962). An alternative explanation, suggested by Poortmans and his colleagues, is that during exercise the increased release of adrenalin and noradrenalin produces vasoconstriction of the arterioles of the renal glomerulus, thereby slowing down the renal plasma flow and glomerular filtration rate and allowing increased diffusion of plasma proteins through the glomerulus; after the termination of the exercise, the glomerular filtrate—which returns to its pre-exercise output or even higher—washes down the proteins from the tubules (Poortmans, 1970).

The proteins excreted in exercise proteinuria have been extensively studied by Poortmans and his colleagues (see Poortmans, 1970). The major part of the proteins is derived from the plasma. Agar gel electrophoresis shows predominantly albumin, and a well-marked β_1-globulin fraction consisting mainly of transferrin. Immunoelectrophoresis shows that a greater variety of plasma proteins occurs in exercise urine than in normal urine. The urinary output of proteins per unit time does not reach the high levels sometimes found in postural proteinuria (Poortmans, 1970).

Immunochemical estimation of urine/serum concentration ratios of a range of serum proteins of different molecular weights has shown that exercise proteinuria is moderately selective and postural proteinuria is poorly selective (Rowe and Soothill, 1961).

Chyluria, in which the urine may become white and milky, is an uncommon type of proteinuria, not renal in origin, but resulting from abnormal communication between the intestinal chyle ducts and the urinary tract, via the lymphatic vessels. The protein content of chyluric urine may vary from traces to several grams per litre. Electrophoretic analysis shows a similar pattern to that of the plasma proteins, except that the albumin peak obtained with chyle is relatively larger than that for serum. The material excreted has a high lipid content, mainly neutral fat and phospholipids. It also contains fibrinogen, which may clot and produce ureteral and urethral obstructions. The condition has been studied by Ray and Rao (1939), Lazarus and Marks (1946), Löwgren (1953), and Sonnet and Brisbois (1956), among others.

Finally, it may be noted that significant proteinuria is a common feature of a variety of skin disorders (Trotter and Fairburn, 1967; Cotterill *et al.*, 1971), though whether it is of clinical importance is unknown. An increase in capillary permeability has been demonstrated in patients with extensive skin disease (Shuster and Marks, 1970), and, in keeping with this, further work on patients with skin diseases has shown that the urinary protein seems to be of glomerular origin (private communication from Dr. J. A. Cotterill).

IMMUNOLOGICAL ASPECTS OF RENAL DISEASES

There is a considerable body of evidence indicating that various types of nephritis are caused by the deposition in the glomerulus of immune complexes. Studies of renal biopsies by the immunofluorescence technique suggest that complement is involved in many types of glomerulonephritis (Lachmann *et al.*, 1962; Berger *et al.*, 1971; McCluskey, 1971; Morel-Maroger *et al.*, 1972; Peters, 1974). Deposition of the third component of complement (C3, β_{1C}-globulin) is usually demonstrable in acute exudative glomerulonephritis, various types of proliferative nephritis, membranoproliferative nephritis, lupus nephritis, and the nephritis due to antiglomerular-basement-membrane antibody (see below), although a proportion of patients with Goodpasture's syndrome have no detectable C3 in the glomeruli. It should be noted that in some circumstances, for example in acute post-streptococcal nephritis and in membranoproliferative nephritis, C3 may be present in the kidney in the absence of detectable amounts of immunoglobulin (Berger *et al.*, 1971). While this failure to detect immunoglobulin might be due to a lack of sensitivity of the immunofluorescence techniques, or to a steric effect leading to the concealment of the immunoglobulin by the β_{1C}-globulin (*Lancet*, 1974), it does suggest the need for caution in attributing the pathological picture and clinical condition to the deposition of antigen–antibody complexes within the kidney. On the other hand, deposition of β_{1C}-globulin may possibly be an early sequel of glomerular damage, rendering the glomerulus more susceptible to the effect of immune complexes (Fish *et al.*, 1970).

A reduction in the serum concentration of one or more complement components is often found in patients with various forms of nephritis, and the estimation of β_{1C}-globulin (C3) and β_{1E}-globulin (C4) may be of value in differential diagnosis.

It appears to have been established that a proportion of patients with glomerulonephritis show a state of humoral and/or cell-mediated allergy to antigens derived from the glomerular basement membrane (Lerner *et al.*, 1967; Macanovic *et al.*, 1974). Soluble glomerular antigens that react with antisera prepared by immunizing sheep with particulate human glomerular basement membrane have been detected in urine, but the significance of this finding is uncertain. Indeed, it is not established that the glomerular basement membrane is the only source of these antigens, since they share antigenic determinants with the basement membranes of other organs (Lerner *et al.*,

1970). Fractionation of collagenase-solubilized glomerular basement membrane and immunochemical studies have shown that the membrane possesses a complex antigenic structure (Macanovic *et al.*, 1974).

Experimental support for the suggestion that antigens from the glomerular basement membrane may play a part in the causation of renal disease is afforded by the development of glomerulonephritis in rabbits injected with sheep antisera to rabbit glomerular basement antigen (Hawkins and Cochrane, 1968) or with crude or partially purified fractions of autologous or homologous urine (Lerner and Dixon, 1968). It may be that native or altered antigen from the glomerular basement membrane comes into contact with immunocompetent cells and initiates the formation of autoantibodies (Lerner *et al.*, 1970), thereby producing damage to the glomerulus.

For detailed information on immunological aspects of renal disease the reader is referred to the reviews by Wilson and Dixon (1973), Peters (1974), and Peters and Williams (1975).

PROTEINURIA AS AN INDEX OF TRANSPLANT REJECTION

Mention has been made above of the increases in serum concentrations of β_2-microglobulin, lambda light chain, and lysozyme that are found in patients with renal failure, and the return of these to near normal concentrations after successful renal transplantation and the resumption of an adequate flow of urine. In particular, measurement of serum and urinary concentrations of β_2-microglobulin has been suggested as possibly providing a sensitive index of the viability of homografts (Bernier and Post, 1973).

A number of other protein measurements have been suggested from time to time, as providing an early warning of rejection. These may conveniently be classified under the headings: fibrin/fibrinogen degradation products, other protein products, and enzymes.

Fibrin/fibrinogen degradation products

As a result of the enzymic break-down of fibrinogen and fibrin a number of soluble fragments are released which are antigenically similar to the parent molecule and are referred to as fibrin/fibrinogen degradation products (FDP) (Nussenzweig and Seligmann, 1960; Fletcher *et al.*, 1962). Fibrin-like protein has been found in the urine of patients with heavy proteinuria (Yatzidis, 1964), and FDP were found by immunodiffusion and immunoelectrophoresis in the urine of patients who had received a renal transplant (Braun and Merrill, 1968; Antoine *et al.*, 1969). By means of the more sensitive tanned red cell haemagglutination-inhibition immunoassay (Merskey *et al.*, 1966) urinary FDP excretion has been shown to rise significantly during periods of clinical rejection and to fall when renal function improves as a result of increased immunosuppressive therapy (Clarkson *et al.*, 1970); and it has been suggested that the regular monitoring of urinary FDP may help in the management of recipients of renal transplants. A number of rapid tests for the detection of FDP in urine have appeared (see, for example, Hulme and Pitcher, 1973; Clarkson, 1973; Cash *et al.*, 1973; Semeraro *et al.*, 1973).

According to Zühlke and Hermann (1971), the excretion of FDP does not appear to be such a sensitive indicator of impending rejection as abnormal 'histuria'.

Other protein fragments

In the post-transplantation period, the demonstration of a γ-globulin fragment with α_2-mobility was found by Zühlke and Hermann (1971) to be of value in indicating the onset of a rejection crisis, this abnormality appearing before clinical signs in about half the patients studied. IgG light chains are also secreted in significantly large amounts during a rejection crisis (A. Schafmayer, cited by Hermann, 1974).

The excretion of tissue proteins ('histuria') has been studied by Antoine and his colleagues (for summary see Antoine, 1974) and by Hermann and his colleagues (see Hermann, 1974). By the use of appropriate antisera the excretion of renal tissue proteins can be followed in transplant recipients, and the appearance of multiple, poorly defined precipitin lines corresponding to these proteins is stated to be a most sensitive indication, and in 50 per cent of cases an early sign of an impending rejection crisis (Hermann, 1974; see also Hermann and Zühlke, 1971).

Enzymes

Enzymes form a group of urinary proteins derived either from the renal tissue or from the serum. A number of these have been investigated, including esterases (de Vaux Saint-Cyr *et al.*, 1962) and leucine aminopeptidases (Burstone and Falk, 1956; Glenner, 1962; Klaus, 1962; Hermann and Zühlke, 1971). Raised urinary levels of *N*-acetyl-β-D-glucosaminidase and β-galactosidase were found in patients with renal disease (Price *et al.*, 1970; Dance *et al.*, 1970); and Ellis and his colleagues (1973), in experiments with dogs and rats, found that after the production of renal damage with selective nephrotoxic agents the urinary levels of these two enzymes, and of lactate dehydrogenase, alkaline phosphatase, and β-glucosidase, rose before any change in other indices of renal function. The urinary excretion of several enzymes, including lactate dehydrogenase (Prout *et al.*, 1964; Ringoir *et al.*, 1968), lysozyme (Noble *et al.*, 1965), β-glucuronidase, acid phosphatase and alkaline phosphatase (Ballantyne *et al.*, 1968), and glutaminase and carbonic anhydrase (Carter, 1970), by patients with transplanted kidneys has been studied, with a view to obtaining early warning of rejection, but the results have generally been disappointing. More encouraging results were reported by Wellwood and his colleagues (1973) in the case of *N*-acetyl-β-D-glucosaminidase, the urinary output of which was abnormally high in 16 out of 17 episodes of acute rejection, becoming raised at least 3 days and indeed up to 21 days before acute rejection was recognized by established methods. The estimation of urinary *N*-acetyl-β-D-glucosaminidase was also found to be a useful confirmatory test for chronic rejection. Later reports, however, while agreeing that urinary estimations of this enzyme are useful in monitoring the progress of patients who have received a renal transplant, have failed to confirm such early rises in enzyme excretion in rejection as were found by Wellwood and his colleagues (Sandman *et al.*, 1973; Keyser *et al.*, 1976). It should be noted that the concentration of this enzyme is particularly high in kidney tissue, and other causes of renal cell damage may therefore be expected to result in a raised urinary output. It is also present in high concentration in the extrarenal tissues of the human urogenital tract, and in semen. Hence, during an uncomplicated post-operative period a rise in enzyme output may indicate renal cell damage (whether associated with rejection, acute tubular necrosis, or renal vascular complications); or it may indicate damage to some other part of the urogenital tract, such as the ureter (Wellwood *et al.*, 1973).

Mention has been made above of the raised urinary output of *N*-acetyl-β-glucosaminidase and β-galactosidase in patients with renal disease. The excretion of these two enzymes, and also of aryl sulphatase A, α-glucosidase, and β-glucuronidase—all five of which appear to be mainly of lysosomal origin—was studied by Gielow and his coworkers (1974) in patients with essential hypertension, in which the conventional tests of renal function reveal an impairment only in the late stages of the disease. Three of these enzymes, *viz.* *N*-acetyl-β-glucosaminidase, β-galactosidase, and β-glucuronidase, were found to be excreted in significantly raised amounts in hypertensive patients as a group, as compared with healthy control subjects. There was, however, considerable overlapping of results for the hypertensive and control groups. The urinary excretion of these enzymes, which have molecular weights ranging from 97,000 (α-glucosidase) to 230,000 (β-glucuronidase), suggests that they might originate chiefly from the kidney tissue itself, or from the lower urogenital tract, rather than by glomerular filtration.

Plasma enzymes

Plasma enzyme concentrations after renal transplantation appear to have been studied to a lesser extent than urinary enzymes, possibly because of the consideration that enzymes released from renal tissue would be almost certain to appear in the urine. Lehmann and his coworkers (1970) measured γ-glutamyl transferase in a number of patients who had received renal transplants. They found that although each episode of graft rejection was accompanied by raised plasma activity of the enzyme, the value of the determination as a means of detecting rejection was diminished by the fact that rises also occurred as a result of infection, surgical operation, or liver disease; however, if these complicating factors can be excluded, raised plasma activity of γ-glutamyl transferase is suggestive of rejection, especially if the transaminase activity is normal. The plasma activity of γ-glutamyl transferase is generally raised in the immediate post-transplantation period.

Monitoring of immunosuppression

The lack of specificity of the immunosuppressive agents used in patients with renal allografts has often given rise to fatal infections and toxicity (Hill *et al.*, 1967). An association between low serum IgG concentrations and septic complications in patients who had received renal allografts was reported by Harris and his colleagues (1971); they noted low IgG concentrations in 6 and leucopaenia in all of 7 patients who had late infections, at least 6 weeks after transplantation, and had recently been receiving increased levels of immunosuppressive therapy. A study of serum IgG concentrations after renal allotransplantation was made by Ku and his colleagues (1973), who concluded that monitoring the IgG concentration, especially in the immediate post-transplant period, is useful in allowing the dosage of immunosuppressive drugs to be controlled; they recommended frequent measurement of serum IgG, in addition to haematological counts, when the creatinine clearance is less than 25 ml/min and when high-dose immunosuppression is used; they also recommended that the serum IgG concentration should probably be kept above 5 g/l, since below this concentration fatal sepsis occurred in 3 of their patients. The suggestion has also been made that measurement of serum immunoglobulin concentrations before transplantation is performed may offer a means of predicting the likelihood of success (de Bono and Franglen, 1973).

PLASMA PROTEIN CHANGES IN RENAL DISEASE

A reduction in the serum concentration of one or more complement components in many patients with various forms of nephritis has already been referred to, and the value of estimating the C3 and C4 components is discussed below in the section dealing with laboratory investigations.

On electrophoresis of the serum, the nephrotic syndrome is typically associated with a lowered albumin and raised α_2-globulin and often a lowered γ-globulin concentration.

Changes in the serum concentration of certain low molecular weight proteins such as lysozyme and β_2-microglobulin are discussed on pages 76–80.

LABORATORY INVESTIGATION OF PROTEINS IN RENAL DISEASE

As in the case of liver disease, the investigation of proteins in patients with diseases of the kidney usually forms only part of a wider range of tests. As well as a simple assessment of the amount of proteinuria, these may involve examination of the urinary deposit and an estimation of the number of erythrocytes, leucocytes, and casts (Addis count) in the urine; bacteriological examination;

measurement of the glomerular filtration rate and of the concentrating ability of the kidney; isotopic and radiological studies; and estimation of the plasma urea, creatinine, proteins, electrolytes, and so on. Most of the functional abnormalities revealed by such studies could form a basis for the classification of renal disease; however, the most useful classification of renal lesions, according to Brod (1963, 1971), is based on correlation of glomerular filtration rate and concentrating ability.

It is clear that the presence or absence of significant proteinuria, when considered together with the results of other tests and with the clinical findings, can be of value in differential diagnosis.

Urinary proteins

In spite of the considerable amount of work that has been done on the differentiation between glomerular and tubular proteinuria, analysis of the urinary proteins with this object in view is seldom required. However, the demonstration of tubular proteinuria is of value in assessing recovery from acute tubular necrosis and the extent of renal damage in cadmium poisoning. In this connection the estimation of low molecular weight proteins, and especially of lysozyme clearances, may be of value.

Pesce and his coworkers (1976) have described a rapid method for measuring semiquantitatively the concentration of urinary low molecular weight proteins, and of albumin, in the urine. After concentration 100-fold in a 'Minicon' concentrator (Amicon) the urine is examined by polyacrylamide gel electrophoresis in the presence of sodium dodecyl sulphate, the stained gel being scanned with a densitometer for assessment of the relative amounts of the various proteins present. In glomerular proteinuria the ratio of albumin to low molecular weight proteins is about 20 : 1, whereas in tubular proteinuria it is about 1:1.

As outlined above (p. 71), measurement of certain proteins in both urine and plasma, in order to obtain an assessment of the selectivity of the kidney in excreting proteins of various molecular weights, may provide information of prognostic value.

Plasma proteins

The nephrotic syndrome, which may appear in some 60 to 70 per cent of patients with diabetic glomerulosclerosis and 80 to 90 per cent of patients with renal amyloidosis, as well as in various forms of glomerulonephritis, is one of the few conditions associated with a characteristic serum protein electrophoretic pattern. As mentioned earlier, this typically shows a lowered albumin and raised α_2-globulin and often a lowered γ-globulin concentration. Electrophoretic findings in other conditions are not so characteristic.

Measurements of serum complement concentrations are of importance in distinguishing between the benign, self-limiting acute glomerulonephritis with low concentrations of C3, and sometimes C4, that return to normal within a few months, and the serious membranoproliferative glomerulonephritis (mesangio-capillary glomerulonephritis). In the latter condition low concentrations of C3 may continue for long periods (Michael *et al.*, 1969); the concentrations of C4 and the other early components of the complement system, however, are normal.

REFERENCES

Antoine, B. (1974), in *Protides of the Biological Fluids: Proceedings of 21st Colloquium, Bruges, 1973* (Ed. H. Peeters), Pergamon Press, Oxford, p. 347.

Antoine, B., J. Neveu, and P. D. Ward (1969), *Transplantation*, **8**, 98.

Ballantyne, R., W. G. Wood, and P. M. Meffan (1968), *Brit. Med. J.*, **ii**, 667.

Barratt, T. M., M. W. Turner, and S. G. O. Johansson (1971), *Lancet*, **ii**, 402.

Beetham, R., R. J. Mills, D. N. Raine, and R. H. R. White (1974), *Ann. Clin. Biochem;* **11**, 59.

Berger, J., H. Yaneva, and N. Hinglais (1971), in *Advances in Nephrology*, Vol. 1. (Eds. J. Hamburger, J. Crosnier, and M. H. Maxwell), Year Book Medical Publishers, Chicago, p. 11.

Berggård, I. (1961), *Clin. Chim. Acta*, **6**, 413.

Berggård, I. (1965), in *Protides of the Biological Fluids: Proceedings of 12th Colloquium, Bruges, 1964* (Ed. H. Peeters), Elsevier, Amsterdam, p. 285.

Berggård, I. (1970), in *Proteins in Normal and Pathological Urine* (Eds. Y. Manuel, J. P. Revillard, and H. Betuel), Karger, Basel, p. 7.

Berggård, I., and A. G. Bearn (1968), *J. Biol. Chem.*, **243**, 4095.

Berggård, I., and H. Bennich (1967), *Nature*, **214**, 697.

Berggård, I., and G. M. Edelman (1963), *Proc. Nat. Acad. Sci.*, **49**, 330.

Berggård, I., and P. Peterson (1967), *Nobel Symp. 3: γ-Globulins*, Almqvist and Wiksell, Stockholm, p. 71.

Berggård, I., H. Cleve, and A. G. Bearn (1964), *Clin. Chim. Acta*, **10**, 1.

Bernier, G. M., and R. S. Post (1973), *Transplantation*, **15**, 176.

Bernier, G. M., E. A. Fermin, C. A. Johnson, and M. W. Fanger (1974), in *Protides of the Biological Fluids: Proceedings of 21st Colloquium, Bruges, 1973* (Ed. H. Peeters), Pergamon Press, Oxford, p. 477.

Bienenstock, J., and T. B. Tomasi, Jr. (1968), *J. Clin. Invest.*, **47**, 1162.

Bing, J. (1936), *Acta Med. Scand.*, Suppl. 76, 1.

Biserte, G., R. Havez, and A. Hayem-Levy (1959), *Path. Biol.*, **7**, 123.

Blainey, J. D., D. B. Brewer, J. Hardwicke, and J. F. Soothill (1960), *Quart. J. Med.*, **29**, 235.

Braun, W. E., and J. P. Merrill (1968), *New Engl. J. Med.*, **278**, 1366.

Brod, J. (1963), *Postgrad. Med. J.*, **39**, 121.

Brod, J. (1971), *Brit. Med. J.*, **ii**, 135.

Burstone, M. S., and J. E. Falk (1956), *J. Histochem. Cytochem.*, **4**, 217.

Butler, E. A., and F. V. Flynn (1958), *Lancet*, **ii**, 978.

Butler, E. A., and F. V. Flynn (1961), *J. Clin. Path.*, **14**, 172.

Butler, E. A., F. V. Flynn, H. Harris, and E. B. Robson (1962), *Clin. Chim. Acta*, **7**, 34.

Cameron, J. S. (1966), *Proc. Roy. Soc. Med.*, **59**, 512.

Cameron, J. S., and G. Blandford (1966), *Lancet*, **ii**, 242.

Cameron, J. S., and R. H. R. White (1965), *Lancet*, **i**, 463.

Carter, B. A. (1970), Publication from Dept. of Biochemical Sciences, Univ. of Surrey (cited by Wellwood *et al.*, 1973).

Cash, J. D., M. S. Hoq, M. Cunningham, and J. L. Anderton (1973), *Lancet*, **i**, 154.

Clarkson, A. R. (1973), *Lancet*, **i**, 109.
Clarkson, A. R., J. B. Morton, and J. D. Cash (1970), *Lancet*, **ii**, 1220.
Cotterill, J. A., W. J. Cunliffe, and L. Bulusu (1971), *Lancet*, **ii**, 403.
Dance, N., R. G. Price, W. R. Cattell, J. Landsell, and B. Richards (1970), *Clin. Chim. Acta*, **27**, 87.
de Bono, D. P., and G. Franglen (1973), *Lancet*, **i**, 207.
de Vaux Saint-Cyr, Ch., G. Hermann, and N. Talal (1962), *Verh. Deut. Ges. Inn. Med.*, **68**, 335.
de Vaux Saint-Cyr, Ch., H. Clève, and G. Hermann (1963), *Rev. franç. Etudes clin. biol.*, **8**, 485.
Dunker, A. K., and R. R. Rueckert (1969), *J. Biol. Chem.*, **244**, 5074.
Ellis, B. G., R. J. Price, and J. C. Topham (1973), cited by Wellwood *et al.*, 1973.
Fish, A. J., R. C. Herdman, A. F. Michael, R. J. Pickering, and R. A. Good (1970), *Amer. J. Med.*, **48**, 28.
Fleming, A. (1922), *Proc. Roy. Soc.*, **B**, **93**, 306.
Fleming, A., and V. D. Allison (1922), *Brit. J. Exp. Path.*, **13**, 252.
Fletcher, A. P., N. Alkjaersig, and S. Sherry (1962), *J. Clin. Invest.*, **41**, 896.
Franklin, E. C. (1959), *J. Clin. Invest.*, **38**, 2159.
Friberg, L. (1950), *Acta Med. Scand.*, Suppl. 240, 138.
Gielow, L., D. Maruhn, I. Fuchs, G. Mues, and K. D. Bock (1974), in *Protides of the Biological Fluids: Proceedings of 21st Colloquium, Bruges, 1973* (Ed. H. Peeters), Pergamon Press, Oxford, p. 547.
Glenner, G. G. (1962), *J. Histochem, Cytochem.*, **10**, 257.
Goddard, P. F., and J. R. Hobbs (1968), *Proc. Roy. Soc. Med.*, **61**, 335.
Grant, A. M. S., L. R. I. Baker, and A. Neuberger (1973), *Clin. Sci.*, **44**, 377.
Grant, G. H. (1957), *J. Clin. Path.*, **10**, 360.
Hall, P. W., and M. Vasiljević (1974), in *Protides of the Biological Fluids: Proceedings of 21st Colloquium, Bruges, 1973* (Ed. H. Peeters), Pergamon Press, Oxford, p. 501.
Hardwicke, J. (1965), *Clin. Chim. Acta*, **12**, 89.
Hardwicke, J. (1974), in *Protides of the Biological Fluids: Proceedings of 21st Colloquium, Bruges, 1973* (Ed. H. Peeters), Pergamon Press, Oxford, p. 341.
Hardwicke, J., J. S. Cameron, J. F. Harrison, B. Hulme, and J. F. Soothill (1970), in *Proteins in Normal and Pathological Urine* (Eds. Y. Manuel, J. P. Revillard, and H. Betuel), Karger, Basel, p. 111.
Hardwicke, J., R. J. Mills, and R. H. R. White (1974), in *Protides of the Biological Fluids: Proceedings of 21st Colloquium, Bruges, 1973* (Ed. H. Peeters), Pergamon Press, Oxford, p. 449.
Harris, J. A., A. G. Diethelm, K. N. Mason, and C. G. Cobbs (1971), *Alabama J. Med. Sci.*, **8**, 105.
Harrison, J. F., J. D. Blainey, J. Hardwicke, D. S. Rowe, and J. F. Soothill (1966), *Clin. Sci.*, **31**, 95.
Harrison, J. F., G. S. Lunt, P. Scott, and J. D. Blainey (1968), *Lancet*, **i**, 371.
Hawkins, D., and C. G. Cochrane (1968), *Immunology*, **14**, 665.
Hayslett, J. P., P. E. Perillie, and S. C. Finch (1968), *New Engl. J. Med.*, **279**, 506.
Heremans, J. F. (1958a), *Rev. Belge Pathol. Méd. Exptl.*, **26**, 264.
Heremans, J. F. (1958b), *Clin. Chim. Acta*, **3**, 34.
Heremans, J. F., J. P. Vaerman, and M.-Th. Heremans (1959), *Nature*, **183**, 1606.
Heremans, M.-Th., J. P. Vaerman, and J. F. Heremans (1960) in *Protides of the Biological Fluids: Proceedings of the 7th Colloquium, Bruges, 1959* (Ed. H. Peeters), Elsevier, Amsterdam, p. 396.
Hermann, G. (1974), in *Protides of the Biological Fluids: Proceedings of 21st Colloquium, Bruges, 1973* (Ed. H. Peeters), Pergamon Press, Oxford, p. 379.
Hermann, G., and V. Zühlke (1971), *Z. ges. exp. Med.*, **154**, 101.
Hill, R. B., B. E. Dahrling, T. E. Starzl, and D. Rifkind (1967), *Amer. J. Med.*, **42**, 327.

Hitzig, W. H., S. Auricchio, and J.-L. Benninger (1965), *Klin. Woch.*, **43**, 1154.
Hochwald, G. M., and G. J. Thorbecke (1962), *Proc. Soc. Exp. Biol. Med.*, **109**, 91.
Hulme, B., and P. M. Pitcher (1973), *Lancet*, **i**, 6.
Jayle, M.-F., and G. Boussier (1954), *Bull. Soc. Chim. Biol.*, **36**, 959.
Jayle, M.-F., J. Vialatte, G. Boussier, and G. Lagrue (1953), *J. Urol. Med. Chir.*, **59**, 800.
Joachim, G. R., J. S. Cameron, M. Schwartz, and E. L. Becker (1964), *J. Clin. Invest.*, **43**, 2332.
Johansson, B. G., and U. Ravnskov (1972), *Scand. J. Urol. Nephrol.*, **6**, 249.
Kanai, M., A. Raz, and D. S. Goodman (1968), *J. Clin. Invest.*, **47**, 2025.
Keyser, J. W., G. L. Watkins, and J. R. Salaman (1976), *Clin. Chem.*, **22**, 925.
King, S. E. (1959), *N. Y. State Med. J.*, **59**, 825.
Klaus, D. (1962), *Ärtzl. Forsch.*, **16**, 18.
Ku, G., Z. Varghese. O. N. Fernando, R. Baillod, J. P. Hopewell, and J. F. Moorhead (1973), *Brit. Med. J.*, **iv**, 702.
Lachmann, P. J., H. J. Müller-Eberhard, H. G. Kunkel, and F. Paronetto (1962), *J. Exp. Med.*, **115**, 63.
Lancet (1974), **i**, 787.
Lazarus, J. A., and M. S. Marks (1946), *J. Urol.*, **56**, 246.
Lehmann, D., M. Prentice, and S. B. Rosalki (1970), *Ann. Clin. Biochem.*, **7**, 148.
Lerner, R. A., and F. J. Dixon (1968), *J. Immunol.*, **100**, 1277.
Lerner, R. A., R. J. Glassock, and F. J. Dixon (1967), *J. Exp. Med.*, **126**, 989.
Lerner, R. A., J. J. McPhaul, Jr., and F. J. Dixon (1970), in *Proteins in Normal and Pathological Urine* (Eds. Y. Manuel, J. P. Revillard, and H. Betuel), Karger, Basel, p. 63.
Löwgren, E. (1953), *Acta Med. Scand.*, **144**, 375.
Macanovic, M., A. de Bats, and D. K. Peters (1974), in *Protides of the Biological Fluids: Proceedings of 21st Colloquium, Bruges, 1973* (Ed. H. Peeters), Pergamon Press, Oxford, p. 473.
MacLean, P. R., and J. S. Robson (1967), *Lancet*, **i**, 539.
Marnay, A. (1961), *Nature*, **191**, 74.
McCluskey, R. T. (1971), *J. Exp. Med.*, **134**, 242.
McGarry, E., A. H. Sehon, and B. Rose (1955), *J. Clin. Invest.*, **34**, 832.
McKay, E., and R. J. Slater (1962), *J. Clin. Invest.*, **41**, 1638.
McQueen, E. G. (1962), *J. Clin. Path.*, **15**, 367.
Merskey, C., G. J. Kleiner, and A. J. Johnson (1966), *Blood*, **28**, 1.
Michael, A. F., R. C. Herdman, A. J. Fish, R. J. Pickering, and R. L. Vernier (1969), *Transplantation Proc.*, **1**, 925.
Mills, R. J., D. N. Raine, and R. H. R. White (1973), *Lancet*, **i**, 373.
Misra, R. P. (1964), *Chemical Composition of the Glomerular Basement Membrane* (Thesis, McGill University, Montreal), cited by Misra, 1972.
Misra, R. P. (1971), in *Pathobiology Annual*, vol. 1 (Ed.H. L. Ioachim), Appleton-Century-Crofts, New York, p. 325, cited by Misra, 1972.
Misra, R. P. (1972), in *Renal Disease* (Ed. D. Black), 3rd edn., Blackwell, Oxford, p. 187.
Morel-Maroger, L., A. Leathem, and G. Richet (1972), *Amer. J. Med.*, **53**, 170.
Noble, R. E., J. S. Najarian, and H. D. Brainerd (1965), *Proc. Soc. Exp. Biol. Med.*, **120**, 737.
Nussenzweig, V., and M. Seligmann (1960), *Rev. Hémat.*, **15**, 451.
Osserman, E. F. (1970), in *Proteins in Normal and Pathological Urine* (Eds. Y. Manuel, J. P. Revillard, and H. Betuel), Karger, Basel, p. 260.
Osserman, E. F., and D. P. Lawlor (1966), *J. Exp. Med.*, **124**, 921.
Patte, J.-C., G. Baldassaire, and J. Loret (1958), *Rev. franç. Etudes clin. biol.*, **3**, 960.
Pesce, A. J., M. Gaiyutis, and V. E. Pollak (1970), *J. Lab. Clin. Med.*, **75**, 586.
Pesce, A. J., I. Boreisha, and V. E. Pollak (1972), *Clin. Chim. Acta*, **40**, 27.
Pesce, A. J., A. Hsu, C. Kornhauser, K. Sethi, B. S. Ooi, and V. E. Pollak (1976), *Clin. Chem.*, **22**, 667.

Peters, D. K. (1974), in *Clinical Aspects of Immunology*, 3rd ed. (Eds. P. G. H. Gell, R. R. A. Coombes, and P. J. Lachmann) Blackwell, Oxford, p. 1217.
Peters, D. K., and D. G. Williams (1975), in *Pediatric Nephrology* (Eds. M. I. Rubin and T. M. Barratt), Williams and Wilkins, Baltimore.
Peterson, P. A. (1969), *Abstracts of Uppsala Dissertations in Medicine*, 75, cited by Rask and Peterson (1973).
Peterson, P. A., and I. Berggård (1971), *J. Biol. Chem.*, **246**, 25.
Peterson, P. A., P.-E. Evrin, and I. Berggård (1969), *J. Clin. Invest.*, **48**, 1189.
Piscator, M. (1962), *Arch. Environ. Health*, **4**, 607.
Poortmans, J. R. (1967), *Arch. Int. Physiol.*, **75**, 346.
Poortmans, J. R. (1970), in *Proteins in Normal and Pathological Urine* (Eds. Y. Manuel, J. P. Revillard, and H. Betuel), Karger, Basel, p. 229.
Poortmans, J. R., K. Bloch, and R. W. Jeanloz (1967a), *Clin. Chim. Acta*, **17**, 229.
Poortmans, J. R., R. W. Jeanloz, and K. Schmid (1967b), *Biochim. Biophys. Acta*, **133**, 363.
Price, R. G., N. Dance, B. Richards, and W. R. Cattell (1970), *Clin. Chim. Acta*, **27**, 65.
Prockop, D. J., and W. D. Davidson (1964), *New Engl. J. Med.*, **270**, 269.
Prout, G. R., E. V. Macalalag, and D. M. Hume (1964), *Surgery*, **56**, 283.
Rask, L., and P. A. Peterson (1973), in *Protides of the Biological Fluids: Proceedings of 21st Colloquium, Bruges, 1973* (Ed. H. Peeters), Pergamon Press, Oxford, p. 485.
Ravnskov, U., and B. G. Johansson (1974), in *Protides of the Biological Fluids: Proceedings of 21st Colloquium, Bruges, 1973* (Ed. H. Peeters), Pergamon Press, Oxford, p. 513.
Ray, P. N., and S. S. Rao (1939), *Brit. J. Urol.*, **11**, 48.
Revillard, J. P. (1964), *Les protéinuries au cours des maladies rénales*, Thesis (Lyon), Gatheron, Pont-de-Veyle, p. 39.
Ringoir, S., R. J. Wieme, and F. Derom (1968), *Excerpta Medica International Congress Series*, No. 179, p. 270.
Robinson, R. R. (1970), in *Proteins in Normal and Pathological Urine* (Eds. Y. Manuel, J. P. Revillard, and H. Betuel), Karger, Basel, p. 224.
Robinson, R. R., S. N. Glover, P. J. Phillippi, F. R. Lecocq, and P. R. Langelier (1961a), *Amer. J. Path.*, **39**, 291.
Robinson, R. R., C. T. Ashworth, S. N. Glover, P. J. Phillippi, F. R. Lecocq, and P. R. Langelier (1961b), *Amer. J. Path.*, **39**, 405.
Rowe, D. S. (1956), *J. Physiol.*, **134**, 1*P*.
Rowe, D. S. (1957), *Biochem. J.*, **67**, 435.
Rowe, D. S., and J. F. Soothill (1961), *Clin. Sci.*, **21**, 75.
Sandman, R., R. M. Margules, and S. L. Kountz (1973), *Clin. Chim. Acta*, **45**, 349.
Schultze, H. E., and J. F. Heremans (1966), *Molecular Biology of Human Proteins*, Vol. 1, Elsevier, Amsterdam.
Semeraro, N., M. B. Donati, and J. Vermylen (1973), *Lancet*, **i**, 1058.
Shapiro, A. L., E. Vinuela, and J. V. Maizel, Jr. (1967), *Biochem. Biophys. Res. Comm.*, **28**, 815.
Shehadeh, I. H., C. B. Carpenter, C. H. Montorio, and J. P. Merrill (1968), *Clin. Res.*, **16**, 324.
Shuster, S., and J. Marks (1970), *Systemic Effects of Skin Disease*, Heinemann, London.
Sonnet, J., and P. Brisbois (1956), *Acta Clin. Belg.*, **11**, 42.
Tamm, I., and F. L. Horsfall, Jr. (1950), *Proc. Soc. Exp. Biol. Med.*, **74**, 108.
Tamm, I., and F. L. Horsfall, Jr. (1952), *J. Exp. Med.*, **95**, 71.
Trotter, M. D., and E. A. Fairburn (1967), *Lancet*, **ii**, 231.
Turner, M. W., and D. S. Rowe (1966), *Nature*, **210**, 130.
Vaughan, J. H., R. F. Jacox, and B. A. Gray (1967), *J. Clin. Invest.*, **46**, 266.
Vere, D. W., and A. Walduck (1966), *Clin. Sci.*, **30**, 315.
Virella, G., and M. T. Pires (1974), in *Protides of the Biological Fluids: Proceedings of 21st Colloquium, Bruges, 1973* (Ed. H. Peeters), Pergamon Press, Oxford, p. 407.

Virella, G., M. T. Pires, and I. M. Coelho (1974), *Clin. Chim. Acta*, **50**, 63.
Waldmann, T. A., W. Strober, and R. P. Mogielnicki (1972), *J. Clin. Invest.*, **51**, 2162.
Walravens, P., E. C. Laterre, and J. F. Heremans (1968), *Clin. Chim. Acta*, **19**, 107.
Weber, K., and M. Osborn (1969), *J. Biol. Chem.*, **244**, 4406.
Wellwood, J. M., B. G. Ellis, J. H. Hall, D. R. Robinson, and A. E. Thompson (1973), *Brit. Med. J.*, **i**, 261.
Wibell, L., and P.-E. Evrin (1974), in *Protides of the Biological Fluids: Proceedings of 21st Colloquium, Bruges, 1973* (Ed. H. Peeters), Pergamon Press, Oxford, p. 519.
Wilson, C. B., and F. J. Dixon (1973), in *Renal Disease* (Ed. D. Black), Blackwell, Oxford, p. 275.
Yatzidis, H. (1964), *Nature*, **201**, 187.
Zühlke, V., and G. Hermann (1971), *Transplantation Proc.*, **3**, 361.

CHAPTER 5

Cardiovascular disease and lipoproteins

Historical*

Since about the middle of the century a variety of serum lipid measurements have in turn been proposed to aid in the diagnosis and management of coronary artery disease. The demonstration that *cholesterol* is a prominent constituent of atherosclerotic plaques, and the production of atherosclerotic-like lesions in experimental animals by feeding with cholesterol, were followed by innumerable studies of the relationship of cholesterol to cardiovascular disease. The clinical association of hypercholesterolaemia with conditions characterized by premature vascular disease (Piper and Orrild, 1956), numerous epidemiological observations (Keys *et al.*, 1958; Keys and Fidanza, 1960; Keys *et al.*, 1963; Keys, 1967), and several long-term prospective studies (Dawber *et al.*, 1957; Doyle *et al.*, 1959; Stamler *et al.*, 1960; Paul *et al.*, 1963) have established a strong association between ischaemic heart disease and hypercholesterolaemia (Kannel *et al.*, 1962; Epstein *et al.*, 1965). The experiments of Duff and McMillan (1949), which suggested that the physicochemical state of the cholesterol in the blood rather than its concentration might be the important factor, led to a series of physicochemical studies by Gofman and Lindgren and their coworkers (Gofman *et al.*, 1949; Jones *et al.*, 1951; Lindgren *et al.*, 1956). Beginning with the fact that cholesterol, together with phospholipid and triglyceride, is an integral part of the *lipoproteins*, those investigators were able with the aid of the ultracentrifuge to define a series of discrete classes of lipoproteins. They, and subsequently Fredrickson and his coworkers (1967), proposed that increases in the concentration of certain lipoprotein classes are associated with specific clinical syndromes; an example is the increase in the S_f 0–20 fraction of lipoproteins characteristic of familial hypercholesterolaemia, a condition that has been shown to be closely associated with premature vascular disease (Guravich, 1959). Application of ultracentrifugal lipoprotein analysis (Tamplin *et al.*, 1954) to the serum of subjects in the Framingham study† led to the suggestion that the susceptibility of a person to atherosclerosis might be estimated by calculation of an 'atherogenic index' (Gofman *et al.*, 1953) derived by assigning weighting factors to two particular lipoprotein classes, though the provisional nature of these factors was emphasized. A

*This account is based upon the review by Brown (1969).

†A major epidemiological and biochemical study of heart disease (see Kannel and Gordon, 1974).

Table 5.1 Properties of the various classes of lipoproteins. (Reproduced from J. W. Winkelman and D. R. Wybenga, *Clinical Chemistry: Principles and Technics*, 2nd edn. (Eds. R. J. Henry, D. C. Cannon and J. W. Winkelman), Harper & Row, Hagerstown, Md., 1974, by permission of Harper & Row, Inc., and the authors.)

	LP class*						
	Chylomicrons	VLDL (pre-β)	LDL (β)	HDL (α)	HDL_2	HDL_3	VHDL
Density range (g/ml)	< 0.95	0.95–1.006	1.006–1.063	1.063–1.21	1.063–1.125	1.125–1.21	> 1.21
Size (diameter)	1200–11,000 Å	300–700 Å	170–260 Å	74–98 Å			< 100 Å
Electrophoretic behaviour							
Paper	Origin	Pre-β	β	α			
Cellulose acetate	Origin	Pre-β	β	α			
Agarose	Origin	Pre-β	β	α			
Starch block	α_2, β	α_2	β_1	α_1			
Disc	Origin (loading gel)	α_2	β_1	α_1			
Flotation characteristics†							
S_f	>400	20–400	0–20				
F_{1-21}				0–9			
N-Terminal amino acids‡							
Major	Ser, Thr	Ser, Ala, Val	Ser	Gln, Thr			
Minor	Gln, Asp	Gln, Thr	Ala	Ala, Val			
Apoprotein	Apo-B Apo-A (secondary)	Apo-A Apo-B Apo-C (?)	Apo-B Apo-C (?)	Apo-A			Apo-A
Approximate molecular weight (in millions)	10^3–10^4	5–100	2–3	0.25			

*These abbreviations are as follows: VLDL, very-low-density lipoproteins; LDL, low-density lipoproteins; HDL, high-density lipoproteins; VHDL, very-high-density lipoprotein.

†S_f designates the negative sedimentation coefficient in Svedbergs in density 1.063 g/ml NaCl solution at 26° C. F_{1-21} is also a negative sedimentation coefficient at density 1.21 g/ml and at 26° C.

‡Major, > 30% of detectable end groups; minor, 10%–30% of detectable end groups.

large-scale study of lipoproteins and cholesterol concentrations as possible predictors of the clinical complications of atherosclerosis (Technical Group of the Committee on Lipoproteins and Atherosclerosis, 1954) led to the conclusion, however, that a simple determination of serum cholesterol was as useful as the more difficult, time-consuming, and expensive lipoprotein analysis.

In 1959 Albrink and Man focussed attention on the *triglyceride* content of serum, concluding that ischaemic heart disease is more closely associated with raised triglyceride concentrations than with hypercholesterolaemia. A relationship between hypertriglyceridaemia and ischaemic heart disease was subsequently confirmed (Carlson, 1960; Nicolaysen and Westlund, 1963; Hayes and Neil, 1964; Brown *et al.*, 1965); however, it has been emphasized that since both cholesterol and triglyceride are always present in serum as integral parts of lipoproteins, it is neither feasible nor desirable to relate either of these lipids independently to the atherosclerotic process (Brown *et al.*, 1966).

The development of a relatively simple paper electrophoretic technique by Lees and Hatch (1963) for the separation and identification of the major lipoprotein classes led to the classification of lipid disorders by Lees and Fredrickson which, with minor modifications, is widely used at the present time. The publications of Fredrickson and his coworkers have supported the concept of Gofman and Lindgren referred to above and suggest that many of the studies previously carried out would have been more fruitful if lipoprotein measurements rather than cholesterol and/or triglyceride determinations had been employed (Brown, 1969).

LIPOPROTEINS IN PLASMA

It has been known for a long time that many of the plasma proteins—especially those occurring in the electrophoretic α- and β-globulin regions—are rich in cholesterol and triglycerides. Several different systems of characterization of these lipoproteins have developed from studies of their physical, chemical, and other properties, and there are a number of nomenclatures based on the various methods of investigation employed. Table 5.1 summarizes the properties of the various classes of lipoproteins.

An important feature of lipoproteins is that they are particulate, the size, density, and mobility of the particles being related to their lipid/protein ratio. Although variations in chemical composition, for example in respect of triglyceride, phospholipid, cholesterol, and protein, do occur, there does not appear to be a continuous spectrum in the composition or properties either among the lipoproteins in general or within any particular class of lipoprotein (Winkelman and Wybenga, 1974).

From the clinical aspect the most important of these classes at present appear to be the α- or high-density lipoproteins, the β- or low-density lipoproteins, the pre-β- or very-low-density lipoproteins, and the chylomicrons. The distribution of these four classes in plasma as segregated by paper electrophoresis and by the ultracentrifuge is illustrated in Figure 5.1.

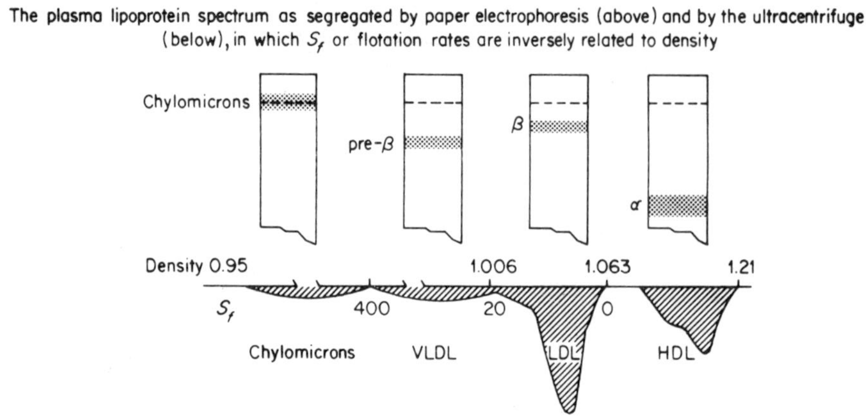

Figure 5.1. The plasma lipoprotein spectrum as segregated by paper electrophoresis (above) and by the ultracentrifuge (below), in which S_f or flotation rates are inversely related to density. (Reproduced, by permission of World Health Organization, from *Bull. Wld. Hlth. Org.*, 1970, **43**.)

α-Lipoproteins (high-density lipoproteins)

These lipoproteins on ultracentrifugation are mostly isolated between the densities of 1.063 and 1.21. They contain about 45 per cent of protein and the lipid component consists mainly of cholesterol and phospholipid.

β-Lipoproteins (low-density lipoproteins)

β-Lipoproteins are isolated between densities 1.006 and 1.063 and have S_f values of 0–20. They consist mainly of cholesterol and cholesteryl esters and contain also phospholipids, protein, and small amounts of glyceride. In man, β-lipoproteins are the major cholesterol-bearing lipoproteins and together the α- and β-lipoproteins normally account for about 90 per cent of the cholesterol and phospholipid in the plasma.

Pre-β-lipoproteins, or *very-low-density lipoproteins*

These are isolated in the ultracentrifuge in the fraction of density 0.96–1.006 and have S_f values of 20–400. They consist mainly of glycerides that are of 'endogenous' origin, i.e. either newly synthesized or derived from body stores rather than directly from the diet (see, however, p. 104). They also contain cholesterol, triglyceride, and a small amount of protein. Pre-β-hyperlipoproteinaemia renders the plasma opalescent but not creamy.

There is much evidence indicating that the liver is the main site of synthesis of endogenous triglyceride and presumably of many if not all of the circulating pre-β-lipoproteins. Conditions in which there is increased release of free fatty acids are potential causes of raised plasma concentrations of pre-β-lipoproteins (Fredrickson *et al.*, 1967).

Chylomicrons

These large particles, which have a density of about 0.9 and a correspondingly high S_f value (> 400), collect at the top of plasma when it is allowed to stand, and they remain at the origin on paper or agarose electrophoresis. The term chylomicron was originally coined to denote the visible particles that appear in lymph and blood in response to fat feeding and contain the fed glycerides (Gage and Fish, 1924). Subsequently the term was applied to all particulate lipid material in the plasma, but it is sometimes restricted to particles resulting from *exogenous* fat. It should be noted that endogenous particles may also have flotation rates greater than 400 (Fredrickson *et al.*, 1967), and also that some dietary triglycerides appear, soon after ingestion, in particles having the properties of very-low-density lipoproteins; moreover, some very-low-density lipoproteins have the immobility of chylomicrons on electrophoresis (Beaumont *et al.*, 1970). Chylomicrons consist mainly of triglycerides, with small amounts of phospholipid, cholesterol and protein. The protein content of chylomicrons is very low—usually between 0.5 and 2.5 per cent of their total weight.

Abnormal lipoproteins

A few apparently abnormal lipoproteins have been reported, such as β-lipoproteins that behave anomalously on centrifugal analysis; 'lipoprotein-X', found in patients with obstructive liver disease (see below); complexes of 'normal' lipoproteins with other globulins; the abnormal 'X_T-lipoproteins' found in persons homozygous for Tangier disease (p. 108); and a number of others (see Beaumont *et al.*, 1970).

Lipoprotein-X

Patients with obstructive jaundice have increased serum concentrations of unesterified cholesterol and phospholipids, and these changes are associated with the presence of a low-density lipoprotein of abnormal composition and properties (Eder *et al.*, 1955; Switzer, 1967; Picard and Veissiere, 1970; Seidel, 1971). This abnormal lipoprotein, called lipoprotein-X, differs from the normally occurring lipoproteins in composition, and in migrating towards the cathode instead of the anode on electrophoresis in agar gel at the usual pH—a property which forms the basis for its separation from the other lipoproteins (Seidel, 1971). The presence of lipoprotein-X is regarded as a specific and sensitive indicator of cholestasis; however, a positive result in the qualitative test does not differentiate between intra- and extrahepatic obstruction (Seidel *et al.*, 1973a; Ritland *et al.*, 1973), though quantitative determinations may be useful (Ritland, 1975; Magnani and Alaupovic, 1976). It has been suggested that combined determinations of the enzyme lecithin:cholesterol acyltransferase and of lipoprotein-X may help in differentiating between intra- and extrahepatic cholestasis (Wengeler *et al.*, 1972).

Table 5.2. Classification of apolipoproteins. (Reproduced from A. Chait, *Recent Advances in Clinical Biochemistry*, No. 1 (Ed. K. G. M. M. Alberti), Churchill Livingstone, Edinburgh, 1978, by permission of Churchill Livingstone Ltd. and Dr. Chait.)

ABC nomenclature	Lipoprotein	C-Terminal	Synonyms	
Apo-A-I	HDL	Glutamine	Fraction III	apo-LP-Gln-I
Apo-A-II	HDL	Glutamine	Fraction IV	apo-LP-Gln-II
Apo-B	LDL,VLDL	Serine		apo-LP-Ser
Apo-C-I	HDL,VLDL	Serine	Fraction V	apo-LP-Ser
Apo-C-II	HDL,VLDL	Glutamic acid	Fraction V	apo-LP-Glu
Apo-C-III	HDL,VLDL	Alanine	Fraction V	apo-LP-Ala
Apo-D	HDL		Thin line polypeptide	
Apo-E	HDL,VLDL	Alanine	Arginine-rich peptide	

APOLIPOPROTEINS

The proteins that form complexes with lipids presumably serve to facilitate lipid transport and metabolism. This non-lipid portion of the lipoprotein is called an apolipoprotein or more simply an apoprotein.

No type of hyperlipidaemia has hitherto been recognized as being due to an abnormality of apoprotein structure. The occurrence of such abnormalities, especially if they were to arise by mutation, would offer a basis for the possible aetiology of some forms of hyperlipidaemia (Beaumont *et al.*, 1970).

Nevertheless, the study of apolipoproteins is of considerable importance, since the nature of the apoprotein determines the lipid-binding characteristics of the molecule and the metabolic fate of the lipoprotein.

Each lipoprotein class contains one or more of these protein components. Various classifications have been proposed, but the one that has gained general acceptance derives from that originally suggested by Alaupovic (1968, 1971), known as the 'ABC' nomenclature (Table 5.2).

The major apolipoprotein of the high-density lipoprotein class is *apolipoprotein A (apo-A)*, which consists of two non-identical peptides, apo-A-I and apo-A-II (Shore and Shore, 1968), each of which has glutamine as the carboxy-terminal amino acid. *Apolipoprotein B (apo-B)* is probably the only apoprotein in the low-density lipoproteins, and it also occurs as a major component of the very-low-density lipoproteins. These also contain significant amounts of the three low molecular weight peptides of the *apolipoprotein C* family (*apo-C-I*, *apo-C-II*, and *apo-C-III*), the carboxy-terminal amino acids of which are serine, glutamic acid, and alanine respectively (Herbert *et al.*, 1971). These three peptides also occur as minor components of the high-density lipoproteins. Little is known of the apoprotein composition of the chylomicrons, except that they contain all the classes mentioned above. *Arginine-rich apoprotein* (*apo-E*) (Shore and Shore, 1972; Havel and Kane, 1973; Shore *et al.*, 1974) is found in very-low-density lipoproteins, high-density lipoproteins, and the intermediate-density lipoprotein formed during the catabolism of very-low-density to low-density lipoproteins; however, it is not found in low-density lipoproteins themselves. Yet another apoprotein, *apo-D*, has been described (McConathy and Alaupovic, 1973) and partially characterized (McConathy and Alaupovic, 1976). It occurs in a subgroup of the high-density lipoproteins.

Little is known of the precise function of the apolipoproteins, except that they serve to transport triglyceride from the sites of absorption or storage to the sites of utilization. *Apo-A-I* and *apo-D* have been thought to activate lecithin:cholesterol acyltransferase; the presence of *apo-B* seems to be essential for the formation of chylomicrons and very-low-density and low-density lipoproteins, which are absent in patients with abetalipoproteinaemia (p. 107), a condition in which *apo-B* is absent from the plasma (Gotto *et al.*, 1971).

ABNORMALITIES OF THE PLASMA LIPOPROTEIN PATTERN

The first classification of lipoprotein abnormalities appears to have been that of Fredrickson and Lees (1965), and this formed the basis of a fuller classification which was published in 1967 and which was later modified by a committee of the World Health Organisation (Beaumont *et al.*, 1970). Another classification—apparently not used nowadays to any great extent—was proposed by Strisower *et al.* (1968); and yet a third, based on a method of analysis which separates the lipoproteins according to particle size, was proposed by Stone and Thorp (1966; Stone *et al.*, 1970).

Although the classification of Fredrickson and his coworkers is widely used, some prefer a simpler scheme. According to Lewis (1973), the recognition of three categories is probably sufficient to distinguish groups for purposes of treatment and prognosis: these are hyper-β-lipoproteinaemia, endogenous hypertriglyceridaemias, and exogenous hypertriglyceridaemia. (For a discussion of this classification and its relationship to that of Fredrickson see Lewis (1973) and Chait (1978).)

The following brief account of the main features of the hyperlipoproteinaemias follows the classification of Fredrickson and his colleagues, which, as indicated above, is based upon electrophoretic analysis of the plasma lipoprotein pattern (Lees and Hatch, 1963) and the associated clinical picture. Correlation of the lipoprotein patterns or phenotypes with the clinical manifestations and with genetic information indicates that each type probably represents a different genotype, though this does not yet appear to have been proved. It may be noted that the numbering of lipoprotein patterns according to type in the Fredrickson system is arranged in a mnemonically convenient way, beginning at the origin on the electrophoretic strip, with Type I referring to the presence of chylomicrons, Type II to hyper-β-lipoproteinaemia, and so on.

Type I

The serum of patients in this group is characterized by the presence of chylomicrons in high concentration, even as long as 14 hours or more after the last meal, when the patient is on a normal fat intake. This chylomicronaemia is believed to be due to a deficiency of lipoportein lipase (Havel and Gordon, 1960; Kuo *et al.*, 1965; Fredrickson and Lees, 1966). The plasma is creamy in appearance, and on standing a creamy supernatant layer is formed (Figure 5.2). The cholesterol and triglyceride concentrations are raised. A number of clinical abnormalities develop (Table 5.3), but Type I hyperlipoproteinaemia is not thought to predispose to atherosclerotic disease. The syndrome is due to a rare abnormal allele appearing in the homozygous state.

Type II

Here the β-lipoproteins and cholesterol concentrations are raised, but the triglyceride concentration is usually normal or only slightly raised. The condition has been recognized for a long time and is known as essential familial hypercholesterolaemia (Wilkinson *et al.*, 1948). A subgrouping of Type II into Types IIa and IIb was proposed by Beaumont and his collaborators, (1970): in Type IIa there is a raised concentration of β-lipoproteins; Type IIb shows in addition an increase in the pre-β-lipoproteins, as well as a moderate increase in the triglyceride concentration. The plasma is clear or only slightly turbid (Figure 5.2). According to Beaumont and his collaborators (1970) the importance of identifying a Type IIb hyperlipoproteinaemia—i.e. of distinguishing it from Type IIa—is that treatment additional to that recommended for the 'pure' hypercholesterolaemia of Type IIa may be indicated. (Type IIa corresponds to the original Fredrickson Type II.) Type II hyperlipoproteinaemia, unlike Type I, is often associated with accelerated development of ischaemic heart disease. It may be secondary to hypothyroidism, the nephrotic syndrome, and a number of other diseases (see p. 105). The basic defect in familial Type II hyperlipoproteinaemia remains to be established.

Type III

This group probably includes most of the patients previously described as having 'mixed' familial hypercholesterolaemia and hyperlipaemia, in whom xanthomatosis, ischaemic heart disease, and mild diabetes are frequently present. Characteristically there is an increase in both β- and pre-β-lipoproteins; the electrophoretic strip may show either a broad, indistinct, heavily stained β-band or else completely separated, heavily stained β- and pre-β-bands. The plasma is lipaemic. There is some uncertainty as to whether both electrophoretic patterns definitely represent Type III hyperlipoproteinaemia, and additional supportive evidence—such as the typical schlieren pattern obtained by ultracentrifugal analysis, or the characteristic presence of a β-migrating band among the very-low-density lipoproteins—may be needed (Fredrickson and Levy, 1970). Fredrickson and his associates (1975) have recommended measurement of the ratio of very-low-density lipoprotein cholesterol to plasma

Classification of hyperlipoproteinaemia according to Frederickson.

	Normal Serum	Type I	Type IIa	Type IIb	Type III	Type IV	Type V

Fasting-serum after standing 12 hours

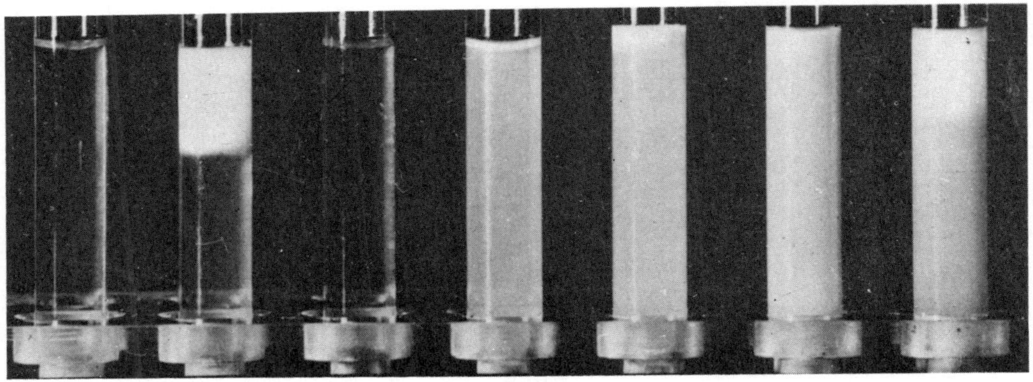

	Normal Serum	Type I	Type IIa	Type IIb	Type III	Type IV	Type V
Cholesterol	180–250mg/100ml	n–↑	↑↑↑	↑↑↑	↑↑	n–↑	n–↑
Triglycerides	74–172mg/100ml	↑↑↑	n	↑↑	↑↑	↑↑↑	↑↑↑

n = normal ↑ = slightly increased ↑↑ = increased ↑↑↑ = very high

Figure 5.2. Appearance of plasma, on standing, in the various types of hyperlipoproteinaemia. (Reproduced by permission of The Boehringer Corporation (London) Ltd.)

triglyceride concentration for the diagnosis of Type III hyperlipoproteinaemia. (Very-low-density lipoprotein cholesterol was calculated as the difference between the whole plasma cholesterol and that in the ultracentrifugal fraction having a density greater than 1.006.) When the plasma triglyceride concentration is between 1.5 and 10 g/l, Fredrickson and his coworkers regard ratios of over 0.30 as diagnostic of Type III hyperlipoproteinaemia, and advise that the diagnosis should be suspected if the ratio falls between 0.25 and 0.29.

In Type III hyperlipoproteinaemia there is an excess of lipoproteins having β-mobility but abnormally low density, i.e. less than 1.006. The predominant abnormalities are: subnormal concentrations of S_f 0–12 lipoproteins, moderate increases in S_f 12–20, and marked increases in the S_f 20–100 and often the S_f 100–400 subclasses (Fredrickson *et al.*, 1967). The plasma often shows lipaemia, which remains homogeneously dispersed even on standing in the refrigerator, apart from a slight 'creaming' that occurs if chylomicrons are present (Figure 5.2).

Tentative evidence indicates that the disorder may be due to accumulation of a normal intermediate in the conversion of pre-β- to β-lipoprotein (Levy *et al.*, 1971).

The genetics of Type III hyperlipoproteinaemia have been the subject of much speculation and study (see Fredrickson and Lees, 1965; Morganroth *et al.*, 1975; Hazzard *et al.*, 1975).

Type IV

Patients with this condition have increased plasma pre-β-lipoprotein and triglyceride, and normal or increased cholesterol concentrations. The concentrations of α- and β-lipoproteins are usually below normal and there is no chylomicronaemia. As in Type III, the plasma is turbid, and the turbidity remains evenly distributed in the tube after storage at 4 °C for up to 24 hours (Figure 5.2).

The Type IV lipoprotein pattern has been described as 'the hallmark of endogenous hyperlipaemia' (Fredrickson *et al.*, 1967). This endogenous hyperlipaemia is typically carbohydrate-inducible. It may be caused by the excretion of endogenous glycerides into the plasma at rates exceeding the capacity of the tissues to remove them. Another possibility is that there is a decrease in the ability of the adipose tissue to remove glyceride that is entering the plasma at a normal rate; and a third possible abnormality is the formation of abnormal lipoproteins that are resistant to the normal processes of removal (Fredrickson *et al.*, 1967). Of these possibilities, the second—i.e. defective removal of triglyceride from the plasma—appears to be the underlying lesion in many patients (Havel *et al.*, 1970; Boberg *et al.*, 1972).

Type IV hyperlipoproteinaemia almost certainly predisposes to coronary heart disease (Carlson and Böttiger, 1972). It is often secondary to other diseases, especially diabetes mellitus and pancreatitis (see p. 105).

Table 5.3. Summary of the most consistent features of the Fredrickson classification of the hyperlipidaemias as described in the W.H.O. memorandum of 1970.*(Reproduced, with permission, from *J. Clin. Path.*, 1973, **26**, Suppl. (Ass. Clin. Path.), **5**, 26.)

Fredrickson Type	Chylomicrons (immobile) Mainly triglyceride	LDL (β-mobility) Mainly cholesterol	VLDL (pre-β-mobility) Mainly triglyceride	'Floating' β (VLDL)	Plasma cholesterol	Plasma triglyceride	Fasting plasma on standing	Incidence	Clinical features: general	Clinical features: xanthomas	Commoner causes of secondary hyperlipidaemia
I Hyperchylomicronaemia	+		N or slightly +		Usually +	+	Clear with cream	Rare	Hepatosplenomegaly Attacks of abdominal pain (including pancreatitis)	Eruptive	Diabetes Dysglobulinaemia
IIA Hyper-β-lipoproteinaemia		+			+		Clear	Second most common	Arterial disease	Tendinous Tuberous Xanthelasma Planar	Hypothyroidism Nephrosis Dysglobulinaemia Biliary obstruction
IIB Hyper-β-lipoproteinaemia (with pre-β)		+	+		+	+	Clear or slightly milky				
III 'Broad' or 'floating' β-lipoproteinaemia	N or slightly +			+	+	+	Milky with a little cream	Rare		Tuberous Tubero-eruptive Planar Xanthelasma	Dysglobulinaemia
IV Hyper-pre-β-lipoproteinaemia			+		N or +	+	Clear or milky (no cream)	Most common	Arterial disease Attacks of abdominal pain (including pancreatitis)	Tubero-eruptive	Diabetes Nephrosis Dysglobulinaemia Alcohol, gout Hypothyroidism Pancreatitis
V 'Mixed' hyperchylomicronaemia + hyper-pre-β-lipoproteinaemia	+		+		+	+	Milky with cream	Rare	Attacks of abdominal pain	Eruptive	Diabetes Nephrosis Dysglobulinaemia Pancreatitis

*Beaumont *et al.*, (1970). N = Normal level; + = raised level.

Type V

The lipoprotein pattern here suggests a mixture of Types I and IV. Chylomicrons are present, and the plasma on standing shows a creamy layer at the top, with turbid plasma underneath (Figure 5.2). (This is a particularly useful test when the presence of extremely high concentrations of pre-β-lipoprotein makes it difficult to demonstrate chylomicrons by electrophoretic analysis.) The plasma concentration of pre-β-lipoprotein is increased, and so is that of cholesterol and triglyceride.

The Type V pattern is often regarded as indicating a combination of exogenous and endogenous hyperlipaemia. It may thus represent simply a stage of Type IV, produced by the imposition of a large amount of dietary fat on clearing mechanisms burdened by endogenous glycerides; or it may appear when the exogenous hyperlipaemia of Type I is clearing on a low-fat diet, which causes 'carbohydrate induction' in such patients, with an abnormal accumulation of pre-β-lipoproteins.

As with the other types of hyperlipoproteinaemia, Type V can be separated into primary and secondary forms. It is uncertain whether patients with the condition are more liable to atherosclerotic diseases.

The characteristics of the hyperlipoproteinaemia phenotypes are summarized in Table 5.3.

Lewis (1973) expresses reservations about Type V hyperlipoproteinaemia as an entity. The pattern can vary in a given patient, some serum samples merely showing hyper-pre-β-lipoproteinaemia without an excess of chylomicrons. Secondly, affected families may show either the Type V pattern of hyper-pre-β-lipoproteinaemia alone (i.e. as in Type IV) (Nixon *et al.*, 1969; Fredrickson, 1969). Finally, there is evidence, cited by Lewis (1973), that the physical properties that define chylomicrons on electrophoresis and ultracentrifugation do not provide proof of the origin of the triglyceride they carry. Thus Mancini and his coworkers (1973) have shown that chylomicron-like particles containing fat of endogenous origin appear in the plasma of normal subjects on high carbohydrate diets; and although pre-β-lipoprotein is known to transport endogenous triglyceride, there is evidence that dietary fat also appears in this lipoprotein and acutely raises its plasma concentration (February *et al.*, 1972; Lewis *et al.*, 1973). It may be that the physical properties—for example, density—of triglyceride-containing lipoproteins are affected by the quantity of lipid requiring transport as well as by its origin (Lewis *et al.*, 1973).

Other recent work has shown that the diagnosis of primary hyperlipoproteinaemia, Types I–V, does not imply the recognition of a defined metabolic defect in lipid of lipoprotein metabolism; in other words, a specific type of hyperlipoproteinaemia, as assessed by clinical symptoms, together with the lipoprotein electrophoresis pattern and lipid analyses, could represent a heterogeneous group of lipid disorders. Conversely, different lipoprotein patterns (corresponding to Types IIa, IV, and IIb—associated with hypercholesterolaemia, hypertriglyceridaemia, or both) may occur in a single family in the disorder known as *familial combined hyperlipidaemia* (Goldstein *et al.*, 1973).

Hyper-α-lipoproteinaemia

A rare condition has been described in which the concentration of serum α-lipoprotein is markedly increased (Naito and Lewis, 1973; Glueck *et al.*, 1974; Naito *et al.*, 1975). In the absence of any obvious metabolic, hormonal, or other aetiological factors, it is regarded as a primary or familial condition. It does not appear to be associated with ill health. Immunological studies suggest that the high-density lipoproteins in these subjects have the properties of normal high-density lipoproteins, these simply being present in excessive concentration.

SECONDARY HYPERLIPIDAEMIA

It must be emphasized that *secondary hyperlipidaemia* may account for a high percentage of the cases of lipid abnormality seen. Common causes of secondary hyperlipidaemia are: diabetes mellitus, alcoholism, hypothyroidism, the nephrotic syndrome, chronic renal failure, gout, and obstructive liver disease. Other causes are: steroid therapy, Cushing's syndrome, hypopituitarism, pregnancy, oral contraceptive therapy, lipodystrophy, acromegaly, dysglobulinaemias, systemic lupus erythematosus, porphyria, idiopathic hypercalcaemia, vitamin D intoxication, glycogen storage disease, and anorexia. It is important to diagnose the condition, because, in most cases, the lipid abnormality responds to treatment of the primary disorder (Chait, 1973); however, exceptions to this are the hyperlipidaemias associated with gout and chronic renal failure (Chait, 1973).

Almost any lipoprotein pattern may be found in any of these conditions, and the pattern may even vary from time to time in the same patient (Chait, 1973). Possible mechanisms have been reviewed by Chait (1973).

LIPOPROTEINS AND THE PATHOGENESIS OF ATHEROSCLEROSIS

Histologically, atherosclerosis is characterized by the accumulation of lipids in the arterial wall and by a variable connective-tissue reaction. Evidence from a number of sources suggests that sclerosis of the arterial wall is followed by an accumulation of lipids, among which cholesterol, particularly esterified cholesterol, predominates. Although experimental evidence shows that cholesterol enters the wall of the normal vessel mainly in the free form, it has been suggested that damage to the endothelium in established atheroma permits the entry of significant amounts of lipoprotein. This would imply that atheroma or atherosclerosis is a self-perpetuating process once it has exceeded a certain critical phase. The subject has been reviewed by Adams (1973).

From the work of several groups of investigators it would seem that the concentration of α- or high-density lipoproteins in the plasma is inversely related to the risk of acquiring coronary heart disease (Lewis *et al.*, 1974; Carlson and Ericsson, 1975; Rhoads *et al.*, 1976; Berg *et al.*, 1976; Miller *et al.*, 1977; Gordon *et al.*, 1977). One study suggested that the association is not a causal one but simply reflects the reciprocal relationship between the plasma concentrations of high-density-lipoprotein-cholesterol and triglyceride (Carlson and Ericsson, 1975); however, an inverse correlation has since been shown to exist between the concentration of plasma high-density-lipoprotein-cholesterol and coronary heart disease in the absence of a correlation between this disease and plasma triglyceride concentration (Rhoads *et al.*, 1976).

The mechanism of the apparently protective effect of high-density lipoproteins is not known with certainty. Interaction between high-density lipoproteins and lechithin:cholesterol acyltransferase has been suggested (Glomset, 1968) as a mechanism whereby unesterified cholesterol is removed from peripheral tissues and transported to the liver, where it undergoes catabolism. The enhancement of the release of cholesterol from skin fibroblasts *in vitro* by high-density lipoprotein (Stein *et al.*, 1976) provides additional support for its rôle as an acceptor of tissue cholesterol.

New evidence for the regulation of tissue cholesterol pools by high-density lipoproteins was presented by Miller and Miller (1975), who showed that the size of the body cholesterol pool increases with decreasing plasma concentrations of high-density lipoprotein but is unrelated to the plasma concentrations of other lipoproteins and of cholesterol. An additional explanation for the apparently protective effect of high-density lipoprotein is suggested by the work of Carew and his associates (1976). They investigated the interaction between porcine lipoproteins and cultured smooth-muscle cells derived from the arterial wall, and found that the extent to which these cells accumulated cholesterol when incubated with low-density lipoproteins was greatly diminished by the presence of high-density lipoproteins in the incubation medium. This effect was due to a reduction in the amount of low-density lipoproteins bound to smooth-muscle cells; since the latter form one of the major sites of accumulation of low-density lipoproteins within the arterial wall, these experimental findings suggest that high-density lipoproteins may, by competing with low-density lipoproteins for receptors on the cell surface, play a part in limiting the deposition of cholesterol and in promoting its removal from the arterial wall.

The views that high-density lipoproteins are primarily a means for the carriage of tissue cholesterol back to the liver, and that they 'compete' with low-density lipoproteins in the manner described above, have been questioned by Cramp and Tickner (1977). They point out how, in terms of a model previously proposed (Cramp *et al.*, 1976), low concentrations of high-density lipoproteins may be a by-product of the atherogenic process rather than its cause.

INHERITED LIPOPROTEIN DEFICIENCY STATES

There are two genetically determined disorders in which the normal β- or α-lipoproteins, respectively, are absent from the plasma, namely abetalipoproteinaemia and familial α-lipoprotein deficiency (Tangier disease). In the latter condition small amounts of α-lipoproteins are in fact present, but they appear to differ immunologically from the normally occurring α-lipoproteins.

Abetalipoproteinaemia

The earliest description of this condition appears to have been that of Bassen and Kornzweig (1950), who investigated two patients with neurological abnormalities and 'crenated' red blood corpuscles (acanthocytes). In addition to acanthocytosis a very low plasma concentration of cholesterol and absence of β-lipoproteins were subsequently recognized as features of the condition, for which the name abetalipoproteinaemia was suggested (Salt *et al.*, 1960). The disease is usually associated in infancy with steatorrhoea and retarded growth. Malabsorption becomes less pronounced in late childhood and neurological abnormalities develop. The key features may be summarized as follows: hypolipidaemia and clear plasma, malabsorption, cerebellar ataxia, peripheral neuropathy, acanthocytosis, retinitis pigmentosa, and autosomal recessive inheritance (Fredrickson *et al.*, 1967). In a study of 6 patients from four kindreds, the absence of plasma β-lipoprotein was confirmed by sensitive immunochemical methods capable of detecting less than one ten-thousandth of the normally occurring amounts (Levy *et al.*, 1966b).

Abetalipoproteinaemia is one of the rare instances in which, on ultracentrifugal analysis of the plasma, α-lipoproteins appear in the density region of 1.019 to 1.063—a region usually occupied exclusively by the β-lipoproteins. This lowering of the density of the α-lipoproteins is attributed to the presence of an abnormally large amount of lipid, the apoprotein ('A' protein) being normal in respect of both immunochemical behaviour and amino acid composition (Levy *et al.*, 1966b).

Patients with abetalipoproteinaemia digest fats and absorb the resulting monoglycerides and free fatty acids into the cells of the intestinal mucosa, reforming them into triglycerides; however, chylomicrons are not released (Fredrickson *et al.*, 1967).

When the patients are given diets with a high carbohydrate content, designed to induce the production of endogenous glycerides and the release of pre-β-lipoprotein, the plasma glyceride concentration is not increased and pre-β-lipoproteins do not appear (Levy *et al.*, 1966b). It would seem that in patients with abetalipoproteinaemia the liver is able to produce and store glycerides but not to transfer the lipid into the plasma. The condition is associated with an absence of apolipoprotein B from the plasma.

Hypobetalipoproteinaemia

A familial deficiency of β-lipoproteins has been reported in a few patients (Kuo and Basset, 1962; van Buchem *et al.*, 1966; Lewis *et al.*, 1966). Plasma β-lipoprotein concentrations were from 10 to 50 per cent of normal, and there were comparable decreases in cholesterol, phospholipids and glycerides. Although some patients were found to have abnormally fragile red cells or acanthocytes, and progressive neuromuscular difficulties developing in adulthood, fat absorption and chylomicron formation are not abolished. Familial hypo-β-lipoproteinaemia is differentiated from that secondary to acute infections, other severe debilitating illnesses, or malabsorption caused by gastro-intestinal lesions.

Familial α-lipoprotein deficiency (Tangier disease)

This condition has been named Tangier disease, since it was first discovered in two siblings who resided in Tangier Island in Chesapeake Bay, USA. The characteristic abnormality is the great size and peculiar orange colour of the tonsils, associated with gross deposition of cholesterol esters in the reticulo-endothelial tissues. Sometimes there is also enlargement of the liver, spleen, and lymph nodes. Deposition of lipids is widespread and may occur in cutaneous lesions and in the cornea, in blood vessels, and in the reticuloendothelial cells of the rectal mucosa.

The primary inheritable defect appears to be a mutation in an allele regulating the synthesis of one of the major apoproteins of α-lipoprotein, as a result of which the concentration of α-lipoprotein in the plasma is greatly reduced (Lux *et al.*, 1972). The presence of a single abnormal autosomal gene results in abnormally low plasma concentrations of α-lipoprotein and no significant deposition of lipid in the tissues (Fredrickson, 1964), but the homozygous abnormal genotype is expressed by an almost complete absence of all plasma high-density or α-lipoproteins and by the accumulation of cholesterol esters in the tissues. On electrophoretic or immunoelectrophoretic analysis the plasma of the homozygote usually appears to be devoid of α-lipoproteins, though with appropriate antisera and under suitable experimental conditions a small amount of α-lipoprotein can be detected. Although this has similarities to normal α-lipoprotein it has been shown not to be antigenically identical (Levy and Fredrickson, 1966) and has been called Tangier α-lipoprotein ('α_T-lipoprotein'). The heterozygous relatives of patients have both α_T-lipoprotein and normal α-lipoprotein in their plasma.

Patients with Tangier disease absorb fat normally from the intestine, and chylomicrons are released into the circulation. This contrasts with the situation in abetalipoproteinaemia, and so does their unimpaired ability to release endogenous glyceride into the circulation in response to a dietary carbohydrate load (Levy *et al.*, 1966a). This endogenous hyperlipidaemia is associated with the presence of triglyceride-rich lipoproteins having a density of less than 1.006, and these appear as a broad β-band on electrophoresis. The fact that they do not appear in the pre-β-position normally occupied by very low-density lipoproteins is good evidence that the latter owe their pre-β-mobility to the presence of a α-lipoproteins in the complex (Levy *et al.*, 1966a).

It is evident that α-lipoproteins are not essential for the transfer of endogenous and exogenous glyceride into the plasma.

LABORATORY TESTS IN THE INVESTIGATION OF LIPOPROTEIN DISORDERS

These tests will usually be for the diagnosis and typing of hyper- rather than hypolipoproteinaemia. Some simple screening tests should first be applied before more complicated procedures are adopted. An estimation of the serum cholesterol concentration, together with inspection of the serum for turbidity (Figure 5.2), may suffice. According to Fredrickson and his colleagues (1967) the best combination of tests is the measurement of both cholesterol and glyceride concentrations: if both are clearly within the normal range, hyperlipoproteinaemia is ruled out.

In reviewing an extensive series of 'lipid profiles' Iammarino (1975) concluded that routine lipoprotein electrophoresis is superfluous in the vast majority of cases, sufficient information generally being obtained from the serum cholesterol and triglyceride concentrations. He recommends that lipoprotein electrophoresis should be restricted to those specimens in which the concentration of triglyceride exceeds 3.50 g/l; according to St. Clair (1975), however, the decisive concentration should be set somewhat lower, *viz*. at 1.50–2.00 g/l.

It should be emphasized that before primary hyperlipidaemia or primary hyperlipoproteinaemia may be diagnosed certain secondary causes must be excluded. As mentioned above, certain disease states not primarily related to alterations of lipid metabolism—hyperthyroidism, uraemia, the nephrotic syndrome, obstructive liver disease, etc.—may be associated with increases in serum lipid concentrations and abnormal lipoprotein patterns; so may pregnancy. In addition, contraceptive pills and other drugs have been reported to cause hyperlipidaemia.

Probably the most convenient method for routine laboratory phenotyping of hyperlipoproteinaemias is electrophoresis on cellulose acetate followed by lipid staining, the pattern being compared visually with known normal and abnormal patterns. A suitable technique is described by Winkelman and Wybenga (1974). The same authors discuss critically the various methods available and give criteria for determining whether the cholesterol and triglyceride results are consistent with the electrophoretic pattern.

A method based on the precipitation by polyanion of serum lipoproteins *in situ* after electrophoresis in gels has been described (Seidel *et al.*, 1973b). An application of this technique involving selective precipitation in the gel (Wieland and Seidel, 1973) appears to offer a rapid method for the diagnosis of Type III hyperlipoproteinaemia without the necessity for ultracentrifugal analysis.

It is important to standardize the conditions under which blood is taken. The patient should be resting and in the fasting state, i.e. the specimen should be taken 10–14 hours after the last meal. Venostasis should be avoided. Either plasma or serum may be used.

With regard to the stability of specimens, conflicting reports have appeared, for example as to whether freezing has an effect on the electrophoretic pattern; Fredrickson and his coworkers (1967) reported that freezing brought about irreversible changes in the paper electrophoretic pattern, whereas other workers found that storage in the frozen state for several months had no such effect (Adlersberg *et al.*, 1955; Dangerfield and Smith, 1955). Mills and Wilkinson (1962) found that in most samples with a 'normal' distribution of lipoproteins very little decay occurs during the first 12 months at $-15\,^{\circ}C$; however, when the plasma contains high concentrations of lipoproteins degradation often occurs; and Mills (1977) has reiterated the warning against freezing plasma for lipoprotein studies. According to Gottfried and his colleagues (1955), storage either at $37\,^{\circ}C$ or in the refrigerator brings about decreases in the β-lipoprotein to the extent of 10, 20, and 25 per cent after 1, 2, and 3 days' storage, respectively. On the other hand, Winkelman and his associates (1970) found that samples kept at room temperature for 3 days were suitable for lipoprotein analysis by cellulose acetate electrophoresis; stability was satisfactory after storage at refrigerator temperature for at least 28 days, or at freezer temperature for 14 days provided that only one freeze–thaw cycle occurred. It is clearly necessary, unless the analysis can be performed on the day the specimen is taken, for each laboratory to establish the effect of delay, and of conditions of storage, for the method employed in that particular laboratory.

For the determination of cholesterol and triglycerides, samples should similarly be collected 10–14 hours after a meal. The patient should if possible be allowed to rest on a bed for at least half an hour before blood is taken, since changes of the order of 10 to 15 per cent in the concentration of serum lipids may occur with changes of posture (Stoker *et al.*, 1966). Venous stasis should be avoided, as this can cause errors due to haemoconcentration (Koerselman *et al.*, 1961). Freezing of samples has no effect on the result of either analysis.

α_2-ANTITHROMBIN, β-THROMBOGLOBULIN, AND CLOTTING

As mentioned in the Preface, the various proteins involved in blood clotting have, in the main, been excluded from consideration in this book. Exceptions are made, however, in the cases of *α_2-antithrombin* and *β-thromboglobulin*, which are discussed briefly below.

α_2-Antithrombin

α_2-Antithrombin (also called antithrombin III) is one of the plasma antagonists of thrombin, as well as other clotting enzymes (Rosenberg, 1975), and hence is concerned in the regulation of blood clotting. Patients with a deficiency of α_2-antithrombin are highly susceptible to venous thrombosis (Egeberg, 1965; Van der Meer *et al.*, 1973; Marciniak *et al.*, 1974).

Measurements of plasma α_2-antithrombin in women taking oral contraceptives have given varying results, depending on the methods of assay used (von Kaulla and von Kaulla, 1970; Hender and Nilsson, 1973; Gitel and Wessler, 1975). Most investigators, however, would probably agree that a causal relationship between the use of oral contraceptives and deep-vein thrombosis in previously healthy women has been established by several studies (M.R.C. Sub Committee, 1967; Vessey *et al.*, 1970; Royal College of General Practitioners Study Group, 1974; Sagar *et al.*, 1976a,b.). Using a functional assay for antithrombin, Sagar and his coworkers (1976a) showed that, in a series of women undergoing emergency surgical operation, patients with the lowest plasma antithrombin activity were those who developed post-operative deep-vein thrombosis; and the same group showed that patients undergoing total hip replacement were also more liable to this complication if their pre-operative plasma antithrombin activity was low (Sagar *et al.*, 1976b).

It should be noted that normal plasma concentrations of antithrombin in patients with thrombosis have been reported (Hedner and Nilsson, 1973; Donati *et al.*, 1973; Korvald *et al.*, 1974); it would seen that immunological measurement of the concentration of antithrombin is of less value in predicting thrombosis than measurement of its biological activity, as in the studies of Sagar and his associates referred to above. This is borne out by the observations of Sas and his coworkers (1974), who found that in a Hungarian family with a high incidence of spontaneous thromboembolism immunological measurement indicated normal concentrations of antithrombin, but that this had a marked diminution of antithrombin activity.

β-Thromboglobulin

Aggregation of platelets occurs during thrombus formation (French, 1969) and is followed by the release of β-thromboglobulin, a recently isolated platelet-specific protein (Moore *et al.*, 1975; Ludlam *et al.*, 1975a). Using a radioimmunoassay, Ludlam and his coworkers (1975b) found markedly raised plasma concentrations of β-thromboglobulin in patients with proven deep-vein thrombosis, and proposed this measurement as a rapid screening test. Other causes of intravascular platelet aggregation can result in raised plasma concentrations of the protein, and these have been observed in patients with rheumatic heart-disease, prosthetic cardiac valves, or arterial thrombosis (Ludlam *et al.*, 1975a).

Estimation of β-thromboglobulin has also been proposed as an aid to the diagnosis of arterial thrombosis: in patients with myocardial infarction a very high plasma concentration of the protein at or shortly after admission, associated with a negative ^{125}I-fibrinogen leg scan or ultrasound test, is strongly indicative of mural thrombosis (Denham *et al.*, 1977).

Release of β-thromboglobulin from platelets during clotting necessitates great care during venepuncture and preparation of the plasma; a carelessly collected blood sample can contain a high concentration of β-thromboglobulin (Ludlam *et al.*, 1975b).

REFERENCES

Adams, C. W. M. (1973), in *Atherogenesis: Initiating Factors* (Ciba Foundation Symposium 12 (N.S.), Eds. R. Porter and J. Knight), Elsevier-Excerpta Medica-North-Holland, Amsterdam, p. 5.

Adlersberg, D., E. T. Bossak, I. H. Sher, and H. Sobotka (1955), *Clin. Chem.*, **1**, 18.

Alaupovic, P. (1968), *Progr. Biochem. Pharmacol.*, **4**, 91.

Alaupovic, P. (1971), *Atherosclerosis*, **13**, 141.

Albrink, M. J., and E. B. Man (1959), *Arch. Int. Med.*, **103**, 4.

Bassen, F. A., and A. L. Kornzweig (1950), *Blood*, **5**, 381.

Beaumont, J. L., L. A. Carlson, G. R. Cooper, Z. Fejfar, D. S. Fredrickson, and T. Strasser (1970), *Bull. Wld. Hlth. Org.*, **43**, 891.

Berg, K., A.-L. Børresen, and G. Dahlén (1976), *Lancet*, **i**, 499.

Boberg, J., A. L. Carlson, U. Freyschuss, B. W. Lassers, and M. L. Wahlqvist (1972), *Europ. J. Clin. Invest.*, **2**, 454.

Brown, D. F. (1969), *Amer. J. Med.*, **46**, 691.

Brown, D. F., J. T. Doyle, and S. H. Kinch (1965), *New Engl. J. Med.*, **273**, 947.

Brown, D. F., S. H. Kinch, and J. T. Doyle (1966), *J. Atheroscler. Res.*, **6**, 232.

Carew, T. E., T. Koschinsky, S. B. Hayes, and D. Steinberg (1976), *Lancet*, **i**, 1315.

Carlson, L. A. (1960), *Acta Med. Scand.*, **167**, 399.

Carlson, L. A., and L. E. Böttiger (1972), *Lancet*, **i**, 865.

Carlson, L. A., and M. Ericsson (1975), *Atherosclerosis*, **21**, 435.

Chait, A. (1973), *J. Clin. Path.*, **26**, Suppl. (Assoc. Clin. Path.) **5**, 68.

Chait, A. (1978), in *Recent Advances in Clinical Biochemistry* (Ed. K. G. M. M. Alberti), No. 1, Churchill Livingstone, Edinburgh, p. 73.

Cramp, D. G., and T. R. Tickner (1977), *Lancet*, **ii**, 1086.

Cramp, D. G., T. R. Tickner, and M. R. Wills (1976), *Lancet*, **ii**, 176.

Dangerfield, W. G., and E. B. Smith (1955), *J. Clin. Path.*, **8**, 132.

Dawber, T. R., F. E. Moore, and G. V. Mann (1957), *Amer. J. Pub. Health*, **47**, Suppl. 4, 4.

Denham, M. J., M. Fisher, G. James, and M. Hassan (1977), *Lancet*, **i**, 1154.

Donati, M. B., K. Vandenberghe, A. Molla, M. De Roo, and M. Verstraete (1973), *Lancet*, **i**, 726.

Doyle, J. T., S. Heslin, H. E. Hilleboe, and P. F. Formel (1959), *New Engl. J. Med.*, **261**, 1096.

Duff, G. L., and G. C. McMillan (1949), *J. Exp. Med.*, **89**, 611.

Eder, H. A., E. M. Russ, R. A. R. Pritchett, M. M. Wilber, and D. P. Barr (1955), *J. Clin. Invest.*, **34**, 1147.

Egeberg, O. (1965), *Thromb. Diath. Haemorrh.*, **13**, 516.

Epstein, F. H., T. Francis, Jr., N. H. Hayner, B. C. Johnson, M. O. Kjelsberg, J. A. Napier, L. D. Ostrander, Jr., N. W. Payne, and H. J. Dodge (1965), *Amer. J. Epidemiol.*, **81**, 307.

February, A., M. Mattock, A. Chait, and B. Lewis (1972), *Clin. Sci.*, **43**, 4P.

Fredrickson, D. S. (1964), *J. Clin. Invest.*, **43**, 228.

Fredrickson, D. S. (1969), *Trans. Assoc. Amer. Phycns.*, **82**, 68.

Fredrickson, D. S., and R. S. Lees (1965), *Circulation*, **31**, 321.

Fredrickson, D. S., and R. S. Lees (1966), in *The Metabolic Basis of Inherited Disease* (Eds. J. B. Stanbury, J. B. Wyngaarden, and D. S. Fredrickson), 2nd edn., McGraw Hill, New York, p. 429.

Fredrickson, D. S., and R. I. Levy (1970), *Lancet*, **i**, 191.

Fredrickson, D. S., R. I. Levy, and R. S. Lees (1967), *New Engl. J. Med.*, **276**, 34, 94, 148, 215, 273.
Fredrickson, D. S., J. Morganroth, and R. I. Levy (1975), *Ann. Int. Med.*, **82**, 150.
French, J. E. (1969), in *Thrombosis* (Eds. S. Sherry, K. M. Brinkhouse, E. Genton, and J. M. Stengle), National Academy of Sciences, Washington, D. C., p. 300.
Gage, S. H., and P. A. Fish (1924), *Amer. J. Anat.*, **34**, 1.
Gitel, S. N., and S. Wessler (1975), *Thrombosis Res.*, **7**, 5.
Glomset, J. A. (1968), *J. Lipid Res.*, **9**, 155.
Glueck, C. J., R. W. Fallat, F. Millett, W. V. Brown, and D. Puppione (1974), *Circulation*, **50**, Suppl. III, 20.
Gofman, J. W., F. T. Lindgren, and H. Elliott (1949), *J. Biol. Chem.*, **179**, 973.
Gofman, J., B. Strisower, O. DeLalla, A. Tamplin, H. Jones, and F. Lindgren (1953), *Mod. Med.*, **21**, 119.
Goldstein, J. L., H. G. Schrott, W. R. Hazzard, E. L. Bierman, and A. G. Motulsky (1973), *J. Clin. Invest.*, **52**, 1544.
Gordon, T., W. P. Castelli, M. C. Hjortland, W. B. Kannel, and T. R. Dawber (1977), *Amer. J. Med.*, **62**, 707.
Gottfried, S. P., R. H. Pope, N. H. Friedman, I. B. Akerson, and S. Di Mauro (1955), *Clin. Chem.*, **1**, 253.
Gotto, A. M., R. I. Levy, K. John, and D. S. Fredrickson (1971), *New Engl. J. Med.*, **284**, 813.
Guravich, J. L. (1959), *Amer. J. Med.*, **26**, 8.
Havel, R. J., and R. S. Gordon, Jr. (1960), *J. Clin. Invest.*, **39**, 1777.
Havel, R. J., and J. P. Kane (1973), *Proc. Nat. Acad. Sci.*, **70**, 2015.
Havel, R. J., J. P. Kane, E. O. Balasse, N. Segal, and L. V. Basso (1970), *J. Clin. Invest.*, **49**, 2017.
Hayes, D., and D. Neil (1964), *Clin. Sci.*, **26**, 185.
Hazzard, W. R., T. F. O'Donnell, and Y. L. Lee (1975), *Ann. Int. Med.*, **82**, 141.
Hedner, U., and I. M. Nilsson (1973), *Thrombosis Res.*, **3**, 631.
Herbert, P., R. I. Levy, and D. S. Fredrickson (1971), *J. Biol. Chem.*, **246**, 7068.
Iammarino, R. M. (1975), *Clin. Chem.*, **21**, 300.
Jones, H., J. W. Gofman, F. Lindgren, T. Lyon, D. Graham, and B. Strisower (1951), *Amer. J. Med.*, **11**, 358.
Kannel, W. B., and T. Gordon (1974), *The Framingham Study*, U.S. Govt. Printing Office, Washington, D.C.
Kannel, W. B., A. Kagan, T. R. Dawber, and N. Revotskie (1962), *Geriatrics*, **17**, 675.
Keys, A. (1967), *J. Chron. Dis.*, **6**, 552.
Keys, A., and F. Fidanza (1960), *Circulation*, **22**, 1091.
Keys, A., N. Kimura, A. Kusukawa, B. Bronte-Stewart, N. Larsen, and M. H. Keys (1958), *Ann. Int. Med.*, **48**, 83.
Keys, A., H. L. Taylor, H. Blackburn, J. Brozek, J. T. Anderson, and E. Simonson (1963), *Circulation*, **28**, 381.
Koerselman, H. B., B. Lewis, and T. R. E. Pilkington (1961), *J. Atheroscler. Res.*, **1**, 85.
Korvald, E., U. Abildgaard, and M. K. Fagerhol (1974), *Thrombosis Res.*, **4**, 147.
Kuo, P. T., and D. R. Basset (1962), *Circulation*, **26**, 660.
Kuo, P., D. Bassett, A. DiGeorge, and G. Carpenter (1965), *Circulation Res.*, **16**, 221.
Lees, R. S., and F. T. Hatch (1963), *J. Lab. Clin. Med.*, **61**, 518.
Levy, R. I., and D. S. Fredrickson (1966), *Circulation*, **34**, Suppl. 3, 156.
Levy, R. I., R. S. Lees, and D. S. Fredrickson (1966a), *J. Clin. Invest.*, **45**, 63.
Levy, R. I., D. S. Fredrickson, and L. Laster (1966b), *J. Clin. Invest.*, **45**, 531.
Levy, R. I., D. W. Bilheimer, and S. Eisenberg (1971), in *Plasma Lipoproteins: Biochemical Society Symposium No. 33* (Ed. R. M. S. Smellie), Academic Press, London and New York, p. 3.
Lewis, B. (1973), *J. Clin. Path.*, **26**, Suppl., (Assoc. Clin. Path.) **5**, 26.

Lewis, B., A. Chait, A. W. February, and M. Mattock (1973), *Atherosclerosis*, **17**, 455.
Lewis, B., A. Chait, C. M. O. Oakley, I. D. P. Wootton, D. M. Krikler, A. Onitiri, G. Sigurdsson, and A. February (1974), *Brit. Med., J.*, **iii**, 489.
Lewis, L. A., A. Robertson, H. Mars, and G. Williams, Jr. (1966), *Circulation*, **34**, Suppl. 3, 19.
Lindgren, F., T. Freeman, K. Norman, A. V. Nichols, and J. W. Gofman (1956), in *Blood Lipids and the Clearing Factor: Third International Conference on Biochemical Problems of Lipids*, Konikl. Vlaam. Acad. Wetenschappen, Brussels, p. 224.
Ludlam, C. A., S. Moore, A. E. Bolton, D. S. Pepper, and J. D. Cash (1975a), *Thrombosis Res.*, **6**, 543.
Ludlam, C. A., A. E. Bolton, S. Moore, and J. D. Cash (1975b), *Lancet*, **ii**, 259.
Lux, S. E., R. I. Levy, A. M. Gotto, and D. S. Fredrickson (1972), *J. Clin. Invest.*, **51**, 2505.
Magnani, H., and P. Alaupovic (1976), *Gastroenterology*, **71**, 87.
Mancini, M., M. Mattock, E. Rabaya, A. Chait, and B. Lewis (1973), *Atherosclerosis*, **17**, 445.
Marciniak, E., C. H. Farley, and P. A. DeSimone (1974), *Blood*, **43**, 219.
McConathy, W. J., and P. Alaupovic (1973), *FEBS Lett.*, **37**, 178.
McConathy, W. J., and P. Alaupovic (1976), *Biochemistry*, **15**, 515.
Miller, G. J., and N. E. Miller (1975), *Lancet*, **i**, 16.
Miller, N. E., O. H. Førde, D. S. Thelle, and O. D. Mjøs (1977), *Lancet*, **i**, 965.
Mills, G. L. (1977), *Lancet*, **ii**, 133.
Mills, G. L., and P. A. Wilkinson (1962), *Clin. Chim. Acta*, **7**, 685.
Moore, S., D. S. Pepper, and J. D. Cash (1975), *Biochim. Biophys. Acta*, **379**, 360.
Morganroth, J., R. I. Levy, and D. S. Fredrickson (1975), *Ann. Int. Med.*, **82**, 158.
M. R. C. Sub-Committee (1967), *Brit. Med. J.*, **ii**, 355.
Naito, H. K., and L. A. Lewis (1973), *Clin. Chem.*, **19**, 644 (abstract).
Naito, H. K., L. A. Lewis, L. J. McCormack, G. Hofstetter, and J. Mihanovic (1975), *Clin. Chem.*, **21**, 641.
Nicolaysen, R., and K. Westlund (1963), *Scand. J. Clin. Lab. Invest.*, **15**, 291.
Nixon, J. C., W. G. Martin, M. Kalab, and G. J. Monahan (1969), *Clin. Biochem.*, **2**, 389.
Paul, O., M. H. Lepper, W. H. Phelan, G. W. Dupertuis, A. MacMillan, H. McKean, and H. Park (1963), *Circulation*, **28**, 20.
Picard, J., and D. Veissiere (1970), *Clin. Chim. Acta*, **30**, 149.
Piper, J., and L. Orrild (1956), *Amer. J. Med.*, **21**, 34.
Rhoads, G. G., C. L. Gulbrandsen, and A. Kagan (1976), *New Engl. J. Med.*, **294**, 293.
Ritland, S. (1975), *Scand. J. Gastroent.*, **10**, 5.
Ritland, S., J. P. Blomhoff, K. Elgjo, and E. Gjone (1973), *Scand. J. Gastroent.*, **8**, 155.
Rosenberg, R. D. (1975), *New Engl. J. Med.*, **292**, 146.
Royal College of General Practitioners Study Group (1974), cited by Sagar *et al.*, 1976a.
Sagar, S., J. D. Stamatakis, D. P. Thomas, and V. V. Kakkar (1976a), *Lancet*, **i**, 509.
Sagar, S., D. Nairn, J. D. Stamatakis, F. H. Maffei, A. F. Higgins, D. P. Thomas, and V. V. Kakkar (1976b), *Lancet*, **i**, 1151.
Salt, H. B., O. H. Wolff, J. K. Lloyd, A. S. Fosbrooke, A. H. Cameron, and D. V. Hubble (1960), *Lancet*, **ii**, 325.
Sas, G., G. Blaskó, D. Bánhegyi, J. Jákó, and L. Á. Pálos (1974), *Thromb. Diath. Haemorrh.*, **32**, 105.
Seidel, D. (1971), *Clin. Chim. Acta*, **31**, 225.
Seidel, D., H. Gretz, and C. Ruppert (1973a), *Clin. Chem.*, **19**, 86.
Seidel, D., H. Wieland, and C. Ruppert (1973b), *Clin. Chem.*, **19**, 737.
Shore, B., and V. Shore (1968), *Biochemistry*, **7**, 2773.
Shore, B., V. G. Shore, and R. G. Hart (1974), *Biochemistry*, **13**, 1579.
Shore, V. G., and B. Shore (1972), in *Blood Lipids and Lipoproteins: Quantitation, Composi-*

tion, and Metabolism (Ed. G. J. Nelson), Wiley–Interscience, New York, p. 789. (Cited by Chait, 1978.)

Stamler, J., H. A. Lindberg, W. H. Berkson, A. Shaffer, W. Miller, and A. Poindexter (1960), *J. Chron. Dis.*, **11**, 405.

St. Clair, R. W. (1975), *Clin. Chem.*, **21**, 307.

Stein, O., J. Vanderhoek, and Y. Stein (1976), *Biochim. Biophys.Acta*, **431**, 347.

Stoker, D. J., V. Wynn, and G. Robertson (1966), *Brit. Med. J.*, **i**, 336.

Stone, M. C., and J. M. Thorp (1966), *Clin. Chim. Acta*, **14**, 812.

Stone, M. C., J. M. Thorp, G. L. Mills, and T. B. S. Dick (1970), *Clin. Chim. Acta*, **30**, 809.

Strisower, E. H., G. Adamson, and B. Strisower (1968), *Amer. J. Med.*, **45**, 488.

Switzer, S. (1967), *J. Clin. Invest.*, **46**, 1855.

Tamplin, A. R., B. Strisower, O. DeLalla, J. Gofman, and F. Glazier (1954), *J. Gerontol.*, **9**, 403.

Technical Group of the Committee on Lipoproteins and Atherosclerosis (1954), *Circulation*, **14**, 725.

van Buchem, F. S. P., G. Pol, J. de Gier, C. J. F. Böttcher, and C. Pries (1966), *Amer. J. Med.*, **40**, 794.

Van der Meer, J., E. A. Stoepman-Van Dalen, and J. M. S. Jansen (1973), *Abstracts, IVth International Congress on Thrombosis and Haemostasis, Vienna*, p. 226. (Cited by Sas *et al.*, 1974.)

Vessey, M. P., R. Doll, A. S. Fairbairn, and G. Glober (1970), *Brit. Med. J.*, **iii**, 123.

von Kaulla, E., and K. N. von Kaulla (1970), *Lancet*, **i**, 36.

Wengeler, H., H. Greten, and D. Seidel (1972), *Europ. J. Clin. Invest.*, **2**, 372.

Wieland, H., and D. Seidel (1973), *Clin. Chem.*, **19**, 1139.

Wilkinson, C. F., E. A. Hand, and M. T. Fliegelman (1948), *Ann. Int. Med.*, **29**, 671.

Winkelman, J. W., and D. R. Wybenga (1974), in *Clinical Chemistry: Principles and Technics*, 2nd ed. (Eds. R. J. Henry, D. C. Cannon, and J. W. Winkelman), Harper and Row, Hagerstown, Md., p. 1495.

Winkelman, J. W., D. R. Wybenga, and F. A. Ibbott (1970), *Clin. Chim. Acta*, **16**, 507.

CHAPTER 6

Hypersensitivity reactions and immune-complex diseases

It will be clear from earlier chapters that the immune system plays an active part in many disease processes. Such disease processes may arise either because of hypofunction of the system or because of inappropriate function. The former results in the immunodeficiency syndromes discussed in Chapter 1. Inappropriate immunological function, on the other hand, is associated with allergic and autoimmune (autoallergic) diseases. These are produced by exposure to certain extrinsic agents to which an immune response develops; on re-exposure to the extrinsic agent, immunological reactions take place which produce the clinical symptoms.

TYPES OF HYPERSENSITIVITY REACTIONS

Four types of hypersensitivity have been defined by Coombs and Gell (1975). A full discussion of these cannot be given here, but the essential features are summarized in Table 6.1.

The present chapter is limited to brief discussions of the role of IgE in Type I reactions and the clinical application of IgE estimations; and the formation of antigen–antibody complexes and their significance in certain disease processes. The phenomenon of autoimmunity is discussed in the next chapter.

Type I hypersensitivity reactions occur, as indicated in the Table, when antigens interact with tissue mast-cell-bound IgE antibodies, causing release of histamine and other vasoactive amines. Such reactions may occur as the result of the absorption of naturally occurring allergens through mucous surfaces, causing hay fever or asthma; sensitivity to certain drugs or foodstuffs can also be the result of Type I reactions.

IgE

Antibodies involved in hypersensitivity of the atopic type (the so-called *reaginic* or *homocytotrophic* antibodies) have been shown to belong to a particular immunoglobulin class (IgE) (Ishizaka *et al.*, 1966a,b), and persons with atopic allergy usually have high plasma concentrations of this immunoglobulin.

The principal value of estimating plasma IgE is in the investigation of atopic disorders such as extrinsic asthma, allergic rhinitis, and atopic eczema. In these conditions plasma concentrations are abnormally high, especially during periods of exacerbation. High concentrations are also found in various kinds

Table 6.1. Hypersensitivity reactions. (Reproduced from R. A. Thompson, *The Practice of Clinical Immunology*, 2nd edn., Arnold, London, 1978, by permission of Edward Arnold (Publisher) Ltd. and Dr. Thompson.)

Type	Nature of immunological mechanism	Associated clinical conditions
I	Antigen reacting with specific IgE antibody found on basophils and tissue mast cells, causing release of histamine and other vasoactive amines	Allergic asthma, hay fever, acute urticarial skin rashes and some drug reactions
II	Antibody reacting with antigen, either adsorbed on to or forming an intrinsic part of a cell surface; in the presence of complement, cell death ensues	Some haemolytic anaemias and thrombocytopaenia, induced by drugs, as well as autoimmune haemolytic anaemia
III	Reaction between antibody and soluble antigen in capillaries and tissue spaces, resulting in complement fixation, with vascular stasis, the attraction and disruption of phagocytes, and the histological picture of the Arthus reaction. If antigen–antibody complexes are formed in antigen excess, these fix complement relatively poorly, but persist in the circulation and are deposited in small end-arterioles of the skin, serous surfaces, and glomeruli	Serum sickness, systemic lupus erythematosus, many types of nephritis, some types of gastrointestinal food intolerance, allergic extrinsic alveolitis, and features of some infective illnesses
IV	Reaction between antigen and antigen-sensitive cells, causing release of lymphokines and the manifestations of the delayed hypersensitivity response	Contact dermatitis, due to drugs, metals, materials, etc.; some pathological features of mycobacterial infection

of parasitic infestations (for example, ascariasis, trichinosis, and leishmaniasis), and sometimes after an episode of drug hypersensitivity; certain kinds of bullous skin disorders are also associated with significantly raised concentrations (Reeves *et al.*, 1976).

A method for the detection of antigen-specific IgE antibody was described by Wide and his colleagues (1967) and called the 'radioallergosorbent test' (RAST). In this test reaginic (IgE) antibodies react with the specific allergen which has been chemically coupled to an insoluble matrix; the bound reagins are then detected by their ability to bind ^{125}I-labelled antibodies directed against IgE, and the uptake of labelled antibodies, measured in terms of radioactivity on the solid phase, gives a direct indication of the amount of antigen-specific IgE in the patient's plasma. Common allergens such as those of pollen, mites, and so on can readily be coupled to a solid phase like cellulose or cross-linked dextran ('Sephadex'); the solid phase may be in the form of either fine particles or a paper disc (Wide *et al.*, 1971).

A number of studies (reviewed by Wide, 1973) have shown, in most cases, good correlation between the RAST and skin and provocation tests.

LABORATORY INVESTIGATION OF ALLERGIES

The possibility of an allergic disorder will generally be suggested by the clinical history, and a high serum IgE concentration will support the diagnosis. RAST assays may be of value in identifying the offending antigen when other methods of investigation have failed or are not readily available.

The radioimmunoassay of IgE and IgE antibodies and its clinical application has been reviewed by Johansson (1975).

If hereditary angioneurotic oedema is suspected, the serum *C1-esterase inhibitor* should be measured. Patients with this condition have low concentrations of the protein. They also usually have low concentrations of total haemolytic complement and of C4 and C2.

ANTIGEN–ANTIBODY COMPLEXES

As indicated in Table 6.1, hypersensitivity reactions of Type III involve a reaction between an antibody and soluble antigen in the capillaries and tissue spaces. This may give rise to an acute inflammatory reaction. If complement is fixed, the release of histamine and chemotactic factors will lead to changes in vascular permeability and an intensification of the inflammation.

The consequences of immune-complex formation *in vivo* depend both on the absolute amounts of antigen and antibody involved and on their relative proportions. If there is gross *antibody excess* the complexes are rapidly precipitated and so tend to remain near the site of introduction of the antigen. In conditions of *antigen excess*, however, soluble immune complexes are formed which may cause systemic reactions and be widely deposited in kidneys, joints, and skin. Slow complement fixation occurs at the sites of deposition of the complexes, causing local vasodilation and tissue damage. The clinical picture, which is relatively subacute, is typified by serum sickness following therapy with heterospecific serum such as horse anti-tetanus serum—a condition in which, as long ago as 1905, Von Pirquet and Schick postulated the presence of toxic antigen–antibody complexes in the circulation. More than half a century later, definite evidence was presented that such antigen–antibody complexes may play a part in many disease processes (Weigle, 1961; Dixon, 1963; Cochrane and Dixon, 1969; Cochrane and Koffler, 1973). Mechanisms of this kind are believed to operate in certain forms of glomerulonephritis (see Chapter 4); in systemic lupus erythematosus complexes of DNA and anti-DNA are deposited at a number of sites (skin, joints, serous surfaces, kidneys), which is in keeping with the clinical features of the disease. There is evidence that immune complexes may play a significant rôle in the pathogenesis of lesions in rheumatoid arthritis (Broder *et al.*, 1972). The rôle of immune complexes in human diseases has been reviewed by Roy and his associates (1972), Nakamura (1974), and Jones (1975), among others.

Not all immune complexes are damaging: sensitive methods of detection show that low concentrations may be present in apparently healthy persons.

Sera from patients with immune-complex disease are often found to contain immunoglobulins that precipitate on incubation at 4 °C. Many of these *cryoglobulins* have the ability to fix complement and initiate an inflammatory reaction similar to that of the 'classical' antigen–antibody complexes; they probably play a significant rôle in viral diseases and in producing the lesions of vasculitis and glomerulonephritis (Wager *et al.*, 1968; Barnett *et al.*, 1970; Grey and Kohler, 1973).

Two examples of immune-complex disease will be briefly mentioned. The first, systemic lupus erythematosus, is called by Nakamura and Tucker (1975) a 'primal model of immune-complex disease in humans'.

Systemic lupus erythematosus (SLE)

Although the cause of this disease is unknown, it may be classified, together with rheumatoid arthritis and other collagen diseases, under the category of non-organ-specific autoimmune disease (Chapter 7). In SLE, antibodies are produced to many cellular constituents, including DNA, and it is thought that the antigen–antibody complexes of DNA and anti-DNA are the agents responsible for the nephritis that may develop. The evidence for this has been presented by Barnett and his colleagues (1969). Not only are immunoglobulins and complement deposited within the glomerular membrane, as in serum sickness, but antinuclear antibodies can be specifically eluted from glomeruli in greater concentrations than in serum; furthermore, DNA and other nuclear antigens have been demonstrated in the glomeruli by the immunofluorescence technique; finally, very low serum complement concentrations and high titres of complement-fixing antibodies to DNA are associated particularly with active renal disease (Schur and Sandson, 1968).

Immunofluorescence studies of the skin in systemic lupus erythematosus by several groups of workers have demonstrated deposition of immunoglobulins and complement components at the dermal–epidermal junction, lending support to the hypothesis that this is the site of an antigen–antibody complex (see Percy and Smyth, 1969). Also at the dermal–epidermal junction, widespread deposits of aggregates containing DNA complexed with γ-globulin have been demonstrated (Tan and Kunkel, 1966).

Cold-insoluble complexes (cryoglobulins) have been found in the plasma of a number of patients with SLE. These cryoglobulins may, as mentioned above, possess similar biological properties to the immune complexes.

Serum concentrations of total complement are lowered in active SLE, but the low concentrations of the C3 component are reported to be due largely to decreased synthesis (Sliwinski and Zvaifler, 1972). The presence of properdin in the kidneys of patients with SLE (Rothfield *et al.*, 1972) suggests that the alternative pathway of complement activation as well as the classical pathway is involved in the pathogenesis of the disease (Hunsicker *et al.*, 1972; Rothfield *et al.*, 1972).

Rheumatoid arthritis

There is much evidence that γ-globulin complexes are involved in the immunopathological mechanisms associated with the synovial lesions occurring in this disease (Winchester *et al.*, 1971; Zvaifler, 1971, 1973; Broder *et al.*, 1972). Thus a lowered concentration of complement and a high concentration of γ-globulin complexes have been found in the synovial fluid, and immunofluorescence studies have demonstrated the deposition of immunoglobulin and complement in the synovium. There is synthesis of immunoglobulins in the synovium, and deposition of immunoglobulins and complement in leukocytes.

Cryoprecipitable complexes containing IgG, IgA, and IgM have been identified in the synovial fluid of patients who had detectable amounts of *rheumatoid factor* in their serum (Marcus and Townes, 1971; Zvaifler, 1973).

Rheumatoid factor

This collective term includes both 7S and 19S immunoglobulins with antibody specificity to certain determinants on the γ-globulin molecule. Some of these factors combine with IgG and circulate in the blood as 22–29S IgM–IgG complexes, which can sometimes be detected as cryoglobulins. Rheumatoid factor is detectable in the serum of some 70 to 80 per cent of patients with rheumatoid arthritis (Kellgren, 1968). It is also found in a proportion of patients with other diseases (systemic lupus erythematosus, scleroderma, polymyositis, chronic liver disease, subacute bacterial endocarditis, etc.); however, since the large majority of patients with rheumatoid arthritis do have detectable amounts of rheumatoid factor in the serum, a positive finding is of considerable diagnostic significance. Statistically, high titres of rheumatoid factor are associated with progressive arthritis; however, a positive test is of no prognostic value in the individual patient (Duthie *et al.*, 1957; Ragan and Farrington, 1962). The major application of the test is to distinguish rheumatoid arthritis from other conditions associated with symptomatic arthritis (osteoarthritis, post-infective arthritis, psoriatic arthritis, systemic lupus erythematosus, etc.); the test is nearly always negative in rheumatic fever.

What part, if any, rheumatoid factor plays in the pathogenesis of the disease is not clear. Intra-articular injection of autologous IgG in patients with rheumatoid arthritis produced synovitis in patients with a positive rheumatoid factor test, but not in those without the factor (Restifo *et al.*, 1965). On the other hand, prolonged infusion of 'rheumatoid' plasma into normal subjects had no harmful effect (Vaughan and Harris, 1959); moreover, definite or 'classical' rheumatoid arthritis may, as indicated above, occur in patients without detectable amounts of rheumatoid factor in their serum, and a high incidence of rheumatoid arthritis in patients with agammaglobulinaemia has been reported (Good and Rotstein, 1960; Bridges and Good, 1960). In Good's series of 27 agammaglobulinaemic patients, no less than eight had various classical manifestations of rheumatoid arthritis, and no demonstrable rheumatoid factor in the serum. Janeway and his collaborators (1956) have likewise reported a high incidence of 'collagen disease' in children with congenital agammaglobulinaemia. Good and Rotstein comment that the very high incidence of rheumatoid arthritis and collagen disease among patients with agammaglobulinaemia makes the participation of antibodies and γ-globulins in the pathogenesis of the diseases a remote possibility. They suggest a number of alternative hypotheses, including the suggestion that rheumatoid arthritis may be initiated by a direct toxic action of bacteria or viruses, arising from distant sites of infection; the associated deficiency of γ-globulin will ensure frequent and extensive exposure to bacterial products.

γ-Globulin complexes in serum and joint fluid

The complexes found in the serum and joint fluid of patients with rheumatoid arthritis differ in their immunochemical properties, the joint-fluid complexes reacting readily *in vitro* with C1q and polyclonal or monoclonal rheumatoid factor to form a precipitate (Agnello *et al.*, 1970; Winchester *et al.*, 1971). These complexes presumably contribute to the inflammatory destruction of the joint space.

The different properties of the serum complexes in rheumatoid arthritis, which are not associated with a lowering of the serum complement concentration, may help to explain the low incidence of glomerulonephritis in this condition (Nakamura and Tucker, 1975).

Cryoglobulins in synovial fluid

Cryoglobulins are demonstrable in most synovial fluids from patients with rheumatoid arthritis. They contain fibrin products and immunoglobulins, and in their immunoglobulin composition (predominantly IgG and IgM) they resemble the 'mixed-type' cryoglobulins that are found in the serum in a variety of disorders (Meltzer *et al.*, 1966, Marcus and Townes, 1971). Several investigators have reported the presence of cryoprecipitates in the synovial fluid, but not the blood serum, of patients with rheumatoid arthritis (Barnett *et al.*, 1970; Marcus and Townes, 1971; Grey and Kohler, 1973).

C-reactive protein (CRP)

This is usually found in the serum in increased concentration in rheumatic diseases, especially *rheumatic fever*, in which the test is almost always positive in the early untreated disease and serves as a measure of activity during the course of the illness (Tillett and Francis, 1930; Anderson and McCarty, 1950; Ziegra and Kuttner, 1951; Stollerman *et al.*, 1953; Fischel *et al.*, 1958). In *rheumatoid arthritis* the concentration is raised in about 70 to 80 per cent of patients with signs of disease activity; it may remain raised for a long time in patients judged to be 'inactive' clinically (Fischel, 1975). Occasionally, however, the test is negative in the presence of mild, but definite, activity (Hill, 1951; Roantree and Rantz, 1955; Shetlar *et al.*, 1956; Hedlund, 1961).

In reviewing the CRP and erythrocyte sedimentation (ESR) tests, Fischel (1975) concludes that the latter is the more valuable laboratory test for assessing activity in the rheumatic diseases, on account of its ready availability, ease of performance, and general reliability as a screening test, and the long background of experience with it in clinical medicine; and that the CRP test is an auxiliary which may provide useful information, particularly in the early phase of an inflammatory reaction. In rheumatoid arthritis McConkey and his coworkers find measurement of both CRP and ESR to be more helpful than either alone (Amos *et al.*, 1977); serial measurements of CRP and ESR are useful for assessing the progress of the disease and provide a reliable means of discriminating between drugs that afford symptomatic relief only and those with a more profound effect (McConkey *et al.*, 1972; Constable *et al.*, 1975; Amos *et al.*, 1977).

Other plasma protein changes

Serum haptoglobin concentrations are generally increased in inflammatory states, and measurement of this protein has been recommended for assessing the activity of rheumatic diseases (Mathies *et al.*, 1963; Müller *et al.*, 1963). Increases often occur in the concentrations of α_1-acid glycoprotein (Gamp, 1962; Augener, 1965; Cleve and Behrend, 1966) and other glycoproteins (Augener, 1965). In rheumatoid arthritis an increase in the concentration of IgM is frequently found (Cleve and Hartmann, 1957; Krebs *et al.*, 1963).

LABORATORY INVESTIGATION OF IMMUNE-COMPLEX DISEASES

In some forms of renal disease, in the vasculitis group of disorders, and in systemic lupus erythematosus, the detection of immune complexes may be of value diagnostically. Serial studies of circulating immune complexes may also help in evaluating therapy and assessing the development of the disease (Jones *et al.*, 1976).

A variety of tests are available. One of the most sensitive is based on the ability of immune complexes to fix complement, the amount of complement that remains unbound being estimated by the degree of lysis that occurs on addition of sheep red blood cells coated with a horse haemolytic antibody; anticomplementary sera fix guinea pig complement, with the result that the sheep red blood cells do not lyse. Immune complexes with complement already attached may not possess anticomplementary activity and so may be missed in this assay system. They may be detected by first heating the serum under carefully controlled conditions (Johnson *et al.*, 1975). Other tests for immune complexes are based on precipitation with the C1q component of complement or with rheumatoid factor or the Fab portion of an anti-human-IgG. Radioimmunoassays with rheumatoid factor or labelled Fab fraction of an anti-IgG preparation are also available. These and other tests are described by Jones

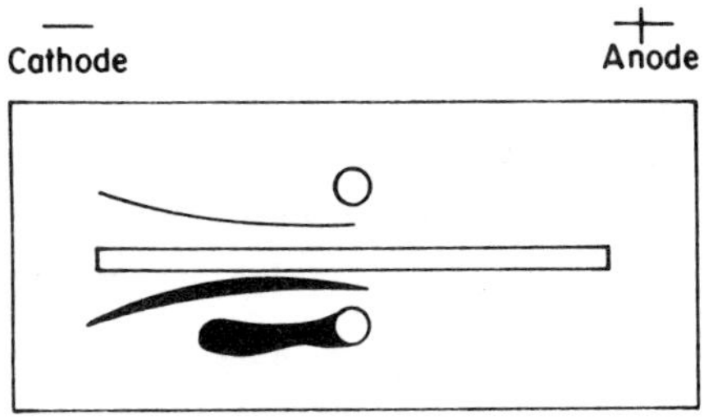

Figure 6.1. Immunoelectrophoretic pattern of serum of patient with systemic lupus erythematosus, containing cryoglobulins and DNA–anti–DNA immune complexes. The immunoelectrophoretic pattern was developed with specific anti-IgG antiserum. Top well: normal; lower well: serum from patient. Note the IgG precipitin arcs and trailing phenomenon extending toward the cathode from the lower well. (Reproduced from R. M. Nakamura, *Immunopathology: Clinical Laboratory Concepts and Methods*, Little, Brown, Boston, 1974, by permission of Little, Brown, Inc., and Dr. Nakamura.)

and Cumming (1977). Standardization of the tests can be difficult, and much experience is required if the results are not to be misleading.

It should be noted that not all methods detect the same immune complexes, and there is evidence that the significance to be attached to a positive finding may depend on which method is used. For example, whereas with most methods of detection the presence of serum antibody to DNA has been associated with the development of nephropathy in patients with systemic lupus erythematosus, the use of a sensitive two-stage electroimmunodiffusion method led to the opposite conclusion, *viz.* that *absence* of the antibody is associated with nephropathy, its presence being correlated with the occurrence of cutaneous vasculitic lesions (Johnson *et al.*, 1973). The rapid development of precipitin arcs in this electroimmunodiffusion method would indicate the presence of high-affinity antibody, and it was suggested that antibody affinity is an important factor in determining the sites of immune-complex-induced lesions (Johnson *et al.*, 1973).

Immune-complex disease may often be suspected on the basis of the serum immunoelectrophoretic analysis. According to Ritzmann and his coworkers (1972), immune complexes may show a marked trailing from the antigen well, usually within the IgG area towards the cathode; this takes the form of a diffuse oblong spot, connected to the antigen well and showing a narrowing just behind the well (Figure 6.1). Opaque spots confined closely to the cathodal side of the well indicate the possible presence of an abnormal immunoglobulin (Ritzmann *et al.*, 1972), but such spots do not show the narrowing referred to above. Although the cathode trailing effect is not given by all immune complexes, a positive result is reported to be very helpful (Nakamura, 1974).

Sera from patients suspected of having immune-complex disease should be tested for cryoglobulins, which precipitate on incubation at 4 °C. These are usually found to be mixtures of immunoglobulins, and in some instances it is possible to detect antigen in the cryoprecipitate (Barnett *et al.*, 1970; Grey and Kohler, 1973). For the detection of cryoglobulins the blood must be collected in a warmed syringe and kept at 37 °C until clotting has taken place. After separation in a centrifuge maintained at 37 °C the serum should be stored at 4 °C for 24 hours or more and then centrifuged and washed in buffered saline at this temperature. It may then be redissolved, in buffer at 37 °C, for analysis (Whitsed and Penny, 1971).

Systemic lupus erythematosus (SLE)

In the various collagen diseases, antibodies to many different nuclear antigens are found, and a variety of tests are available for their detection (reviewed by Nakamura and Tucker, 1975). Of these the most easily performed and practical one is the *indirect immunofluorescence test* (Beck, 1969), in which the patient's serum is reacted with a section of substrate containing nuclei; this is then washed and treated with fluorescein-conjugated anti-human-globulin. A wide variety of antibodies in SLE have been demonstrated by this technique. However, the symptoms and pathological features of SLE are apparently due to circulating complexes of DNA and anti-DNA, and it is probable that some of the antibodies to other nuclear constituents, which are responsible for the positive tests given by the indirect immunofluorescence and other tests, merely accompany the development of anti-DNA antibodies without being directly related to them and to their pathological effects. Certain sera, for example from some patients with chronic active hepatitis, may give strongly positive tests for antinuclear antibodies yet have normal concentrations of the anti-DNA antibodies; and occasionally serum from a patient with SLE gives only a weakly positive test for antinuclear factor but contains significant amounts of anti-DNA antibodies. It follows that tests for anti-DNA antibodies are essential adjuncts to the indirect fluorescence test for antinuclear factor (Thompson, 1978).

Of the various methods available, the most satisfactory is a radioimmunoassay using labelled DNA (Wold *et al.*, 1968). Commercial kits based on this method are available. The test appears to be useful in the diagnosis of SLE and assessment of the course of the disease (Pincus *et al.*, 1969; Hughes *et al.*, 1971).

Response of SLE to treatment with prednisone or immunosuppressive agents, or both, is associated with a reduction of the concentration of DNA antibody; and the specific test for antibodies to native DNA is more useful than the test for antinuclear antibodies in monitoring the clinical course of the disease (Nakamura and Tucker, 1975). Tests for serum cryoglobulins, complement, or immune complexes, as well as immunofluorescence studies on kidney biopsy specimens, may also be used.

It has been suggested that persistent depression of the fourth component of complement (C4) in SLE may be an indication of occult disease activity (Kohler and Ten Bensel, 1969). Detection of C3 conversion products and measurement of the C4 concentration have been thought to be very important in assessing renal involvement and in monitoring treatment, and the C4 concentration alone is a sensitive index of the effectiveness of corticosteroid therapy (Whicher, 1978).

Rheumatoid arthritis

The most commonly used tests for the detection of rheumatoid factor are the human-IgG-coated latex agglutination test and the sensitized sheep cell agglutination test. The former, which was first described by Singer and Plotz (1956), uses latex particles coated with human γ-globulin that are reacted against dilutions of the test serum. The sensitized sheep cell agglutination test (Rose–Waaler test) employs sheep cells coated with subagglutinating amounts of rabbit anti-sheep-red-cell antibody (Waaler, 1940; Rose *et al.*, 1948). Both types of test have been modified for use as slide tests using commercially available kits.

Table 6.2. Serological differentiation of rheumatoid arthritis and systemic lupus erythematosus. (Reproduced from R. A. Thompson, *The Practice of Clinical Immunology*, 2nd edn., Arnold, London, 1978, by permission of Edward Arnold (Publisher) Ltd. and Dr. Thompson.)

Test	RA	SLE
Rheumatoid factor	Positive in 70% of cases	Mostly negative—positive in 10% of cases
ANF*	Commonly negative (if positive usually IgM antibody)	Very rarely negative
LE cell test†	Rarely positive—5% of cases	Positive in 40% of cases
DNA antibodies	Normal levels	Elevated levels
Immunoglobulin levels	Often normal; if elevated no consistent pattern	IgG alone may be elevated
Complement component levels (C3 and C4)	Usually elevated—rarely low	Low levels with renal involvement—if the C3 is normal, the C4 is often at the lower end of the normal range

*Anti-nuclear factor (anti-nuclear antibody).

†The LE cell is a leukocyte, containing a characteristic inclusion body, occasionally found in bone marrow in SLE. LE cells may be formed *in vitro*, by defibrination of blood from the patient, during which cell disruption releases nuclei; these react with antinuclear antibodies and are phagocytosed by polymorphs to form LE cells.

The major application of the test for rheumatoid factor is in distinguishing between rheumatoid arthritis and other conditions associated with symptomatic arthritis (see p. 120).

The possible use, and the limitations, of CRP estimations have been mentioned above.

Table 6.2 summarizes the serological differentiation of rheumatoid arthritis and systemic lupus erythematosus.

REFERENCES

Agnello, V., R. J. Winchester, and H. G. Kunkel (1970), *Immunology*, **19**, 909.
Amos, R. S., T. J. Constable, R. A. Crockson, A. P. Crockson, and B. McConkey (1977), *Brit. Med. J.*, **i**, 195.
Anderson, H. C., and M. McCarty (1950), *Amer. J. Med.*, **8**, 445.
Augener, W. (1965), in *Protides of the Biological Fluids: Proceedings of the 12th Colloquium, Bruges, 1964* (Ed. H. Peeters), Elsevier, Amsterdam, p. 363.
Barnett, E. V., G. Kantor, Y. B. Bickel, R. Forsen, and H. C. Gonick (1969), *Calif. Med.*, **11**, 467.
Barnett, E. V., R. Bluestone, A. Cracchiola, L. S. Goldberg, G. L. Kantor, and R. M. McIntosh (1970), *Ann. Int. Med.*, **73**, 95.
Beck, J. S. (1969), *Mayo Clin. Proc.*, **44**, 600.
Bridges, R. A., and R. A. Good (1960), *Ann. N. Y. Acad. Sci.*, **86**, 1089.
Broder, I., M. B. Urowitz, and D. A. Gordon (1972), *Med. Clin. N. Amer.*, **56**, 529.
Cleve, H., and T. Behrend (1966), *Z. Rheumaforsch.*, **25**, 278.
Cleve, H., and F. Hartmann (1957), *Klin. Woch.*, **35**, 334.
Cochrane, C. G., and F. J. Dixon (1969), in *Textbook of Immunopathology*, Vol. 1 (Eds. P. Miescher and H. J. Müller-Eberhard), Grune and Stratton, New York, p. 94.
Cochrane, C. G., and D. Koffler (1973), in *Advances in Immunology*, Vol. 16 (Eds. F. J. Dixon and H. G. Kunkel), Academic Press, New York, p. 183.
Constable, T. J., R. A. Crockson, A. P. Crockson, and B. McConkey (1975), *Lancet*, **i**, 1176.
Coombs, R. R. A., and P. G. H. Gell (1975), in *Clinical Aspects of Immunology* (Eds. P. G. H. Gell, R. R. A. Coombes, and P. J. Lachmann), Blackwell, Oxford, p. 761.
Dixon, F. J. (1963), *Harvey Lect.*, **58**, 21.
Duthie, J. J. R., P. E. Brown, J. D. E. Knox, and M. Thompson (1957), *Ann. Rheum. Dis.*, **16**, 411.
Fischel, E. E. (1975), in *Laboratory Diagnostic Procedures in the Rheumatic Diseases* (Ed. A. S. Cohen) 2nd edn., Little, Brown, Boston, p. 83.
Fischel, E. E., C. W. Frank, A. J. Boltax, and M. Arcasoy (1958), *Arthr. Rheum.*, **i**, 351.
Gamp, A. (1962), *Z. Rheumaforsch.*, **21**, 128.
Good, R. A., and J. Rotstein (1960), *Bull. Infect. Dis.*, **10**, 203.
Grey, H. M., and P. F. Kohler (1973), *Semin. Hemat.*, **10**, 87.
Hedlund, P. (1961), *Acta Med. Scand.*, Suppl. 361, 1.
Hill, A. G. S. (1951), *Lancet*, **ii**, 807.
Hughes, G. R. V., S. A. Cohen, and C. L. Christian (1971), *Ann. Rheum. Dis.*, **30**, 259.
Hunsicker, L. G., S. Ruddy, C. B. Carpenter, P. H. Schur, J. P. Merrill, H. J. Müller-Eberhard, and K. F. Austin (1972), *New Engl. J. Med.*, **287**, 835.
Ishizaka, K., T. Ishizaka, and M. H. Hornbrook (1966a), *J. Immunol.*, **97**, 75.
Ishizaka, K., T. Ishizaka, and M. H. Hornbrook (1966b), *J. Immunol.*, **97**, 840.
Janeway, C. A., D. Gitlin, J. M. Craig, and D. S. Grice (1956), *Trans. Assoc. Amer. Phycns.*, **69**, 93.
Johansson, S. G. O. (1975), *J. Clin. Path.*, 28, Suppl. (Assoc. Clin. Path.) **6**, 33.

Johnson, G. D., J. P. Edmonds, and E. J. Holborow (1973), *Lancet*, **ii**, 883.
Johnson, A. H., J. F. Mowbray, and K. A. Porter (1975), *Lancet*, **i**, 762.
Jones, J. V. (1975), *Practitioner*, **214**, 481.
Jones, J. V., and R. H. Cumming (1977), in *Techniques in Clinical Immunology* (Ed. R. A. Thompson), Blackwell, Oxford, p. 136.
Jones, J. V., R. H. Cumming, R. C. Bucknall, C. M. Asplin, I. D. Fraser, J. Bothamley, P. Davis, and T. J. Hamblin (1976), *Lancet*, **i**, 709.
Kellgren, J. H. (1968), in *Rheumatic Diseases* (Eds. J. J. R. Duthie and W. R. M. Alexander), Medical Monographs, Baltimore, p. 120. (Cited by Broder *et al.*, 1972.)
Kohler, P. F., and R. Ten Bensel (1969), *Clin. Exp. Immunol.*, **4**, 191.
Krebs, A., M. Hess, and R. Bütler (1963), *Dermatologica*, **127**, 86.
Marcus, R. L., and A. S. Townes (1971), *J. Clin. Invest.*, **50**, 282.
Mathies, H., E. Schleifer, and K. G. Liebrich (1963), *Klin. Woch.*, **41**, 653.
McConkey, B., R. A. Crockson, and A. P. Crockson (1972), *Quart. J. Med.* (N.S.), **41**, 115.
Meltzer, M., E. C. Franklin, K. Elias, R. T. McCluskey, and N. Cooper (1966), *Amer. J. Med.*, **40**, 837.
Müller, W., R. Kluthe, and H. Müller (1963), *Z. Rheumaforsch.*, **22**, 1.
Nakamura, R. M. (1974), *Immunopathology: Clinical Laboratory Concepts and Methods*, Little, Brown, Boston, p. 168.
Nakamura, R. M., and E. S. Tucker (1975), in *Serum Protein Abnormalities: Diagnostic and Clinical Aspects* (Eds. S. E. Ritzmann and J. C. Daniels), Little, Brown, Boston, p. 295.
Percy, J. S., and C. J. Smyth (1969), *J. Amer. Med. Assoc.*, **208**, 485.
Pincus, T., P. H. Schur, J. A. Rose, J. L. Decker, and N. Talal (1969), *New Engl. J. Med.*, **281**, 701.
Ragan, C. A., and E. Farrington (1962), *J. Amer. Med. Assoc.*, **181**, 663.
Reeves, W. G., and D. W. Marriott (1977), in *Techniques in Clinical Immunology* (Ed. R. A. Thompson), Blackwell, Oxford, p. 116.
Reeves, W. G., B. R. Allen, and D. W. Marriott (1976), cited by Reeves and Marriott (1977).
Restifo, R. A., A. J. Lussier, A. J. Rawson, J. H. Rockey, and J. L. Hollander (1965), *Ann. Int. Med.*, **62**, 285.
Ritzmann, S. E., M. C. Lawrence, and J. C. Daniels (1972), in *Selected Topics in Clinical Chemistry* (Ed. J. B. Fuller), American Society of Clinical Pathology, Chicago, p. 148. (Cited by Nakamura, 1974.)
Roantree, R. J., and L. A. Rantz (1955), *Arch. Int. Med.*, **96**, 674.
Rose, H. M., C. Ragan, E. Pearce, and M. D. Lipman (1948), *Proc. Soc. Exp. Biol. Med.*, **68**, 1.
Rothfield, N., H. A. Ross, J. O. Menta, and I. H. Lepow (1972), *New Engl. J. Med.*, **287**, 681.
Roy, L. P., A. J. Fish, A. F. Michael, and R. L. Vernier (1972), in *Progress in Clinical Immunology*, Vol. 1 (Ed. R. S. Schwartz), Grune and Stratton, New York, p. 1.
Schur, P. H., and J. Sandson (1968), *New Engl. J. Med.*, **278**, 533.
Shetlar, M. R., R. W. Payne, J. Padron, F. Felton, and W. K. Ishmael (1956), *J. Lab. Clin. Med.*, **48**, 194.
Singer, J. M., and C. M. Plotz (1956), *Amer. J. Med.*, **21**, 888.
Sliwinski, A. J., and N. Z. Zvaifler (1972), *Clin. Exp. Immunol.*, **11**, 21.
Stollerman, G. H., S. J. Glick, D. J. Patel, I. Hirschfeld, and J. H. Rusoff (1953), *Amer. J. Med.*, **15**, 645.
Tan, E. M., and H. G. Kunkel (1966), *Arthr. Rheum.*, **9**, 37.
Thompson, R. A. (1978), *The Practice of Clinical Immunology*, 2nd edn., Arnold, London.
Tillett, W. S., and T. Francis (1930), *J. Exp. Med.*, **52**, 561.
Vaughan, J. H., and J. Harris, (1959), *Arthr. Rheum.*, **2**, 51.
Waaler, E. (1940), *Acta Path. Microbiol. Scand.*, **17**, 172.

Wager, O., J. A. Rasanen, A. Hageman, and A. Klemola (1968), *Int. Arch. Allergy Appl. Immunol.*, **34**, 345.
Weigle, W. O. (1961), in *Advances in Immunology* (Eds. W. H. Taliaferro and J. H. Humphrey), Academic Press, New York, p. 283.
Whicher, J. T. (1978), *Clin. Chem.*, **24**, 7.
Whitsed, H. M., and R. Penny (1971), *Clin. Exp. Immunol.*, **9**, 183.
Wide, L. (1973), *Clin. Allergy*, **3**, 583.
Wide, L., H. Bennich, and S. G. O. Johansson (1967), *Lancet*, **ii**, 1105.
Wide, L., T. Aronsson, E. Fagerberg, and O. Zetterström (1971), *Excerpta Medica*, **235**, 85.
Winchester, R. J., H. G. Kunkel, and V. Agnello (1971), *J. Exp. Med.*, **134**, Suppl., 286.
Wold, R. T., F. E. Young, E. M. Tan, and R. S. Farr (1968), *Science*, **161**, 806.
Ziergra, S. R., and A. G. Kuttner (1951), *Amer. J. Med. Sci.*, **222**, 516.
Zvaifler, H. J. (1971), *J. Exp. Med.*, **134**, Suppl., 276.
Zvaifler, H. J. (1973), in *Advances in Immunology*, Vol. 16 (Eds. F. J. Dixon and H. J. Kunkel), Academic Press, New York, p. 256.

CHAPTER 7

Autoimmunity and collagen diseases

A natural state of immunological unresponsiveness is recognized, which is believed to develop as the result of direct contact at an early stage between the 'self' constituents of the body and potential antibody-producing cells. The cellular aspects of this unresponsiveness are complicated; it would appear that, in addition to macrophages, the lymphoid cells from the thymus (T-cells) and the antibody-producing or B-cells from the bone marrow are involved (see Nakamura, 1974). Autoimmunity, or the failure of an organism to recognize its own tissue, may be considered as a termination of this natural state of unresponsiveness (Weigle, 1967). It may possibly result from a number of processes. In the case of organs that are often involved in autoimmune diseases (thyroid, testes, adrenals, brain) there is normally a very low concentration of native antigens in the circulation. Such low concentrations may be sufficient to induce unresponsiveness in the thymus-derived cells but not in the bone marrow cells; the unresponsive state will then exist only at the level of the thymus-derived cells and the animal will appear normal. A genetic mutation or viral transformation that resulted in an interaction between thymic cells and altered host antigen would initiate an immune response.

According to Burnet (1969, 1972), autoantibody production may be a normal process which is usually suppressed by the presence of the corresponding autoantigens ('immunoparalysis'): transformation of the antigens, or a decrease in their amount, may lead to increased production of autoimmune antibodies. It is possible that modification of 'self' antigens by inflammation, trauma, viruses, drugs, and so on may start an immune reaction. For information on these and other theories the reader is referred to the accounts by Nakamura (1974) and Roitt (1974).

TYPES OF HUMAN AUTOIMMUNE DISORDERS

The autoimmune diseases may be regarded as forming a spectrum. At one end are 'organ-specific' diseases with organ-specific autoantibodies. Examples are Hashimoto's thyroiditis, thyrotoxicosis, pernicious anaemia, and a number of other disorders. At the other end of the spectrum are the 'non-organ-specific' diseases, in which lesions and autoantibodies are not confined to any one organ. Examples are systemic lupus erythematosus and rheumatoid arthritis. In between these two extremes are those disorders in which the lesion tends to be localized in a single organ but the serum autoantibodies are non-organ-specific.

Table 7.1. Spectrum of autoimmune diseases. (Reproduced from I. Roitt, *Essential Immunology*, 2nd edn., Blackwell, Oxford, 1974, by permission of Blackwell Scientific Publications Ltd. and Prof. Roitt.)

Organ-specific ←				→ Non-organ-specific
Hashimoto's thyroiditis }	Goodpasture's syndrome	Myasthenia gravis	Primary biliary cirrhosis	Systemic lupus erythematosus (SLE)
Primary myxoedema }	Pemphigus vulgaris	Autoimmune haemolytic anaemia	Active chronic hepatitis (some cases)	Discoid LE
Thyrotoxicosis	Pemphigoid	Idiopathic thrombocytopaenic purpura	Cryptogenic cirrhosis (some cases)	Dermatomyositis
Pernicious anaemia	Sympathetic ophthalmia	Idiopathic leucopaenia	Ulcerative colitis	Scleroderma
Autoimmune atrophic gastritis	Phacogenic uvetis		Sjögren's syndrome	Rheumatoid arthritis
Addison's disease				
Premature menopause (few cases)				
Male infertility (few cases)	(??Multiple sclerosis??)			

The major diseases considered to be associated in some way with autoimmunity are shown in Table 7.1.

It should be emphasized that in a number of these diseases the rôle, if any, of immune reactions has not actually been demonstrated. An example is rheumatoid arthritis, in which an IgM antibody ('rheumatoid factor') is present in the serum but does not appear to play a primary rôle in the pathogenesis of the disease. As implied above, rheumatoid factor is a non-organ-specific antibody. The rôle of these antibodies in pathogenesis is, for the most part, even more obscure than that of the organ-specific antibodies.

The conception of *collagen disease* was introduced by Klemperer and his colleagues (1942) in order to focus attention on the changes in the connective tissues that may be seen in systemic lupus erythematosus, scleroderma, and a number of other diseases. The term is now used collectively to include a group of diseases in which changes in the connective tissues are believed to be the primary cause of the symptoms and signs, *viz.* rheumatic fever, rheumatoid arthritis, systemic lupus erythematosus, polyarteritis nodosa, scleroderma, dermatomyositis, Sjøgren's syndrome, and serum sickness. The lesions in all these conditions are widely believed to be caused by the development of autoantibodies against the connective and other tissues, though this appears to have been clearly demonstrated only in rheumatic fever, systemic lupus erythematosus, and polyarteritis nodosa.

From Tables 7.1 and 7.2 it will be seen that the collagen diseases constitute a subclass of those disorders that are believed to have an autoimmune basis.

PATHOGENIC MECHANISMS IN AUTOIMMUNE DISEASE

A brief mention of the effect of antibodies to glomerular basement membrane has been made in Chapter 6; in certain cases of glomerulonephritis linear deposition of IgG and the β_{1C}-component of complement (i.e. C3) along the basement membrane of the glomerular capillaries can be demonstrated by renal biopsy and immunofluorescence staining. The antibodies to the glomerular basement membrane can be eluted with acid; injection of these antibodies into a squirrel monkey has been shown to produce a fatal glomerulonephritis, the antibodies binding to the glomerular basement membrane of the monkey's kidney (Lerner *et al.*, 1967). In systemic lupus erythematosus, glomerulonephritis is often associated with the deposition of complexes of deoxyribonucleic acid and other nuclear antigens with immunoglobulin and complement, and in such cases the staining pattern obtained with a fluorescent anti-IgG or anti-C3 antiserum is 'lumpy' rather than 'linear'.

The presence of anti-deoxyribonucleic acid (anti-DNA) antibody in the serum in systemic lupus erythematosus, referred to above, has formed the basis of a number of tests which may be useful in following the response to therapy of patients with this condition. These tests are discussed in detail by Nakamura (1974).

A discussion of the pathogenic mechanisms involved in autoimmune disease is beyond the scope of this book, and for information on this topic the reader is referred to the accounts by Nakamura (1974) and Roitt (1974). However, it is interesting to note here the suggestion that immunological mechanisms, involving membrane-reactive autoantibodies, may be involved also in the pathogenesis of cardiovascular disorders (Mathews *et al.*, 1974). It is postulated that such autoantibodies combine with autoantigens released by cell turnover or death to form immune complexes, which are themselves the more direct cause of vascular damage and thrombosis. The presence of immune complexes in the sera of patients with various vascular diseases has recently been confirmed (Füst *et al.*, 1977).

There is evidence also that insulin-dependent diabetes is associated with disorders of the immune mechanisms. Apart from a statistical association between insulin-dependent diabetes and certain organ-specific autoimmune diseases (Hashimoto's disease, pernicious anaemia, idiopathic adrenal atrophy, Addison's disease) (Ungar *et al.*, 1968; Irvine *et al.*, 1970; Whittingham *et al.*, 1971; Nerup, 1974), serological work has revealed a high prevalence of humoral, organ-specific autoantibodies in insulin-dependent diabetes (Irvine *et al.*, 1970; Whittingham *et al.*, 1971; Nerup and Binder, 1973). Of particular interest are the reports of islet-cell antibodies in insulin-dependent diabetics with coexistent autoimmune disease (Bottazzo *et al.*, 1974; MacCuish *et al.*, 1974), and in newly diagnosed juvenile diabetics (Lendrum *et al.*, 1975, 1976), and the finding that the appearance of islet-cell antibodies in the serum may precede the onset of diabetes by several years (Lendrum *et al.*, 1975; Irvine *et al.*, 1976).

Table 7.2. Autoantibodies in various autoimmune disorders. (After R. M. Nakamura, *Immunopathology: Clinical Laboratory Concepts and Methods*, Little, Brown, Boston, 1974, by permission of Little, Brown and Co. and Dr. Nakamura.)

Disorders	Antigen involved	Common method of detection of antibody*	Reference
A. *Organ-specific endocrine*			
Hashimoto's thyroiditis Primary myxoedema Thyrotoxicosis	Thyroglobulin	a. IFT—human thyroid tissue fixed in methanol at 56° C for 3 min to fix colloid	Balfour *et al.*, 1961
		b. Passive haemagglutination	Fulthorpe *et al.*, 1961
		c. Latex agglutination	Anderson *et al.*, 1962
	Cytoplasmic microsome	IFT—unfixed human thyroid tissue from patient with thyrotoxicosis is used as substrate.	Holborow *et al.*, 1959
		Complement fixation test with thyroid microsomes	Buchanan *et al.*, 1962
Thyrotoxicosis	Thyroid cell surface antigen	Bioassay—mouse thyroid stimulation *in vivo*	Ochi and DeGroot, 1968
Addison's disease	Adrenal cell cytoplasm	IFT on unfixed human adrenal cortex	Blizzard and Kyle, 1963 Blizzard *et al.*, 1967
Parathyroid	Parathyroid cytoplasmic antigen	IFT—human parathyroid gland	Blizzard *et al.*, 1966
B. *Alimentary Tract*			
Pernicious anaemia and atrophic gastritis	Parietal cell microsomes	IFT—human or mouse gastric mucosa substrate	Irvine, 1963; Muller *et al.*, 1971
Pernicious anaemia	Intrinsic factor	Radioactive vit. B_{12} binding assay	Gottlieb *et al.*, 1965
Sjögren's syndrome	Salivary duct cells	IFT—unfixed human salivary gland	Bertram and Halberg, 1964
Ulcerative colitis	Colon, lipopolysaccharide	IFT—human or rat colon	Broberger and Perlmann, 1959
Coeliac disease	Reticulin	IFT—rat kidney	Seah *et al.*, 1971
Active chronic (or lupoid) hepatitis	Smooth muscle	IFT—rat gastric mucosa; human cervical tissue	Whittingham *et al.*, 1966
Primary biliary cirrhosis	Mitochondrial	IFT—rat kidney unfixed	Deodhar *et al.*, 1969; Doniach *et al.*, 1966

C. *Non-organ-specific diseases*			
Lupus erythematosus Dermatomyositis Periarteritis nodosa Scleroderma Rheumatoid arthritis Sjögren's disease 'Autoallergic' liver diseases	*Nuclear antigens* (a) DNA (b) Nucleoprotein (c) Sm antigen (d) Ribonucleoprotein (e) Nucleolar RNA	IFT—rat kidney substrate Peroxidase enzyme-labelled antibody Haemagglutination Radioactive DNA antigen-binding capacity assay Precipitin test	Tan, 1967 Benson and Cohen, 1970; Dorling *et al.*, 1971 Koffler *et al.*, 1971 Carr *et al.*, 1969 Tan *et al.*, 1966
Rheumatoid arthritis Sjögren's disease Lupus erythematosus Other collagen diseases	Altered γ-globulin	Latex test for rheumatoid factor Rose test, sheep cell agglutination	Rheins *et al.*, 1957 Cathcart, 1975
D. *Other*			
Myasthenia gravis	Skeletal or heart muscle	IFT—rat skeletal muscle and calf thymus	Osserman and Weiner, 1965
Goodpasture's syndrome	Glomerular and lung basement membrane	Peroxidase-labelled antibody IFT—biopsy of patient's kidney IFT—human kidney substrate with patient's serum	Davey and Busch, 1970 Lerner *et al.*, 1967
Pemphigus vulgaris	Prickle cell desmosomes	IFT—human skin Peroxidase-labelled antibody	Beutner *et al.*, 1968, 1970 Fukuyama *et al.*, 1970
Bullous pemphigoid	Epithelial basement membrane	IFT—human skin Peroxidase-labelled antibody	Beutner *et al.*, 1968, 1970 Fukuyama *et al.*, 1970
Dermatitis herpetiformis	Reticulin	IFT—rat kidney	Seah *et al.*, 1971
Autoimmune haemolytic anaemic	Red cell or closely associated antigen	Coombs' antiglobulin test—direct and indirect tests on patient's cells and serum	Pirofsky, 1969

*IFT = indirect fluorescence test.

Table 7.3. Direct pathogenic effects of humoral antibodies. (Reproduced, from I. Roitt, *Essential Immunology*, 2nd edn., Blackwell, Oxford, 1974, by permission of Blackwell Scientific Publications Ltd. and Prof. Roitt.)

Disease	Autoantigen	Lesion
Autoimmune haemolytic anaemia	Red cell	Erythrocyte destruction
Lymphopaenia (some cases)	Lymphocyte	Lymphocyte destruction
Idiopathic thrombocytopaenic purpura	Platelet	Platelet destruction
Male infertility (some cases)	Sperm	Agglutination of spermatozoa
Pernicious anaemia	Intrinsic factor	Neutralization of ability to mediate B_{12} absorption
Hashimoto's disease	Thyroid surface antigen	Cytotoxic effect on thyroid cells in culture
Thyrotoxicosis	? Thyroid surface antigen	Stimulation of thyroid cells
Goodpasture's syndrome	Glomerular basement membrane	Complement-mediated damage to basement membrane

Table 7.3 summarizes the direct pathogenic effects of humoral antibodies in a number of diseases. The precise aetiological factors involved in autoimmune diseases are often unknown; possible mechanisms have been classified by Sell (1969, 1975).

LABORATORY TESTS IN AUTOIMMUNE DISORDERS

Diseases thought to have an autoimmune pathogenesis are often associated with high plasma concentrations of γ-globulins, often greater than 15 g/l, and with the presence of one or more autoantibodies which may be detected in serum or tissues (Table 7.2). The serological diagnosis of an autoimmune disorder depends on the demonstration of such antibodies. A detailed consideration of the techniques employed is outside the scope of this book, but their applications are indicated in Table 7.2.

REFERENCES

Anderson, J. R., W. W. Buchanan, R. B. Goudie, and K. G. Gray (1962), *J. Clin. Path.*, **15**, 462.

Balfour, B. M., D. Doniach, I. M. Roitt, and K. G. Couchman (1961), *Brit. J. Exp. Path.*, **42**, 307.

Benson, M. D., and A. S. Cohen (1970), *Ann. Int. Med.*, **73**, 943.

Bertram, V., and P. Halberg (1964), *Acta Allergol.* (*Kbh.*), **14**, 458.

Beutner, E. H., R. E. Gordon, and T. P. Chorzelski (1968), *J. Invest. Dermatol.*, **51**, 64.

Beutner, E. H., T. P. Chorzelski, and R. E. Jordon (1970), *Autosensitization in Pemphigus and Bullous Pemphigoid*, Thomas, Springfield, Ill.

Blizzard, R. M., and M. Kyle (1963), *J. Clin. Invest.*, **42**, 1653.

Blizzard, R. M., D. Chee, and W. Davis (1966), *Clin. Exp. Immunol.*, **1**, 119.

Blizzard, R. M., D. Chee, and W. Davis (1967), *Clin. Exp. Immunol.*, **2**, 19.

Bottazzo, G. F., A. Florin-Christensen, and D. Doniach (1974), *Lancet*, **ii**, 1279.

Broberger, O., and P. Perlmann (1959), *J. Exp. Med.*, **110**, 657.

Buchanan, W. W., D. A. Koutras, J. Crooks, W. D. Alexander, W. Brass, J. R. Anderson, R. B. Goudie, and K. E. Gray (1962), *J. Endocrinol.*, **24**, 115.

Burnet, F. M. (1969), *Cellular Immunology*, Cambridge University Press, London.

Burnet, F. M. (1972), *Autoimmunity and Autoimmune Disease*, Davis, Philadelphia.

Carr, R. I., D. Koffler, V. Agnello, and H. G. Kunkel (1969), *Clin. Exp. Immunol.*, **4**, 527.

Cathcart, E. S. (1975), in *Laboratory Diagnostic Procedures in the Rheumatic Diseases* (Ed. A. S. Cohen), 2nd edn., Little, Brown, Boston.

Davey, F. R., and G. J. Busch (1970), *Amer. J. Clin. Path.*, **53**, 531.

Deodhar, D. S., A. Yazbek, E. Achkar, and C. H. Brown (1969), *Cleveland Clin. Quart.*, **36**, 95.

Doniach, D., I. M. Roitt, J. G. Walker, and S. Sherlock (1966), *Clin. Exp. Immunol.*, **1**, 237.

Dorling, J., G. D. Johnson, J. A. Webb, and M. E. Smith (1971), *J. Clin. Path.*, **24**, 501.

Fukuyama, K., S. D. Douglas, D. L. Tuffanelli, and W. L. Epstein (1970), *Amer. J. Clin. Path.*, **54**, 410.

Fulthorpe, A. J., I. M. Roitt, D. Doniach, and K. Couchman (1961), *J. Clin. Path.*, **14**, 654.

Füst, G., J. Székely, and S. Gerö (1977), *Lancet*, **i**, 193.

Gottlieb, C., K. S. Lau, L. R. Wasserman, and V. Herbert (1965), *Blood*, **25**, 875.

Holborow, E. J., P. C. Brown, I. M. Roitt, and D. Doniach (1959), *Brit. J. Exp. Path.*, **40**, 583.

Irvine, W. J. (1963), *Quart. J. Exp. Physiol.*, **48**, 427.

Irvine, W. J., B. F. Clarke, L. Scarth, D. R. Cullen, and L. J. P. Duncan (1970), *Lancet*, **ii**, 163.

Irvine, W. J., R. S. Gray, and C. J. McCallum (1976), *Lancet*, **ii**, 1097.

Klemperer, P., A. D. Pollack, and G. Baehr (1942), *J. Amer. Med. Assoc.*, **119**, 331.

Koffler, D., R. Carr, V. Agnello, R. Thoburn, and H. G. Kunkel (1971), *J. Exp. Med.*, **134**, 294.

Lendrum, R., G. Walker, and D. R. Gamble (1975), *Lancet*, **i**, 880.

Lendrum, R., P. G. Nelson, D. A. Pyke, G. Walker, and D. R. Gamble (1976), *Brit. Med. J.*, **i**, 553.

Lerner, R. A., R. J. Glassock, and F. J. Dixon (1967), *J. Exp. Med.*, **126**, 989.

MacCuish, A. C., E. W. Barnes, W. J. Irvine, and L. J. P. Duncan (1974), *Lancet*, **ii**, 1529.

Mathews, J. D., S. Whittingham, and I. R. Mackay (1974), *Lancet*, **ii**, 1423.

Muller, H. K., A. R. McGwen, and R. C. Nairn (1971), *J. Clin. Path.*, **24**, 13.

Nakamura, R. M. (1974), *Immunopathology: Clinical Laboratory Concepts and Methods*, Little, Brown, Boston, p. 201.

Nerup, J. (1974), in *Immunity and Autoimmunity in Diabetes Mellitus* (Eds. P. A. Bastenie and W. Gepts), Excerpta Medica, Amsterdam, p. 149.

Nerup, J., and C. Binder (1973), *Acta Endocrinol. (Kbh.)*, **72**, 279.

Ochi, Y., and L. J. DeGroot (1968), *New Engl. J. Med.*, **278**, 718.

Osserman, K. E., and L. B. Weiner (1965), *Ann. N. Y. Acad. Sci.*, **124 (II)**, 730.

Pirofsky, B. (1969), *Autoimmunization and the Autoimmune Hemolytic Anemias*, Williams and Wilkins, Baltimore.

Rheins, M. S., F. W. McCoy, R. G. Burell, and E. V. Beuhler (1957), *J. Lab. Clin. Med.*, **50**, 113.

Roitt, I. (1974), *Essential Immunology*, 2nd edn., Blackwell, Oxford, p. 211.

Seah, P. P., L. Fry, A. V. Hoffbrand, and E. J. Holborow (1971), *Lancet*, **i**, 834.

Sell, S. (1969), *Bull. Rheum. Dis.*, **19**, 546, 554.

Sell, S. (1975), *Immunology, Immunopathology and Immunity*, 2nd edn., Harper and Row, Hagerstown, Md.

Tan, E. M. (1967), *J. Lab. Clin. Med.*, **70**, 800.

Tan, E. M., P. H. Schur, R. I. Carr, and H. G. Kunkel (1966), *J. Clin. Invest.*, **45**, 1732.

Ungar, B., A. E. Stocks, F. I. R. Martin, S. Whittingham, and I. R. Mackay (1968), *Lancet*, **ii**, 415.

Weigle, W. O. (1967), *Natural and Acquired Immunologic Unresponsiveness*, World, Cleveland.

Whittingham, S., J. Irwin, I. R. Mackay, and M. Smalley (1966), *Gastroenterology*, **51**, 499.

Whittingham, S., J. D. Mathews, I. R. Mackay, A. E. Stocks, B. Ungar, and F. I. R. Martin (1971), *Lancet*, **i**, 763.

CHAPTER 8

Trauma

Trauma, which may result from a variety of causes, is associated with a number of metabolic changes, the extent of which depends partly upon the severity of the damage suffered by the tissues. Among these metabolic effects of trauma there are often an increased loss of nitrogen from the body and changes in the concentrations of many of the plasma proteins, some of which rise while some fall, yet others remaining essentially unchanged.

NITROGEN METABOLISM

The development of a negative nitrogen balance after trauma was first reported by Cuthbertson (1930), and many investigators have since studied this phenomenon. After severe trauma there is typically an increase in the urinary excretion of nitrogen (involving mainly urea), which reaches a maximum between the third and twelfth days. The magnitude of this effect of trauma varies from one person to another. Although the reason for this variation in response to injury is not completely known, it appears to depend in part upon the patient's nutritional state, being greatest in previously well-nourished persons (Browne *et al.*, 1944; Peters, 1946). This is in accord with the results of animal experiments (Munro and Cuthbertson, 1943; Munro and Chalmers, 1945; Calloway *et al.*, 1955; Fleck and Munro, 1963).

The negative nitrogen balance associated with this increased urinary output of nitrogen can lead to considerable losses of body protein if it persists. This is often the case in burned patients, where an additional loss of body protein is incurred in the exudation from the burned surface (Keyser, 1948; Moore *et al.*, 1950). It is quite misleading, however, to suggest that trauma is invariably accompanied by a large increase in urinary nitrogen excretion. In the case of burns, for example, although many of the patients studied by a number of workers (Lucido, 1940; Browne, 1942; Taylor *et al.*, 1943; and Moore *et al.*, 1950) excreted large amounts of nitrogen in the urine, others have reported a lower excretion (Cope *et al.*, 1943; Anderson and Semeonoff, 1945; Keyser, 1948). The subject is reviewed by Sevitt (1957). There are many possible reasons for these variations in reported urinary nitrogen excretion, including, as indicated above, the nutritional state of the patient; additional factors are the extent of the injury, the presence or absence of infection (Cope *et al.*, 1943), and so on.

The observation that the catabolic response increases in proportion to the severity of the injury was made long ago (see Moore and Ball, 1952) and is consistent with more recent studies using labelled albumin and IgG (summarized by Davies, 1970), which show that the catabolic rate of these proteins likewise increases with the severity of the injury.

In patients with burns the rate of synthesis of albumin was found to be about normal during the first week after burning and then subnormal during the next two weeks; the rate of synthesis of IgG was substantially above normal, and that of fibrinogen even higher. Patients with other forms of injury show a similar, though less marked, pattern; albumin synthesis is depressed to below the normal range during the second and third weeks after injury, at which time the synthesis of IgG is about twice normal and that of fibrinogen is just above the expected normal range (Davies, 1970).

Other studies of protein turnover are reviewed by Koj (1974).

PROTEIN CHANGES

The earliest observations on the effect of trauma on the concentration of blood proteins appear to have been those made on a fraction, variously known as 'polypeptides' or 'proteoses', characterized by solubility in trichloroacetic acid and insolubility in tungstic or phosphotungstic acid. The difference between the nitrogen contents of trichloroacetic and tungstic (or phosphotungstic) acid filtrates prepared from blood was thus used as a measure of these substances. Hahn (1921) noted an increased concentration in a patient after surgical operation, and this was confirmed by later investigators, who reported increases both after surgical operations and after burn injuries (Wolff, 1921; Cristol and Puech, 1930; Fiessinger, 1934; Goiffon and Spaey, 1934a,b; Duval *et al.*, 1934). From a consideration of their solubility properties it seems likely that these 'polypeptides' are similar to the carbohydrate-rich seromucoid ('mucoprotein') fraction studied by Winzler and his coworkers in the 1940s (Winzler *et al.*, 1948; Winzler and Smyth, 1948; Mehl *et al.*, 1949a,b; Weimer *et al.*, 1950; Smith *et al.*, 1950).

The seromucoid fraction is increased in concentration after various types of injury (Keyser, 1952), as is also the total glycoprotein concentration of the serum (Shetlar *et al.*, 1949; Keyser, 1952). The finding of an enhanced serum 'tryptophan–perchloric acid reaction' in patients with burn injuries (Keyser, 1949, 1950) was presumably the result of an increase in the concentration of glycoproteins in the plasma, since this reaction is apparently due to the sialic acid contained in the carbohydrate portion of the glycoproteins (Werner and Odin, 1952).

Other early findings were a fall in albumin (Cuthbertson and Tompsett, 1935) and a rise in fibrinogen concentration (Chanutin *et al.*, 1938) after trauma; these observations have been confirmed by many workers and appear to be associated with trauma of all kinds.

The changes that occur in the plasma proteins may conveniently be considered under three headings, *viz.* (a) electrophoretic fractions, (b) certain specific proteins, and (c) enzymes.

Electrophoretic fractions

It has long been known that trauma produces certain well-marked changes in the electrophoretic pattern of the plasma. These comprise an increase in the concentration of the α-globulin fraction (Prendergast *et al.*, 1952; Hoch-Ligeti *et al.*, 1953; and many others) and, as noted above, a fall in plasma albumin concentration.

In man no consistent change was found in the plasma concentration of β-globulin after surgical operation (Hoch-Ligeti *et al.*, 1953) or after burn injuries (Deadrick *et al.*, 1956; Lanchantin and Deadrick, 1958), but increases have been reported after experimental injury in rats (Neuhaus *et al.*, 1961) and in goats (Gillette *et al.*, 1958). Also in man, no consistent changes were found by Hoch-Ligeti and her coworkers (1953) in the plasma concentration of total γ-globulin immediately after surgical operation, and no consistent change was found by Linko and his coworkers (1956) or by Belfrage (1963) after myocardial infarction; however, the two patients with myocardial infarction whose serum proteins were studied by the present writer showed falls in γ-globulin concentration of 30% and 40% respectively, as measured by paper electrophoresis (Keyser and Stephens, 1964). An increase in γ-globulin concentration after burn injuries has been reported (Prendergast *et al.*, 1952), but in at least two of the eight patients investigated this increase was preceded by a fall. A fall in the concentration of γ-globulin in the immediate post-burn period was also noted by Deadrick and his colleagues (1956) in the more severely burned patients. Changes in the immunoglobulin constituents of the electrophoretic γ-globulin fraction are discussed below.

There would appear to be little of practical clinical value attached to the electrophoretic evaluation of the serum proteins after trauma; however, any assessment of an electrophoretic analysis of a patient's serum proteins should take into account the possible effects of any recent trauma.

Specific proteins

The ready availability of specific antisera in more recent years has enabled the behaviour of many individual proteins to be studied. In general, plasma proteins fall into three groups, according to whether their concentration is increased, decreased, or essentially unchanged after trauma (Table 8.1). Strictly speaking, this is an over-simplification, since the changes actually observed do depend to some extent upon the type of injury, or to other circumstances: for example, whereas, in the absence of infection, many surgical operations are not associated with consistent changes in immunoglobulin concentrations, these typically show a pronounced fall immediately after burning (Birke *et al.*, 1969; Arturson *et al.*, 1969; Ritzmann *et al.*, 1969). The initial decrease is due to losses of plasma, partly extravascularly and partly in the exudate, and to this extent burns must be considered as a special type of injury. Sometimes changes in the plasma concentrations of immunoglobulins occur

Table 8.1. Proteins of human plasma after surgical trauma. (After A. H. Gordon, *Plasma Protein Metabolism: Regulation of Synthesis, Distribution, and Degradation* (ed. M. A. Rothschild and T. Waldmann), Academic Press, New York, 1970, by permission of Academic Press, Inc., and Dr. Gordon.)

Effect	Protein	Concentration in plasma (% of pre-operative values)
Concentration increased	Fibrinogen	>200
	Haptoglobin	206
	Orosomucoid (α_1-acid glycoprotein)	>200
	C-reactive protein	>200
	α_1-Antitrypsin	>200
	Slow β-globulin	173
	Inter α-globulin	189
	Complement C3	122
	Caeruloplasmin	124
	Easily precipitable glycoprotein	140
Concentration unchanged	More than 30 other proteins	
Concentration decreased	Thyroxine-binding prealbumin	69
	α-Lipoprotein	
	β-Lipoprotein	77
	Transferrin	78
	Albumin	80

All the patients had undergone minor surgical operations 8 hours or more before the second blood sample was taken. Most of the proteins were measured by quantitative immunoelectrophoresis.

Many of these changes had been described by earlier workers.

after surgical operations, even in the absence of infection, the extent of the changes depending on the severity of the surgical trauma (Cohnen, 1972; Fuller and Keyser, 1975). The finding of increases in immunoglobulin concentrations in some patients in the absence of infection has led to the suggestion that substances liberated from the tissues as a result of trauma may in some way stimulate the production of immunoglobulins (Cohnen, 1972; Fuller and Keyser, 1975). It appears that after trauma the serum immunoglobulin concentrations are subject to multiple, unpredictable influences.

It is clear from the work of numerous investigators that the concentration of certain plasma proteins decreases as a result of those same stimuli that lead to increases in the concentration of others. In this connexion it must be emphasized that the plasma concentration of any protein is the result of both production and degradation (and in some cases loss from the circulation); since these processes may not parallel one another, the net effect may not be the same for different proteins.

Proteins showing an increase in plasma concentration after trauma or in the acute phase of inflammatory states are sometimes called *acute-phase reactants*. (The term is occasionally extended to include certain proteins showing a fall in concentration.) These proteins are all rich in carbohydrate, and all are synthesized mainly if not exclusively in the liver parenchymal cells. Apparently the liver is stimulated in some way as a result of trauma, and produces these glycoproteins more rapidly than normally. Similar increases in the plasma concentration of many plasma proteins are seen also in bacterial infections and in cancer.

Acute myocardial infarction offers a useful clinical model for the study of changes in the concentrations of serum proteins after trauma, and a number of reports on the specific protein changes occurring in patients with this condition have appeared (Schwarz, 1963; Lundh, 1965; Karl and Reißmann, 1967; Jayle *et al.*, 1968; Bachmann *et al.*, 1968; Chakrabarti *et al.*, 1969; Agostoni *et al.*, 1970; Johansson *et al.*, 1972; Jakab *et al.*, 1974, 1976; Snyder *et al.*, 1975). Johansson and his coworkers determined the plasma concentrations of 21 individual proteins during 3 weeks after myocardial infarction, and distinguished three major patterns of response:

1. C-reactive protein, haptoglobin, antichymotrypsin, fibrinogen, orosomucoid (α_1-acid glycoprotein), and α_1-antitrypsin showed a rapid increase with a maximum on about day 5 (day 1 being the day of admission to hospital), with a partial return to normal values by day 21;
2. prealbumin, albumin, α-lipoprotein, transferrin, and IgG showed a rapid decrease to 80 per cent or less of their initial values by day 5, and restoration to normal values by day 21;
3. caeruloplasmin and β_{1C}-globulin showed a moderate increase, with a maximum during the second week.

Only slight changes were found for haemopexin, plasminogen, prothrombin, cold-insoluble globulin, β_{1E}-globulin, and α_2-macroglobulin. The immunoglobulin pattern after 3 weeks was characterized by a small increase, which was most prominent in the case of IgM.

The suggestion has been made that substances released from the infarcted tissue may selectively increase the synthesis of certain proteins or increase their degradation (Snyder *et al.*, 1975).

Significance of acute-phase protein changes

From a study of chronic inflammatory and neoplastic states in man Seibert and her colleagues (1947) suggested that the increased concentration of serum total protein-bound carbohydrate was associated with tissue destruction. On the basis of experimental studies in dogs, Shetlar and his coworkers (1949) put forward an alternative suggestion, that the increase was correlated in some way with tissue proliferation or repair. However, experiments with a particular form of trauma, *viz.* the inflammatory process induced by the intraperitoneal injection of silica into rabbits, showed that elevation of the serum total protein-bound carbohydrate (which is a measure of the concentration of total serum glycoproteins) could be correlated with acute inflammation but not with tissue formation as judged by fibrosis or macrophage response (Heppleston and Keyser, 1957). Neither could any correlation be found between the serum protein-bound hexose (total, and α_2-globulin-, seromucoid-, and non-seromucoid-bound) and the extent of tissue formation or destruction as judged by the amounts of viable and necrotic tumour tissue in rats bearing the Walker 256 carcinoma (Heppleston and Keyser, 1959). These and other findings suggest that increases in the concentration of (total) serum glycoproteins, or of the seromucoid fraction, are not specifically related either to tissue break-down or to tissue proliferation (Keyser, 1960). This conclusion does not, of course, exclude the possibility that changes in the concentration of individual proteins may be so related.

Attempts have been made to assess the significance of the 'acute-phase' reaction after trauma by simultaneous enzyme studies. Björnesjö (1958) studied the problem by simultaneous determination of aspartate transaminase activity and hexosamine concentration in blood serum and urine after surgical operations. Surgical trauma was followed by an early increase in serum aspartate transaminase activity and urinary hexosamine, both with a maximum on the day after operation, with a rapid decrease thereafter. Serum hexosamine concentration, however, increased more slowly to a maximum on the third to the tenth day after operation, by which time serum aspartate transaminase and urinary hexosamine had returned to near the normal levels. These findings were interpreted as supporting the view that the early peak in urinary hexosamine occurring simultaneously with the peak in serum aspartate transaminase activity was due to tissue necrosis and that the later increase in serum concentration depended principally on secondary regenerative processes (Björnesjö, 1958; Björnesjö *et al.*, 1959).

A study of patients with myocardial infarction showed that the peak concentration of seromucoid (and total serum glycoprotein) was reached at the fourth to the eleventh day after the occurrence of infarction, and several days after the serum aspartate transaminase activity had reached its peak and had begun to subside (Figure 8.1) (Keyser and Stephens, 1964). Similar results were reported by Musil (1961).

Time sequence of changes

A number of investigators have studied the time sequence of response of various acute-phase reactants after injury. In man, C-reactive protein and in the rat the α_2-acute-phase globulin* respond most promptly, appearing in the

*A protein, sometimes called 'slow-α_2-globulin', or α-macrofetoprotein, observed in rat serum in a number of physiological and pathological states (Yamada, 1959; Lawford, 1961; Beaton *et al.*, 1961; Riou *et al.*, 1962; Fine *et al.*, 1962; Heim and Kerrigan, 1963) and further studied by Weimer and Benjamin (1965).

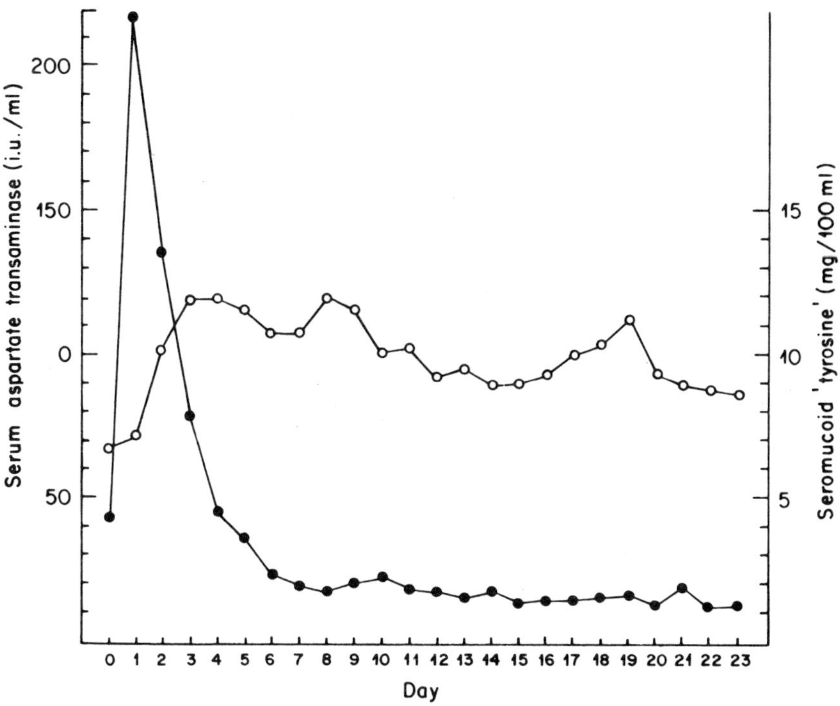

Figure 8.1. Average serum transaminase and seromucoid 'tyrosine' levels in seven patients after myocardial infarction. (From J. W. Keyser and B. T. Stephens, *Clin. Chem.*, 1964, **10**, 736, with the permission of the American Association for Clinical Chemistry.)

plasma usually within 24 hours of injury. Haptoglobin, fibrinogen, seromucoid, and caeruloplasmin concentrations usually increase at a slightly lower rate. The return to normal values also shows some variation (see for example, Crockson *et al.* (1966) and Koj (1970)).

Serum protein changes during the 'acute-phase reaction' are discussed by Werner (1969), who has emphasized the value of studying the response, in man, to operative trauma; this provides an ideal model since both the degree of trauma and the time of onset of the response are known and the effect of trauma can be differentiated from that of infection (Werner and Cohnen, 1969).

Mechanism of acute-phase protein changes

Several investigators have suggested that increases in the concentration of acute-phase plasma proteins after trauma is a response to substances liberated from damaged or necrotic cells (Darcy, 1964; Weimer and Benjamin, 1965). Although Gordon and Darcy (1967) and Sarcione and his colleagues (1965) reported an apparent increase in the rate of synthesis of certain acute-phase plasma proteins when livers isolated from normal rats were perfused with blood from acutely injured rats, subsequent investigations with perfused livers failed to confirm these findings (Schumer *et al.*, 1967; Gordon and Koj, 1968). However, for technical reasons, as Schumer and his colleagues point out, such experiments are inconclusive and do not rule out the presence of 'humoral factors', affecting glycoprotein synthesis, in the plasma of injured animals.

Differences are found between acute-phase reactants in their pattern of response to repeated trauma. Weimer and Humelbaugh (1967) injected rats with turpentine at intervals of several days and found that although plasma fibrinogen reached its maximum concentration after the second injection the α_2-acute-phase globulin concentration was highest after the third injection, while seromucoid showed a similar response each time. These and other experimental findings appear to indicate the existence of systems capable of independently controlling the rate of synthesis of the different proteins. That more than one mechanism may be responsible for controlling the rate of synthesis of certain plasma proteins is suggested by the behaviour of transferrin under various conditions; thus the plasma concentration of this protein, although often decreased after trauma, has been shown to increase (after a preliminary fall) in both rats (Lane, 1948) and man (Laurell, 1947) after acute blood loss; and increases are also found in rats after partial hepatectomy and in conditions of oxygen depletion and excess of plasma iron (Morgan and Brackenridge, 1962; Morgan and Lynch, 1963).

However, as Koj (1974) points out, the difference in the response patterns of individual acute-phase reactants does not necessarily imply that separate stimulatory factors are released from the site of injury, each responsible for the increased rate of synthesis of a specific protein. It may well be that differentiation takes place in the liver by one of several possible mechanisms, such as variations in the rate of formation or stability of specific mRNA, or hormonal control of protein synthesis (Koj, 1974).

Rôle of the adrenal gland

Many investigators have considered the possibility that adrenal steroids are involved in regulating the synthesis of plasma glycoproteins after trauma, since the traumatic stimuli producing this response also stimulate the adrenal cortex. However, experiments in which animals were injected with adrenocortical steroids (Weimer and Redlich-Moshin, 1953; Shetlar and Shetlar, 1955; Keyser, 1959), as well as observations on patients treated with steroids (Keyser *et al.*, 1963), suggest that an adrenocortical mechanism does not by itself bring about the 'acute-phase' response. Others have investigated the effects of adrenalectomy on the plasma glycoprotein response to tissue injury in rats, and the various results of their experiments are summarized in Table 8.2.

The inhibitory effect of adrenalectomy on the response of α_2-acute-phase globulin and seromucoid in rats is restored by small doses of cortisol, while large, pharmacological doses reduce the concentrations of these proteins (Weimer and Coggshall, 1967).

Atencio and Lorand (1970) observed a pronounced rise in fibrinogen synthesis

Table 8.2. Various effects of adrenalectomy on the plasma glycoprotein response to tissue injury in rats.* (After A. Koj, *Energy Metabolism in Trauma* (Eds. R. Porter and J. Knight), Churchill, London, 1970, by permission of Ciba Foundation and Dr. Koj.)

Protein	Effect	Reference
α_2-Acute-phase globulin	Almost total inhibition	Heim and Ellenson, 1967; Weimer and Coggshall, 1967
Haptoglobin	Marked inhibition	Krauss, 1963
Seromucoid	Slight inhibition	Weimer and Coggshall, 1967
Fibrinogen†	No effect	Weimer and Coggshall, 1967
Caeruloplasmin	Probably stimulation	Evans and Wiederanders, 1967
α_1-Acid glycoprotein	Marked stimulation	Darcy, 1965; Gordon and Koj, 1968

*In other species the response of individual acute-phase reactants may be different; for example, Atencio and his colleagues (1969) observed that adrenalectomy in rabbits almost totally abolished the fibrinogen increase after injection of endotoxin.

†Adrenalectomy has no effect on the increase in fibrinogen synthesis following partial hepatectomy (Majumdar *et al.*, 1967).

in rabbits after the injection of adrenocorticotrophic hormone; they suggested that the hormone must have acted by some mechanism other than stimulation of steroid synthesis, since the injection of corticosterone was without effect. It is interesting to compare these with the present writer's earlier finding (Keyser, 1959) that the injection of adrenocorticotrophic hormone into rabbits produced a rise in the concentration of total protein-bound carbohydrate and seromucoid, although the injection of corticosterone or deoxycorticosterone, or an adrenalin-free Swingle–Pfiffner extract of adrenal gland, was without effect. Very large doses of cortisol, however, did raise the concentration of seromucoid.

The view that adrenal steroids do nevertheless play some part in the 'acute-phase' response is supported by the experiments of John and Miller (1969), who were able to induce the enhanced synthesis of fibrinogen, haptoglobin, α_1-acid glycoprotein, and the α_2-acute-phase globulin in the isolated rat liver by supplying it with cortisol and insulin together with a nutritionally complete amino acid mixture.

Koj and Dubin (1974), however, in similar though less prolonged perfusion experiments with rat livers, obtained only insignificant increases in the rate of synthesis of fibrinogen, caeruloplasmin, or the seromucoid fraction by the addition of cortisol, insulin, growth hormone, and amino acids, except in the case of rats previously injected subcutaneously with turpentine. They concluded that the hormones only modify the rate of trauma-induced synthesis of acute-phase reactants, the primary stimulatory factors probably originating from the site of the injury (Gordon and Koj, 1968; Koj, 1970) and the hormones exerting a permissive action. They suggested that the increases observed by John and Miller may have been due to the effects of injury inflicted during the operation and isolation procedure, these effects being manifested only after several hours of perfusion.

Some of the evidence bearing on the hormonal regulation of the hepatic synthesis of acute-phase reactants has been reviewed by Koj (1973).

Amino acids

The importance of amino acids in relation to polyribosomal integrity and the rate of protein synthesis has been demonstrated by a number of workers, both *in vitro* (Baliga *et al.*, 1968; Wannemacher *et al.*, 1970) and in the perfused liver (Jefferson and Korner, 1969). From experiments on rats fed either a low-protein diet or one containing an adequate amount of protein, Wannemacher and his coworkers (1971) concluded that amino acids regulate protein synthesis both by affecting the number of ribosomes that actively synthesize protein and by inhibiting the synthesis of new ribosomes. Neuhaus and his coworkers (Shihabi *et al.*, 1970) demonstrated a two- to fourfold increase in the uptake of the model amino acid, ^{14}C-α-aminoisobutyric acid, by the livers of rats 4–8 hours after laparotomy; and Wannemacher (1972) has concluded that during inflammatory processes there is a rapid movement of amino acids into the liver, these amino acids being then rapidly used for the synthesis of serum proteins, especially glycoproteins. These effects are apparently brought about by a substance, 'leukocytic endogenous mediator' (LEM), which is released from stimulated polymorphonuclear leukocytes (Pekarek *et al.*, 1972). In rats, LEM stimulates a flux of amino acids from plasma to liver (Wannemacher *et al.*, 1972; Pekarek *et al.*, 1974), increases the rate of incorporation of labelled amino acids into serum protein (Pekarek *et al.*, 1972), and raises the plasma concentrations of a number of acute-phase globulins (Eddington *et al.*, 1971, Pekarek *et al.*, 1972, 1974), in addition to other effects. According to Wannemacher and his coworkers (1975), the action of LEM on hepatic amino acid transport appears to be a direct one, without the mediation of other hormones, and to be independent of cyclic AMP; however, the ability of LEM to stimulate the synthesis of RNA and acute-phase globulins may require the presence of physiological amounts of hormones such as adrenal corticoids.

Effect of actinomycin D

Evidence that the increased synthesis of acute-phase reactants depends on an increased transcriptive process at the DNA–RNA level was obtained by Neuhaus and his coworkers (1966), who treated rats with actinomycin D at various times in relation to the trauma (laparotomy). When the actinomycin D was administered 2 hours before, 2 hours after, or at the time of the trauma, a suppression of induced seromucoid synthesis was observed, whereas the usual increase occurred if the actinomycin D was injected 4 hours after operation. These results were interpreted as indicating that the elevation in the concentration of plasma seromucoid in response to trauma is an inductive process involving an increased production of messenger RNA between 2 and 4 hours after trauma.

However, Balegno and Neuhaus (1970) found that rats that had been subjected to laparotomy showed a transient increase in albumin synthesis which was critically dependent on the presence of insulin and was not inhibited by actinomycin D. These experiments seem to differentiate two groups of proteins: on the one hand, stress-responsive glycoproteins (acute-phase reactants), which require the synthesis of new RNA, and on the other hand, proteins such as albumin, which are perhaps synthesized on more stable templates. The transiently increased incorporation of labelled amino acids into albumin may well have reflected a stimulated uptake of amino acids by the liver cells, as discussed above.

Caution has been expressed as to the interpretation of some of the experiments mentioned above, since it would appear that if increased synthesis of mRNA specific for acute-phase proteins does indeed occur after trauma it is apparently not associated with a change of activity of RNA polymerase (Chandler and Neuhaus, 1968). Moreover, as emphasized by Chandler and Neuhaus, actinomycin D may affect various organs, tissues, and subcellular components in different ways; thus it has an effect not only on the synthesis of mRNA and ribosomal RNA but also on the stability of polysomes; and its effect on mitochondria, with consequent depletion of available ATP, would be of particular consequence. Nevertheless, in spite of these reservations, it should be noted that Liu and Neuhaus (1968) confirmed an increased synthesis of protein after trauma by demonstrating a maximally stimulated *in vitro* incorporation of ^{14}C-leucine into protein by microsomal fractions prepared from the livers of rats 18 hours after laparotomy; it was also observed that the polysomal fraction was in a maximal state of aggregation 18 hours after trauma (Liu and Neuhaus, 1968). The evidence suggests that the following sequence of events is initiated by injury:

1. a stimulated uptake of amino acids, maximal at 4–8 hours;
2. an increased synthesis of total hepatic RNA, maximal at 8 hours;
3. a stimulated protein-synthesizing capacity at 18 hours, accompanied by an increased polysomal aggregation; and
4. a maximal concentration of newly synthesized acute-phase proteins in the blood plasma at 24 hours (Liu and Neuhaus, 1968; Prof. O. W. Neuhaus, private communication).

Effects of inhibitors of protein synthesis

Another approach to the problem has been to compare cell-free systems containing microsomes or polyribosomes prepared from the livers of both normal rats and rats after trauma, as well as livers regenerating after partial hepatectomy. (With both the latter a much increased rate of incorporation of radioactive amino acids always occurs.) Skornik and his colleagues (1967) and Von der Decken (1968) found increased rates of incorporation of ^{14}C-labelled leucine by liver polyribosomes and cell sap after these had been passed through columns of 'Sephadex' G25, apparently as a result of the removal of inhibitors. In the presence of added guanosine triphosphate and amino acids the rate of incorporation of labelled leucine by this system became almost as high as that of a similar system prepared from the livers of rats after trauma. Work by Tsukada and his coworkers (1968) has given additional support to the idea that an inhibitor of protein synthesis is normally present and that the increased rates of synthesis that follow tissue damage are brought about by the effective removal of these inhibitors.

Koj and Allison (1969) have postulated that labilization of lysosomes is an early step in the series of events leading to the increased synthesis of acute-phase reactants. The same authors have suggested that, by a kind of 'feedback' mechanism, the acute-phase proteins may inhibit enzymes released from the lysosomes and in this way help to restore homeostasis.

For further information on this complex problem the reader is referred to reviews by Gordon (1970) and Koj (1970, 1974).

ENZYMES AND TRAUMA

In general, injury to tissues results in the release of enzymes from the injured tissue into the circulation. When such leakage of enzymes has begun, three factors affect the rate at which individual enzymes appear in the fluid perfusing the tissues (Moss and Butterworth, 1974). The first of these is the concentration gradient across the cell membrane: for example, the concentration of aspartate and alanine transaminases may be some 10,000 times as high inside liver cells as in the surrounding blood plasma, and even higher concentration ratios are found for alcohol dehydrogenase and sorbitol dehydrogenase.

The second factor is the size of the enzyme molecules, small molecules diffusing more rapidly than larger ones.

The third factor is the intracellular location of the enzymes, those contained in the cytoplasm or cell sap being released more readily than those contained in the mitochondria. This is seen when the cytoplasmic and mitochondrial isoenzymes of aspartate transaminase are studied: the former is released into the perfusing fluid at a rate which correlates well with that of other similar enzymes of similar molecular size, whereas the mitochondrial isoenzyme—although of similar molecular size—is released much more slowly.

Reversible inflammatory processes characterized by increased membrane permeability are more likely to be associated with the release of cell-sap enzymes than those contained within mitochondria, whereas actual destruction—such as occurs in necrotic conditions—leads to the release of both mitochondrial and cell-sap enzymes into the plasma. However, the limitations of this generalization have been emphasized by Wilkinson (1976), who points out that as a disease progresses many of the cells initially involved in an inflammatory lesion will die, and, conversely, that a zone of necrosis may be surrounded by cells that have been adversely affected by ischaemia or pressure. Thus although cell death does lead to a release of enzymes, this can occur also in diseases associated with little tissue necrosis.

Most of the studies of the release of tissue enzymes after trauma appear to have been made in liver diseases and after myocardial infarction, as well as after surgical operation and in other conditions involving trauma to muscle.

Liver

Although, as mentioned above, the nature of the tissue damage—i.e. whether inflammatory or necrotic —does influence the pattern of enzyme release, the nature of the damaging agent itself does not, in the case of the liver, appear to modify greatly the rate or amount of release of enzymes into the circulation. Very high serum transaminase activities were found in liver damage due to such causes as virus infection, chemical or mechanical trauma, hypoxia, and surgical trauma (Pryse-Davies and Wilkinson, 1958).

Reference has been made to the fact that aspartate transaminase occurs in markedly different forms in the cell sap and in the mitochondria. This difference in distribution of the isoenzymes, and the additional finding that alanine transaminase is almost wholly confined to the cell sap, led de Ritis and his coworkers (1955) to suggest the use of the aspartate transaminase:alanine transaminase ratio as a means of distinguishing predominantly inflammatory lesions from necrotic processes. A chromatographic method for separating the two forms of aspartate transaminase was devised by Schmidt and his coworkers (1967b), who were able to demonstrate the presence in serum of significant amounts of the mitochondrial enzyme in several liver diseases, especially in severe hepatitis. Using an electrophoretic method, Fleisher and his coworkers (1960) reported the presence of the cationic form of aspartate aminotransferase in the serum of patients with myocardial infarction. Subsequently Boyde (1968) was able to demonstrate that the cationic (mitochondrial) isoenzyme is a normal constituent of plasma but that after myocardial infarction the plasma concentration usually rises, reaching a peak at 24–48 hours and returning to normal more slowly than the total aspartate aminotransferase activity. However, since this isoenzyme occurs in the serum of patients with liver diseases (Schmidt *et al.*, 1967a), estimation of its serum activity does not afford a specific test for myocardial infarction.

Myocardial infarction

In this condition the serum activities of a number of enzymes are markedly increased, and their measurement is of considerable diagnostic importance. Figure 8.2 shows the average time-course of the changes in the serum activity of creatine kinase, aspartate transaminase, and lactate dehydrogenase. Creatine kinase activity is almost invariably increased at about 12 hours, and sometimes as early as 6 hours, after the onset of symptoms; it reaches a peak after about

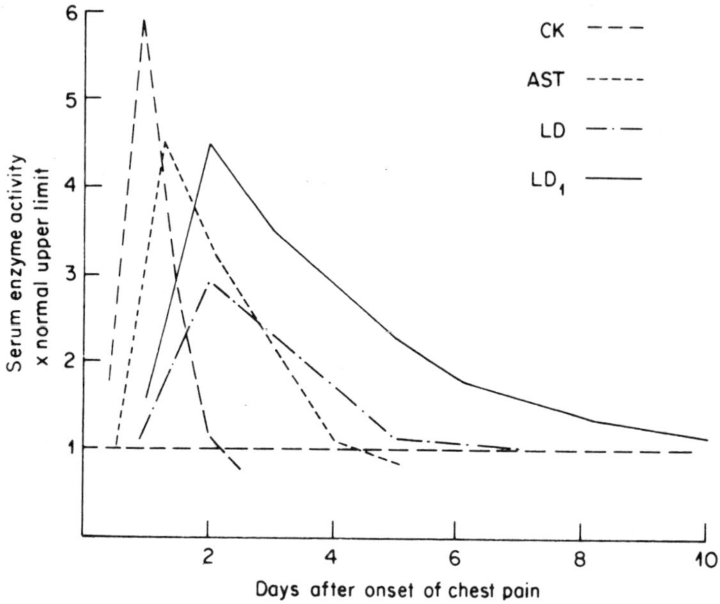

Figure 8.2. Transient elevations (mean values) of the serum creatine kinase, aspartate transaminase, lactate dehydrogenase and lactate dehydrogenase isoenzyme LD_1, as estimated by the 2-hydroxybutyrate dehydrogenase (HBD) reaction, in patients with acute myocardial infarction. (Reproduced, with permission, from J. H. Wilkinson, *The Principles and Practice of Diagnostic Enzymology*, Arnold, London, 1976.)

24 hours and generally returns to normal about the third day (Dreyfus *et al.*, 1960). If a blood specimen can be obtained at an early stage a determination of creatine kinase activity is the enzyme test of choice (Smith, 1967).

The discovery that creatine kinase exists in three forms, with a specific tissue distribution, has added a new tool for the diagnosis of myocardial infarction. Skeletal muscle contains the most cathodal isoenzyme, brain the most anodal, and cardiac muscle the intermediate ('MB') form together with larger amounts of the cathodal, muscle-type isoenzyme (Figure 8.3). Demonstration of the intermediate or 'MB' dimer in the serum is of importance in the diagnosis of myocardial infarction (Figure 8.4) (Konttinen and Somer, 1972, 1973; Wagner *et al.*, 1973).

Acute myocardial infarction occurs in a significant number of patients after major surgical operations and results in an appreciable mortality (Mauney *et al.*, 1970; Driscoll *et al.*, 1961). The detection and measurement of the isoenzymes of lactate dehydrogenase and creatine kinase, especially the cardiac-specific MB isoenzyme, have proved of value in the early recognition of the condition (Dixon *et al.*, 1973).

Changes in the plasma concentration of the mitochondrial isoenzyme of aspartate aminotransferase are discussed above (p. 149).

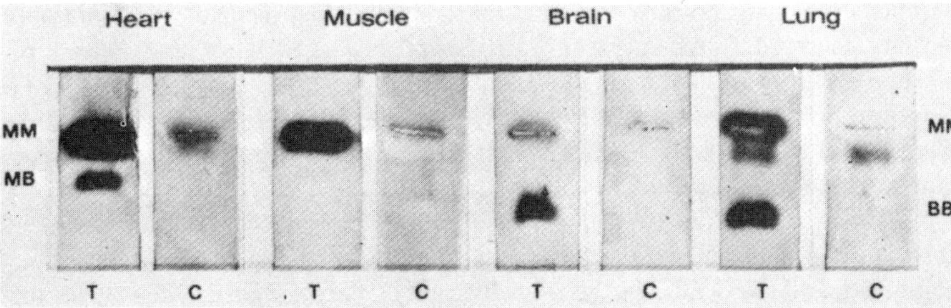

Figure 8.3. The creatine kinase isoenzymes MM, MB, and BB in human myocardium, skeletal muscle, brain, and lung homogenates. C = control slide; T = test slide. (Reproduced from A. Konttinen and H. Somer, *Amer. J. Cardiol.*, 1972, **29**, 817, by permission of Technical Publishing Co. and the authors.)

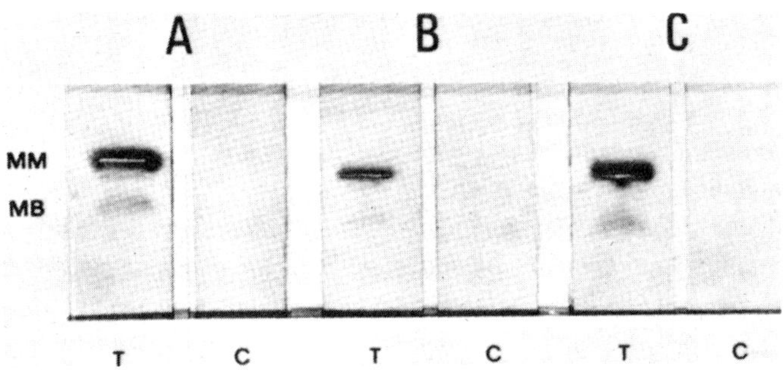

Figure 8.4. Serum creatine kinase isoenzymes in three patients with acute myocardial infarction. (Reproduced from A. Konttinen and H. Somer, *Amer. J. Cardiol.*, 1972, **29**, 817, by permission of Technical Publishing Co. and the authors.)

Surgical operation

Trauma to muscle, whether accidental or associated with surgical operation, or indeed with myocardial infarction, will cause the release of muscle enzymes into the serum. Creatine kinase is the enzyme most frequently raised, increased activity being found after trivial trauma to muscle (Tammisto and Airaksinen, 1966; Marmar *et al.*, 1969) as well as after major surgical operations (Penneys and Wilkinson, 1970; Marmar *et al.*, 1969; Shirey *et al.*, 1970). Serum levels start to rise immediately after the operation, reach a peak at 24 hours and return to normal by the fifth post-operative day (Rosalki, 1976b).

In the investigation of infants for the pre-clinical diagnosis of Duchenne muscular dystrophy, a condition in which a raised serum activity of creatine kinase is found, determination of the enzyme should be avoided in the neonatal period, since trauma sustained during birth may cause temporary increases (Rosalki, 1976a).

Serum aldolase, lactate dehydrogenase, transaminase, and other enzyme activities may also be raised after surgical operation. Aspartate transaminase activity increases after most surgical operations (Lawrence and Schulkins, 1956; Ticktin *et al.*, 1956; Nickell and Allbritten, 1957; Craver *et al.*, 1957; Candura and Minardi, 1957; Person and Judge, 1958); the greatest increases were found to occur after heart operations, especially cardiovascular surgery with extracorporeal circulation (Snyder *et al.*, 1958; Baer and Blount, 1960; Quinn *et al.*, 1960; Werle *et al.*, 1961; Pyörälä *et al.*, 1963). As to the reasons for the increase after cardiac surgery, a number of divergent views have been expressed, and the conflicting results obtained by various workers led Welbourn and her collaborators (1966) to re-examine the problem. They found increases in the serum activity of lactate dehydrogenase, α-hydroxybutyrate dehydrogenase, isocitrate dehydrogenase, and aspartate transaminase in patients after various types of heart operations with extracorporeal circulation; the length of the perfusion was a major factor affecting the rise in post-operative enzyme activities. Hepatocellular damage, the age of the patient, and the type of operation were not considered to be major factors in determining the extent of the increase in enzyme activity, which, in agreement with a concept previously advanced by Hauss and his coworkers (1958), was thought to reflect in some way a response of the whole organism to the perfusion.

The anaesthetic may contribute in some cases to the increased enzyme activities observed after operation. Increased creatine kinase activity is reported to correlate with the duration of anaesthesia and to be associated particularly with the administration of halothane or succinylcholine (Tammisto and Airaksinen, 1966; Innes and Strømme, 1973; Phornphutkul *et al.*, 1974).

LABORATORY INVESTIGATIONS OF PROTEINS AFTER TRAUMA

Most of the investigations of the effect of trauma on protein metabolism have been research projects, and in most cases there would seem to be little of immediate clinical value in evaluating a patient's serum proteins after trauma. However, some investigators have found sequential estimations of acute-phase proteins useful in monitoring the progress of patients with various inflammatory diseases and after surgical operation. A definite increase in the concentration of C-reactive protein and α_1-acid glycoprotein by the fourth or fifth post-operative day (by which time they should be on the downward trend) suggests that a process involving significant tissue damage or inflammation has supervened (Fischer and Gill, 1975). According to Fischer and Gill, such estimations are more useful than the erythrocyte sedimentation rate and white blood cell count.

Kohn (1960) found that the estimation of C-reactive protein may be useful in the management of patients with burns: delayed healing is usually associated with persistence of increased concentrations, and additional complications manifest themselves by secondary peaks. Crockson and his coworkers (1966) also found, in a small series of patients, that a second rise in the concentration

Table 8.3. Sources of error in the interpretation of acute-phase protein concentrations. (After C. L. Fischer and C. W. Gill, *Serum Protein Abnormalities: Diagnostic and Clinical Aspects* (Eds. S. E. Ritzmann and J. C. Daniels), Little, Brown, Boston, 1975, by permission of Little, Brown and Co. and the authors.)

Protein	Cause	Serum concentration
α_1-Acid glycoprotein	Pregnancy (3rd trimester)	Increased
α_1-Antitrypsin	Genetic	Decreased
Caeruloplasmin	Oestrogen	Increased
	Pregnancy	Increased
	Contraceptive pill	Increased
	Severe liver disease	Decreased
	Wilson's disease	Decreased
Haptoglobin	Intravascular haemolysis	Decreased
	Severe liver disease	Decreased
Fibrinogen	Consumptive coagulo-pathies	Decreased
	Severe liver disease	Decreased

of C-reactive protein during the post-operative period was associated with complications.

The concentration of plasma fibrinogen was found by Eastham and Morgan (1963) to be a useful guide in the management of acute myocardial infarction, a raised concentration being a reliable indication of recent infarction; a subsequent return to normal corresponds with clinical recovery. In a small series of patients with thrombophlebitis the plasma fibrinogen concentration remained within normal limits, unless there were complications; and since patients with pulmonary embolism tended to have raised concentrations, it was suggested that measurement of plasma fibrinogen during the treatment of thrombophlebitis might be helpful in detecting pulmonary embolism (Eastham and Morgan, 1963).

In interpreting serum concentrations of acute-phase proteins in patients after trauma it is important to bear in mind the effect of drugs and various conditions (Table 8.3). Conversely, any assessment of the result of either an electrophoretic analysis or a specific protein estimation for diagnostic purposes should take account of the possible effects of recent trauma. For example, a patient who initially had a low serum concentration of haptoglobin caused by a haemolytic state might, after trauma, be found to have a haptoglobin concentration within the normal range.

REFERENCES

Agostoni, A., C. Vergani, R. Stabilini, B. Marasini, R. Arcidiacono, A. Sbaffi, and P. C. Binaghi (1970), *Amer. Heart J.*, **80**, 313.

Anderson, A. B.,and E. Semeonoff (1945), in *Studies of Burns and Scalds*, M. R. C. Special Report Series, No. 249.
Arturson, G., C. F. Högman, S. G. O. Johansson, and J. Killander (1969), *Lancet*, **i**, 546.
Atencio, A. C., P. Y. Chao, A. Y. Chen, and E. B. Reeve (1969), *Amer. J. Physiol.*, **216**, 773.
Atencio, A. C., and L. Lorand (1970), *Amer. J. Physiol.*, **219**, 1161.
Bachmann, G. W., M. E. Weiss, and W. Rapp (1968), *Schweiz. med. Wschr.*, **98**, 1825.
Baer, H., and S. G. Blount, Jr. (1960), *Amer. Heart J.*, **60**, 867.
Balegno, H. F., and O. W. Neuhaus (1970), *Life Sci.*, **9**, 1039.
Baliga, B. S., A. W. Pronczuk, and H. N. Munro (1968), *J. Molec. Biol.*, **34**, 199.
Beaton, G. H., A. E. Selby, M. J. Veen, and A. M. Wright (1961), *J. Biol. Chem.*, **236**, 2005.
Belfrage, S. (1963), *Acta Med. Scand.*, Suppl. 395.
Birke, G., S.-O. Liljedahl, and R. Norberg (1969), *Scand. J. Plast. Reconstr. Surg.*, **3**, 39.
Björnesjö, K. B. (1958), *Abstracts of Communications, 4th International Congress of Biochemistry, Vienna*, p. 166.
Björnesjö, K. B., I. Werner, and L. Odin (1959), *Scand. J. Clin. Lab. Invest.*, **11**, 238.
Boyde, T. R. C. (1968), *Enzym. Biol. Clin.*, **9**, 385.
Browne, J. S. L. (1942), in *Report on Bone and Wound Healing*, Second Meeting, Josiah Macey, Jr., Foundation, p. 50.
Browne, J. S. L., V. Schenker, and J. A. F. Stevenson (1944), *J. Clin. Invest.*, **23**, 932.
Calloway, D. H., M. I. Grossman, J. Bowman, and W. K. Calhoun (1955), *Surgery*, **37**, 935.
Candura, F., and C. Minardi (1957), *Minerva chir.*, **12**, 1077.
Chakrabarti, R., E. D. Hocking, and G. R. Fearnley (1969), *J. Clin. Path.*, **22**, 659.
Chandler, A. M., and O. W. Neuhaus (1968), *Biochim. Biophys. Acta*, **166**, 186.
Chanutin, A., J. C. Hortenstine, W. S. Cole, and S. Ludewig (1938), *J. Biol. Chem.*, **123**, 247.
Cohnen, G. (1972), *Trauma*, **12**, 249.
Cope, O., I. Nathanson, G. M. Rourke, and H. Wilson (1943), *Ann. Surg.*, **117**, 937.
Craver, W. L., G. Johnson, Jr., and J. M. Beal (1957), *Surg. Forum*, **8**, 77.
Cristol, P., and A. Puech (1930), *Languedoc Méd.*, **13**, 434.
Crockson, R. A., C. J. Payne, A. P. Ratcliff, and J. F. Soothill (1966), *Clin. Chim. Acta*, **14**, 435.
Cuthbertson, D. P. (1930), *Biochem. J.*, **24**, 1244.
Cuthbertson, D. P., and S. L. Tompsett (1935), *Brit. J. Exp. Path.*, **16**, 471.
Darcy, D. A. (1964), *Brit. J. Exp. Path.*, **45**, 281.
Darcy, D. A. (1965), *Brit. J. Exp. Path.*, **46**, 155.
Davies, J. W. L. (1970), *J. Clin. Path.*, **23**, Suppl. 4, 56.
Deadrick, R. E., J. L. Morico, E. R. Lozano, F. Tausig, R. P. Hummel, and G. F. Lanchantin (1956), *Clin. Chem.*, **2**, 266.
de Ritis, F., M. Coltorti, and G. Giusti (1955), *Minerva Med.*, **46**, 1207.
Dixon, S. H., Jr., L. E. Limbird, C. E. Roe, G. S. Wagner, H. N. Oldham, Jr., and D.C. Sabiston, Jr. (1973), *Circulation*, **47–48**, Suppl. III, 137.
Dreyfus, J. C., G. Schapira, J. Resnais, and L. Scebat (1960), *Rev. franç. Etud. clin. biol.*, **5**, 386.
Driscoll, A. C., J. H. Hobika, B. E. Etsten, and S. Proger (1961), *New Engl. J. Med.*, **264**, 633.
Duval, P., J.-C. Roux, and R. Goiffon (1934), *Presse med.*, **42**, 1785.
Eastham, R. D., and E. H. Morgan (1963), *Lancet*, **ii**, 1196.
Eddington, C. L., H. F. Upchurch, and R. F. Kampschmidt (1971), *Proc. Soc. Exp. Biol. Med.*, **136**, 159.
Evans, G. W., and R. E. Wiederanders (1967), *Nature*, **215**, 766.
Fiessinger, N. (1934), *Presse méd.*, **42**, 1787.
Fine, J. M., G. A. Boffa, and F. Zajdela (1962), *Compt. rend. Acad. Sci.*, **255**, 1045.

Fischer, C. L., and C. W. Gill (1975), in *Serum Protein Abnormalities: Diagnostic and Clinical Aspects* (Eds. S. E. Ritzmann and J. C. Daniels), Little, Brown, Boston, p. 331.
Fleck, A., and H. N. Munro (1963), *Metabolism*, **12**, 783.
Fleisher, G. A., C. S. Potter, and K. G. Wakim (1960), *Proc. Soc. Exp. Biol. Med.*, **103**, 229.
Fuller, J. M., and J. W. Keyser (1975), *Clin. Chem.*, **21**, 667.
Gillette, R. W., A. R. Mansberger, Jr., J. H. Oppenheimer, B. F. Caldwell, and E. G. Neff (1958), *Surgery*, **43**, 747.
Goiffon, R., and J. Spaey (1934a), *Bull. Soc. Chim. biol.*, **16**, 1675.
Goiffon, R., and J. Spaey (1934b), *Compt. rend. Soc. Biol.*, **115**, 711.
Gordon, A. H. (1970), in *Plasma Protein Metabolism: Regulation of Synthesis, Distribution and Degradation*, (Eds. M. A. Rothschild and T. Waldmann), Academic Press, New York and London, p. 351.
Gordon, A. H., and D. A. Darcy (1967), *Brit. J. Exp. Path.*, **48**, 81.
Gordon, A. H., and A. Koj (1968), *Brit. J. Exp. Path.*, **49**, 436.
Hahn, A. (1921), *Biochem. Z.*, **121**, 262.
Hauss, W., U. Gerlach, and E. Schurmeyer (1958), *Deut. med. Woch.*, **83**, 1310.
Heim, W. G., and S. R. Ellenson (1967), *Nature*, **213**, 1260.
Heim, W. G., and M. J. Kerrigan (1963), *Nature*, **199**, 1100.
Heppleston, A. G., and J. W. Keyser (1957), *Brit. J. Exp. Path.*, **38**, 111.
Heppleston, A. G., and J. W. Keyser (1959), *Brit. J. Exp. Path.*, **40**, 263.
Hoch-Ligetti, E., K. Irvine, and E. P. Sprinkle (1953), *Proc. Soc. Exp. Biol. Med.*, **84**, 707.
Innes, R. K. R., and J. H. Strømme (1973), *Brit. J. Anaesth.*, **45**, 185.
Jakab, L., J. Fehér, I. Siró, E. Szondy, and J. Székely (1974), *Acta. Med. Acad. Sci. Hung.*, **31**, 69.
Jakab, L., J. Fehér, I. Siró, E. Szondy, and J. Székely (1976), *Amer. Heart J.*, **92**, 812.
Jayle, M.-F., P. Choubrac, M. Drosdowsky, and P. Jacot (1968), *Presse méd.*, **76**, 1805.
Jefferson, L. S., and A. Korner (1969), *Biochem. J.*, **111**, 703.
Johansson, B. G., C.-O. Kindmark, E. Y. Trell, and F. A. Wollheim (1972), *Scand. J. Clin. Lab. Invest.*, **29**, Suppl. 124, 117.
John, D. W., and L. L. Miller (1969), *J. Biol. Chem.*, **244**, 6134.
Karl, M., and G. Reißmann (1967), *Z. inn. Med.*, **22**, 720.
Keyser, J. W. (1948), *Ann. Surg.*, **127**, 605.
Keyser, J. W. (1949), *Nature*, **164**, 889.
Keyser, J. W. (1950), *J. Clin. Path.*, **3**, 106.
Keyser, J. W. (1952), *J. Clin. Path.*, **5**, 194.
Keyser, J. W. (1959), *J. Endocrin.*, **18**, 197.
Keyser, J. W. (1960), *J. Oklahoma State Med. Assoc.*, **53**, 769.
Keyser, J. W., and B. T. Stephens (1964), *Clin. Chem.*, **10**, 736.
Keyser, J. W., S. Shuster, and B. T. Stephens (1963), *Proc. Assoc. Clin. Biochemists*, **2**, 172.
Kohn, J. (1960), in *Protides of the Biological Fluids: Proceedings of 8th Colloquium, Bruges, 1960* (Ed. H. Peeters), Elsevier, Amsterdam, p. 315.
Koj, A. (1970), in *Energy Metabolism in Trauma* (Eds. R. Porter and J. Knight), Churchill, London, p. 79.
Koj, A. (1973), in *Hormones, Metabolism and Stress: Recent Progress and Perspectives* (Proceedings of International Symposium, Smolenice, 1972), Publishing House of the Slovak Academy of Sciences, Bratislava, p. 201.
Koj, A. (1974), in *Structure and Function of Plasma Proteins*, (Ed. A. C. Allison), Vol. 1, Plenum Press, London, p. 73.
Koj, A., and A. C. Allison (1969), *Folia biol., Kraków*, **17**, 37. (Cited by Koj, 1970.)
Koj, A., and A. Dubin (1974), *Acta Biochim. Polonica*, **21**, 159.
Konttinen, A., and H. Somer (1972), *Amer. J. Cardiol.*, **29**, 817.
Konttinen, A., and H. Somer (1973), *Brit. Med. J.*, **i**, 386.
Krauss, S. (1963), *Proc. Soc. Exp. Biol. Med.*, **112**, 552.

Lanchantin, G. F., and R. E. Deadrick (1958), *J. Clin. Invest.*, **37**, 1736.
Lane, R. S. (1948), *Brit. J. Haematol.*, **15**, 355.
Laurell, C.-B. (1947), *Acta Physiol. Scand.*, **14**, Suppl. 46.
Lawford, D. J. (1961), *Biochem. Pharmacol.*, **7**, 109.
Lawrence, S. H., and T. H. Schulkins (1956), *Anesthesiology*, **17**, 531.
Linko, E., E. Waris, and M. A. Alkoski (1956), *Acta. Med. Scand.*, **153**, 389.
Liu, A. Y., and O. W. Neuhaus (1968), *Biochim. Biophys. Acta*, **166**, 195.
Lucido, J. (1940), *Ann. Surg.*, **111**, 640.
Lundh, B. (1965), *Acta Univ. Lund*, Section II, No. 24, 1.
Majumdar, C., K. Tsukada, and I. Lieberman (1967), *J. Biol. Chem.*, **242**, 700.
Marmar, J. L., L. Karafin, and A. R. Kendell (1969), *J. Urol.*, **102**, 84.
Mauney, F. M., P. A. Ebert, and D. C. Sabiston (1970), *Ann. Surg.*, **172**, 497.
Mehl, J. W., J. Humphrey, and R. J. Winzler (1949a), *Proc. Soc. Exp. Biol. Med.*, **72**, 106.
Mehl, J. W., F. Golden, and R. J. Winzler (1949b), *Proc. Soc. Exp. Biol. Med.*, **72**, 110.
Moore, F. D., and M. R. Ball (1952), *The Metabolic Response to Injury*, Thomas, Springfield, Illinois.
Moore, F. D., J. L. Langohr, M. Ingebretson, and O. Cope (1950), *Ann. Surg.*, **132**, 1.
Morgan, E. H., and C. J. Brackenridge (1962), *Quart. J. Exp. Physiol.*, **47**, 66.
Morgan, E. H., and W. Lynch (1963), *Quart. J. Exp. Physiol.*, **48**, 181.
Moss, D. W., and P. J. Butterworth (1974), *Enzymology and Medicine*, Pitman, London, p. 141.
Munro, H. N., and M. I. Chalmers (1945), *Brit. J. Exp. Path.*, **26**, 396.
Munro, H. N., and D. P. Cuthbertson (1943), *Biochem. J.*, **37**, xii.
Musil, J. (1961), *Clin. Chim. Acta*, **6**, 508.
Neuhaus, O. W., H. F. Balegno, and A. M. Chandler (1961), *Proc. Soc. Exp. Biol. Med.*, **107**, 960.
Neuhaus, O. W., H. F. Balegno, and A. M. Chandler (1966), *Amer. J. Physiol.*, **211**, 151.
Nickell, W. K., and F. F. Allbritten, Jr. (1957), *Surgery*, **42**, 240.
Pekarek, R. S., M. C. Powanda, and R. W. Wannemacher, Jr. (1972), *Proc. Soc. Exp. Biol. Med.*, **141**, 1029.
Pekarek, R., R. Wannemacher, M. Powanda, J. Abeles, D. Mosher, R. Dinterman, and W. Beisel (1974), *Life Sci.*, **14**, 1765.
Penneys, R., and J. H. Wilkinson (1970), *Surgery*, **67**, 302.
Person, D. A., and R. D. Judge (1958), *Arch. Surg.*, **77**, 892.
Peters, J. P. (1946), *Ann. N. Y. Acad. Sci.*, **47**, 327.
Phornphutkul, K. S., S. Anuras, R. S. Koff, L. B. Seef, D. L. Mahler, and H. J. Zimmerman (1974), *Clin. Chem.*, **20**, 340.
Prendergast, J. J., R. L. Fenichel, and B. M. Daly (1952), *Arch. Surg.*, **64**, 733.
Pryse-Davies, J., and J. H. Wilkinson (1958), *Lancet*, **i**, 1249.
Pyörälä, K., R. Gordin, A. Kontinnen, and L. Telivuo (1963), *Acta med. scand.*, **174**, 361.
Quinn, J. W., H. D. Sirak, E. H. Shabanah, and W. J. Frajola (1960), *Ann. Surg.*, **152**, 45.
Riou, G., R. Truhaut, and C. Paoletti (1962), *Rev. franç. Etud. clin. biol.*, **7**, 618.
Ritzmann, S. E., D. L. Larson, C. McClung, S. Abston, D. Falls, and A. S. Goldman (1969), *Lancet*, **i**, 1153.
Rosalki, S. B., (1976a), in *The Principles and Practice of Diagnostic Enzymology* (Ed. J. H. Wilkinson), Arnold, London, p. 266.
Rosalki, S. B. (1976b), in *The Principles and Practice of Diagnostic Enzymology* (Ed. J. H. Wilkinson), Arnold, London, p. 278.
Sarcione, E. J., M. Bohne, and S. Krauss (1965), *Fed. Proc.*, **24**, 230.
Schmidt, E., F. W. Schmidt, and P. Otto (1967a), *Clin. Chim. Acta*, **15**, 283.
Schmidt, E., F. W. Schmidt, and J. Möhr (1967b), *Clin. Chim. Acta*, **15**, 337.
Schumer, W., J. Molnar, J. N. Dowling, and R. Winzler (1967), *Amer. J. Physiol.*, **212**, 184.
Schwarz, G. (1963), *Das C-Reaktive Protein*, Steinkopf Verlag, Darmstadt.

Seibert, F. B., M. V. Seibert, A. J. Atno, and H. W. Campbell (1947), *J. Clin. Invest.*, **26**, 90.
Sevitt, S. (1957), *Burns: Pathology and Therapeutic Applications*, Butterworth, London.
Shetlar, M. R., and C. L. Shetlar (1955), *Proc. Soc. Exp. Biol. Med.*, **88**, 622.
Shetlar, M. R., R. S. Bryan, J. V. Foster, C. L. Shetlar, and M. R. Everett (1949), *Proc. Soc. Exp. Biol. Med.*, **72**, 294.
Shihabi, Z., H. F. Balegno, and O. W. Neuhaus (1970), *Biochem. Biophys. Res. Comm.*, **38**, 692.
Shirey, E. K., W. L. Proudfit, and F. M. Sones (1970), *Chest*, **57**, 122.
Skornik, O. A., M. B. Hoagland, L. B. Pfefferkorn, and E. A. Bishop (1967), *J. Biol. Chem.*, **242**, 131.
Smith, A. F. (1967), *Lancet*, **ii**, 178.
Smith, E. L., D. M. Brown, H. E. Weimer, and R. J. Winzler (1950), *J. Biol. Chem.*, **185**, 569.
Snyder, D. D., C. N. Barnard, R. L. Varco, and C. W. Lillehei (1958), *Surgery*, **44**, 1083.
Snyder, S., B. C. Durham, A. S. Iskandrian, E. L. Coodley, and J. W. Linhart (1975), *Amer. Heart J.*, **90**, 582.
Tammisto, T., and M. Airaksinen (1966), *Brit. J. Anaesth.*, **38**, 510.
Taylor, F. H. L., S. M. Levenson, C. S. Davidson, M. A. Adams, and H. MacDonald (1943), *Science*, **97**, 423.
Ticktin, H. E., B. H. Ostrow, and J. M. Evans (1956), *Clin. Res. Proc.*, **4**, 102.
Tsukada, K., T. Moriyama, O. Doi, and I. Lieberman (1968), *J. Biol. Chem.*, **243**, 1152.
Von der Decken, A. (1968), *Biochim. Biophys. Acta*, **166**, 487.
Wagner, G. S., C. R. Roe, L. E. Limbird, R. A. Rosati, and A. G. Wallace (1973), *Circulation*, **47**, 263.
Wannemacher, R. W., Jr. (1972), *Biochem. J.*, **129**, 5P.
Wannemacher, R. W., Jr., W. K. Cooper, and K. Muramatsu (1970), *Proc. Soc. Exp. Biol. Med.*, **135**, 180.
Wannemacher, R. W., Jr., C. F. Wannemacher, and M. B. Yatvin (1971), *Biochem. J.*, **124**, 385.
Wannemacher, R. W., Jr., R. S. Pekarek, and W. R. Beisel (1972), *Proc. Soc. Exp. Biol. Med.*, **139**, 128.
Wannemacher, R. W., Jr., R. S. Pekarek, W. L. Thompson, R. T. Curnow, F. A. Beall, T. V. Zenser, F. R. DeRubertis, and W. R. Beisel (1975), *Endocrinology*, **96**, 651.
Weimer, H. E., and D. C. Benjamin (1965), *Amer. J. Physiol.*, **209**, 736.
Weimer, H. E., and V. Coggshall (1967), *Can. J. Physiol. Pharmac.*, **45**, 767.
Weimer, H. E., and C. Humelbaugh (1967), *Can. J. Physiol. Pharmac.*, **45**, 241.
Weimer, H. E., and J. Redlich-Moshin (1953), *Proc. Soc. Exp. Biol. Med.*, **84**, 34.
Weimer, H. E., J. W. Mehl, and R. J. Winzler (1950), *J. Biol. Chem.*, **185**, 561.
Welbourn, N., D. G. Melrose, and D. W. Moss (1966), *J. Clin. Path.*, **19**, 220.
Werle, E., I. Trautschold, A. Gorriz, and R. Zill (1961), *Clin. Chim. Acta*, **6**, 99.
Werner, I., and L. Odin (1952), *Acta Soc. Med. Upsaliensis (Upsala Läkarefören. Förh.)*, **57**, 230.
Werner, M. (1969), *Clin. Chim. Acta*, **25**, 299.
Werner, M., and G. Cohnen (1969), *Clin. Sci.*, **36**, 173.
Wilkinson, J. H. (1976), *The Principles and Practice of Diagnostic Enzymology*, Arnold, London.
Winzler, R. J., and I. M. Smyth (1948), *J. Clin. Invest.*, **27**, 617.
Winzler, R. J., A. W. Devor, J. W. Mehl, and I. M. Smyth (1948), *J. Clin. Invest.*, **27**, 609.
Wolff, E. (1921), *Ann. Méd.*, **10**, 185.
Yamada, T. (1959), *Proc. Soc. Exp. Biol. Med.*, **101**, 566.

CHAPTER 9

Cancer

Changes in plasma protein metabolism in the neoplastic immunoglobulinopathies form the subject of Chapter 2 and will not be discussed further here. Before dealing with the protein changes seen in other types of cancer it will be convenient to review briefly the overall protein and nitrogen metabolism of cancer patients in general.

PROTEIN METABOLISM IN CANCER

Metabolic data have shown that in patients with malignant disease associated with cachexia there is a negative nitrogen balance, and that a protein intake adequate for the maintenance of nitrogen balance in normal, healthy persons may be inadequate in patients with cancer (Mueller, 1889; Wallersteiner, 1914; Bolker, 1953). A possible explanation may be found in the 'nitrogen trap' theory (Mider, 1951). Experiments with rats bearing the Walker 256 carcinoma suggested that during the growth of the tumour there is a shift of nitrogen from normal to neoplastic tissue, the normal tissues providing nitrogenous 'building blocks' for the tumour, which acts as a 'trap' for nitrogen. That this concept is applicable also to cancer in human beings is suggested by the work of Waterhouse and his coworkers (1951), from which it appears that patients in whom a malignant neoplasm is growing rapidly may store nitrogen while the body is wasting and the patient is losing weight.

The question whether the ingestion of large amounts of protein can both satisfy the demands of the tumour and prevent this loss of weight was investigated by Terepka and Waterhouse (1956). After a period on control diets, patients were given some 1000–1500 extra calories and 4–7 g of extra protein each day. Although this was found to result in increases in the weight of the patients, and in nitrogen balance, it appeared that the positive balance approached an equilibrium value and cancer patients did not retain nitrogen to the same extent as individuals with 'simple' starvation. It was suggested that, in the presence of an abundant supply of protein and calories, full repletion of host tissues in the cancer patient cannot occur, 'because of some restraining influence exerted by the growing tumour on the host', the gain in weight appearing to be largely the result of accumulation of intracellular fluid.

That the apparent requirement for a higher protein and caloric intake to maintain the cancer patient in nitrogen balance is not specific for cancer but holds for any grave disease is suggested by the work of Pareira and his coworkers

(1955). These workers compared a group of cancer patients, who were cachetic and who had lost from 8 to nearly 60 per cent of their body weight, with a group of cachetic patients without cancer. Both groups of patients were tube-fed a calorically adequate diet containing 33.6 g of protein nitrogen per day, and the range of weight gains and positive nitrogen balances, as well as the clinical improvement, were found to be essentially the same in both groups. (The only difference observed between the two groups was in the regeneration of serum albumin: all of the seven patients without cancer showed some degree of restoration in serum albumin concentration, whereas 5 of the 14 patients with cancer showed either no increase or a continued fall in serum albumin in spite of significant increases in haemoglobin concentration; the other cancer patients showed roughly the same gain in serum albumin as did the non-cancer patients.) It was concluded that there appeared to be no fundamental specific impairment of protein metabolism in patients with widespread cancer.

PLASMA PROTEINS IN CANCER

The earliest observations on plasma protein changes in cancer were made more than fifty years ago. However, the methods then in use were relatively crude and will not be further discussed here. More detailed analysis became available with the advent of electrophoresis.

Electrophoretic pattern of plasma proteins in cancer

A number of electrophoretic studies have been made of the plasma proteins in cancer of various types (Seibert *et al.*, 1947; Petermann *et al.*, 1948; Mider *et al.*, 1950; Ogryzlo *et al.*, 1960; and others). Although there was disagreement as to the presence of statistically significant increases in the concentration of β- and γ-globulins, most studies have demonstrated that cancer is associated with a decrease in the concentration of albumin and increases in the α-globulins. The magnitude of the changes depends on the progress and extent of the cancer, as is shown, for example, in the study of Mider and his colleagues (1950) (Table 9.1).

These changes do not appear to be specific for cancer or for any particular type of cancer, being found also in other conditions, such as advanced tuberculosis (Seibert *et al.*, 1947). In this respect they differ sharply from the protein patterns found in the paraproteinaemias (Chapter 2), which, though still not entirely specific, are nevertheless not found as frequently and in such a variety of disorders.

Elevations in the serum concentration of α-globulins are generally greater when there are widespread metastases, but this is not invariably the case. Thus in a study of patients with colorectal cancer (Cooper *et al.*, 1975a) the concentration of α_2-globulins was found to be raised in 44 per cent of patients with metastases but in only 9 per cent of patients with primary and apparently localized tumours; the α_2-globulins, however, were raised in 88 per cent of

Table 9.1. Electrophoretic protein fractions (g/l) in plasma of normal individuals and cancer patients. (From data of G. B. Mider, E. L. Alling, and J. J. Morton, *Cancer*, 1950, **3**, 56, with permission.)

	No. of cases	Total protein	Albumin	α_1-Globulin	α_2-Globulin	β-Globulin	Fibrinogen	γ-Globulin
Normal adults		68.3 ± 0.7	40.4 ± 0.5	3.8 ± 0.1	6.6 ± 0.2	7.6 ± 0.2	3.1 ± 0.2	6.6 ± 0.3
Cancer, all cases (varying types and severity)	222	66.0 ± 0.4	29.4 ± 0.4	5.3 ± 0.1	9.0 ± 0.1	8.9 ± 0.1	5.8 ± 0.1	7.5 ± 0.2
Late cancer	35	65.5 ± 1.4	23.8 ± 0.5	6.5 ± 0.3	10.5 ± 0.5	9.9 ± 0.5	8.2 ± 0.9	8.2 ± 0.4

patients with primary tumours and in 75 per cent of those with hepatic metastases.

A fall in the concentration of α_2-globulins in response to therapy has been reported in prostatic cancer (Ablin, 1972) and in gastric cancer (Suga and Tamura, 1972).

Electrophoretic studies such as these, while they may possibly be of use in monitoring therapy and in prognosis, suffer from the disadvantage that they are concerned with groups of proteins which may vary independently within each group; in this way, significant changes in the concentrations of individual proteins may be obscured.

Plasma glycoproteins in cancer

Lustig and Langer in 1931 noted that the concentration of 'protein sugar' associated with the serum proteins was increased in patients with cancer, and similar findings were subsequently reported by Shetlar and his colleagues (1949), who observed increases in other diseases also, such as arthritis, ulcerative colitis, nephritis, and most infections.

One fraction in particular—the *seromucoid* fraction discussed in Chapter 3—has been much studied in relation to its possible value in diagnosis and prognosis. Some of the most striking increases in plasma seromucoid concentration are found in many types of cancer (Winzler and Smyth, 1948). In a series of 114 cases studied by Lockey and her colleagues (1956), the highest values were recorded in patients with widely disseminated cancer; results were particularly striking in the lymphomata, while in malignant disease confined to bone very little elevation was found; and other types of cancer occupied an intermediate position. However, comparable increases are found also in many other conditions (see Table 9.2); and this, together with the fact that normal seromucoid concentrations are found in some patients with cancer, especially when the disease is not far advanced, has led to the estimation's being regarded as of little practical value for detecting cancer (Winzler and Smyth, 1948; Henry *et al.*, 1951; Rhees *et al.*, 1954). This view was disputed by Cameron and his coworkers (1961), who pointed out that most non-malignant conditions associated with a high concentration of plasma seromucoid are easily recognized and do not commonly enter into the diagnosis of cancer; consequently the test may often provide considerable diagnostic and prognostic information. In series of 206 patients in whom malignancy was established, either histologically or at operation, or on the basis of clinical and radiological evidence, the majority (about 90%) had raised seromucoid concentrations at the time of their first attendance at hospital; of those patients with normal concentrations, the majority had small tumours which had attracted attention at an early stage because of their superficial situation, and the diagnosis was apparent on clinical grounds. Normal concentrations are commonly found, for example, in patients with cancer of the breast (cf. Shetlar *et al.*, 1949). There remained another group of patients in whom the test failed to detect cancer: these patients either had tumours of border-line malignancy, with little or no invasiveness, or else had small early tumours of internal organs. In such cases, if other investigations proved unhelpful, repeated estimations of seromucoid at intervals were recommended (Cameron *et al.*, 1961).

Occasionally even patients with advanced cancer may show no rise in seromucoid concentration. This was so with two patients in the terminal stages of gastric cancer, and Cameron and his co-authors suggest that the failure of the seromucoid concentration to increase in these two cases may be attributed to the presence of extensive hepatic metastases. This explanation should be accepted with reserve: in published series (Greenspan *et al.*, 1952; Greenspan and Dreiling, 1953: Greenspan, 1954: Keyser *et al.*, 1962) the great majority of patients with hepatic metastases had raised concentrations of seromucoid, only a few falling within the normal range. Indeed, some of the highest values found were in this group of patients. Nevertheless, it may well be that a certain minimal amount of normal liver tissue is required to produce increased concentrations of seromucoid.

Seromucoid estimations can also be used to assess response to treatment, and in prognosis. Thus Cameron and his colleagues found that successful treatment by radiotherapy, or with hormones or cytotoxic agents, is associated with a return of seromucoid concentrations to normal; and in patients treated surgically a sustained return of seromucoid concentrations to normal is an indication of adequate resection and a favourable prognosis (Cameron *et al.*, 1961).

These observations are in agreement with the writer's earlier finding (Keyser, 1954) that treatment of Hodgkin's disease and similar conditions, when it produces clinical improvement, is generally associated with a fall in the elevated seromucoid towards normal concentrations; a rise in seromucoid concentration may precede clinical relapse by several months (Figure 9.1). In such patients similar fluctuations generally occur in the total serum glycoproteins as measured by serum total protein-bound hexose.

Harshman and his colleagues (1967) found that after surgical operation for the removal of tumours a high seromucoid concentration was associated with incomplete removal or with recurrence of the tumour, whereas a low concentration was correlated with remission, either transient or prolonged. Seromucoid concentrations correlated more closely with tumour recurrence than did the serum activities of the enzymes phosphohexose isomerase, lactate dehydrogenase, and aspartate transaminase (glutamate-oxaloacetate transaminase). In a more recent publication the same group have reaffirmed, with reservations, the usefulness of serial seromucoid determinations as a prognostic aid in patients with cancer (Harshman *et al.*, 1974).

In interpreting the significance of a raised concentration of seromucoid it is particularly important to bear in mind the influence of infection (see Table 9.2).

The principal constituent of the seromucoid fraction is α_1*-acid glycoprotein*, and our own observations suggest that estimation of this protein may be of value in assessing prognosis and in monitoring progress in patients with breast cancer (Roberts *et al.*, 1975).

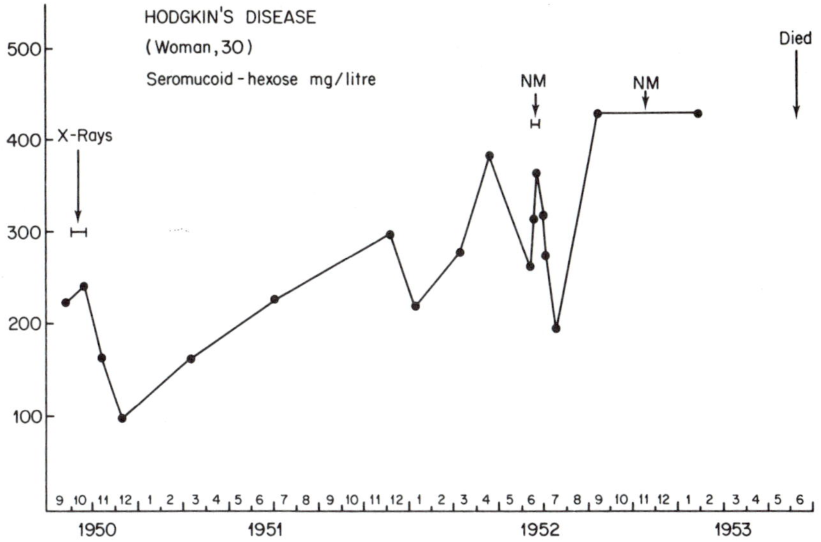

Figure 9.1. Seromucoid concentrations in a patient with Hodgkin's disease. Treatment that produced clinical improvement was associated with a fall towards normal concentrations; a rise preceded clinical relapse by several months. (From data of J. W. Keyser, *Brit. J. Cancer*, 1954, **8**, 238.)

Macbeth and Bekesi (1962b) measured the hexose, hexosamine, *N*-acetylneuraminic acid and fucose of the *non*-seromucoid portion of the serum proteins in a number of diseases, including carcinoma. Patients with clinically localized carcinoma of the breast were found to have concentrations within the normal range, but in metastatic breast carcinoma there were substantial elevations. Similar findings were reported by Almquist and Lausing (1957), and by Shetlar and his colleagues (1949) in respect of total protein-bound hexose.

Other workers (Rosato *et al.*, 1971; Barlow and Dillard, 1972; Evans *et al.*, 1974) have measured serum protein-bound fucose in patients with various types of cancer. Raised fucose concentrations appear to be indicative of disseminated disease. Successful therapy is associated with a fall to normal concentrations.

Table 9.2. Some conditions in which raised blood seromucoid concentrations are commonly found. (Reproduced, by permission of The Postgraduate Medical Journal, from J. W. Keyser, *Postgrad. Med. J.*, 1964, **40**, 184.)

Cancer	Winzler and Smyth, 1948
Rheumatoid arthritis	Shetlar *et al.*, 1953
Rheumatic fever	Kelley *et al.*, 1950, 1953
Pulmonary tuberculosis	Turner *et al.*, 1953
Pneumonia	Winzler and Smyth, 1948
Acute infections	Greenspan, 1955
Trauma (burns, fractures)	Keyser, 1952
Myocardial infarction	Simkin *et al.*, 1949

As with electrophoretic analysis, measurement of protein-bound carbohydrate involves a mixture of proteins. Possibly the sequential measurement of the individual fucose-rich proteins may offer a more useful method of monitoring the extent of the tumour and response to therapy.

The use of specific antisera, and also polyvalent antisera in quantitative immunoelectrophoretic methods such as are described in the Appendices, has allowed the individual proteins to be studied. In general, the changes in cancer are similar to those found in other conditions associated with increases in the concentration of 'acute-phase reactants' (see Chapter 8).

The use of α_1-acid glycoprotein assays in breast cancer has been mentioned above. Measurement of another specific protein, *haptoglobin*, has been found of value in following the course of ovarian carcinoma, and its response to treatment (Mueller *et al.*, 1971).

Among several other specific proteins that have been measured for purposes of cancer diagnosis and monitoring, the *pregnancy-associated α_2-macroglobulin** is of particular interest. This protein occurs in the serum of pregnant women (Stimson, 1972) and has been reported to occur in raised concentrations in patients with mammary, bronchial, intestinal and genitourinary carcinomas, lymphomas, and sarcomas (Stimson, 1975b). Measurement of the plasma concentration of pregnancy-associated macroglobulin appears to be of value in monitoring the progress of patients with cancer and their response to therapy (Stimson, 1975a, b).

Some investigators have found only a small change, or none in the plasma concentration of pregnancy-associated macroglobulin after surgical operation (Horne *et al.*, 1975; Anderson *et al.*, 1976); others have found substantial increases in most cases (Keyser and Ward, 1977).

Another pregnancy-specific glycoprotein, the *pregnancy-specific β_1-glycoprotein* ('SP'$_1$, Chapter 11) has been found in the serum of patients with choriocarcinoma (Tatarinov *et al.*, 1976; Seppälä *et al.*, 1978) and in breast-carcinoma tissue (Horne *et al.*, 1976). Raised serum concentrations of SP_1 are found in a proportion of patients with various other types of carcinoma (Yoshioka *et al.*, 1977; Searle *et al.*, 1978), and in some 13 per cent of healthy subjects (Searle *et al.*, 1978).

Protein 'profile' in cancer

Measurement of 15 serum proteins in two small groups of patients, one with a variety of malignancies at various stages and the other with miscellaneous non-malignant chronic diseases, showed that the mean concentrations of seven proteins (transferrin, α_2-macroglobulin, Gc-globulin, IgA, IgD, IgG, IgM) were not significantly different, in either group, from those for a group of normal

*Variously designated as pregnancy-zone protein, pregnancy-associated α_2-glycoprotein, pregnancy-associated globulin, α_2-pregnoglobulin, α_2 A. P. glycoprotein, pregnancy-associated α_2-macroglobulin, Schwangerschaftsprotein$_3$ (S.P.$_3$), Xh and Pa 1 (see Berne *et al.* (1975), who proposed the standard name pregnancy-associated α_2-glycoprotein).

controls; three (α_1-acid glycoprotein, caeruloplasmin, α_1-antitrypsin) were raised in both the cancer and the non-cancer chronically ill group; two (haptoglobin, haemopexin) were raised in the cancer patients only; and three (α_2 HS-glycoprotein, β_2-glycoprotein I, prealbumin) were decreased in the cancer group and unchanged in the non-cancer chronically ill group (Snyder and Ashwell, 1971). Further studies of this kind on more homogeneous groups of patients may well prove valuable.

TUMOUR-ASSOCIATED PROTEINS AND PEPTIDES

Nearly fifty years ago Hirszfeld and his collaborators showed that antisera obtained by immunizing rabbits with extracts prepared from embryos reacted with tumour extracts more strongly than with extracts of normal tissues (Hirszfeld *et al.*, 1932). This reappearance of embryo-specific materials in tumours was noted also by Stonehill and Bendich (1970), who suggested that it might represent a universal oncological phenomenon, which they called 'retrogenic expression'; this is manifested by the acquisition of properties abnormal for the adult cell, such as the appearance of embryonal gene products and unrestrained growth.

During the past fifteen years or so it has become increasingly recognized that tumours may secrete a variety of peptides or proteins that are not produced in detectable amounts by the corresponding normal adult tissues. Some of these—*the oncofetal antigens*—are found in fetal tissues and occur in the adult in grossly increased amounts in the presence of certain types of tumour; the rôle of these substances in the diagnosis and clinical management of human neoplasms was reviewed by Laurence and Neville (1972) and more recently by Neville and Cooper (1976). Others—*the ectopic hormones*—are secreted by some non-endocrine tumours: examples are the adrenocorticotrophic and parathyroid hormones, normally secreted by endocrine glands, and placental hormones such as human placental lactogen and chorionic gonadotrophin. To date, the ectopic hormones form the best characterized subgroup of tumour-associated proteins and peptides; their biosynthesis has recently been reviewed by Rees (1975), and clinical aspects have been reviewed by Lipsett (1968), Liddle *et al.* (1969), Anderson (1973), Ratcliffe and Rees (1974), Rees and Ratcliffe (1974), and Bodansky (1975).

Carcinoembryonic antigen (CEA)

Many attempts have been made to produce tumour-specific antibodies by immunizing animals with preparations of human tumours. Gold and his colleagues (Gold and Freedman, 1965a,b; Thomson *et al.*, 1969) developed the concept that human neoplasms produce specific antigens, and with the aid of a sensitive radioimmunoassay they were able to measure a specific protein, carcinoembryonic antigen (CEA), which they reported to be present in the plasma in raised concentrations in 35 of 36 patients with colorectal cancer

Table 9.3. Incidence of raised plasma concentrations of carcinoembryonic antigen in various neoplastic and non-neoplastic disorders.* (Reproduced from A. M. Neville and E. H. Cooper, *Ann. Clin. Biochem.*, 1976, **13**, 283, by permission of the Association of Clinical Biochemists and the authors.)

Disorder	Incidence (%) of raised plasma CEA levels
Neoplastic	
Carcinoma of	
Colon and rectum	73
Pancreas	92
Liver	67
Bronchus	72
Breast	52
Uterus	53**
Ovary	36**
Non-neoplastic	
Ulcerative colitis and Crohn's disease	21
Cirrhosis and alcoholic liver disease	42
Chronic bronchitis and emphysema	25
Fibroadenosis	7

*From data compiled by Laurence and Neville (1972) and of Barrelet and Mach (1975).**

and only 3 of 32 patients with cancer of other organs of the digestive system (Thomson *et al.*, 1969); patients with non-cancerous disease of digestive organs, or with cancer of non-enteric organs, had normal concentrations of CEA. Subsequent workers have failed to confirm the sharp discriminations between different groups of patients; the incidence of raised plasma CEA concentrations in various neoplastic and non-neoplastic disorders is shown in Table 9.3. In patients with tumours the plasma concentrations are predominantly related to the extent and site of spread of the tumour or to its volume (Laurence *et al.*, 1972; Barrelet and Mach, 1975; DiSaia *et al.*, 1975). Taken together with the high incidence of raised plasma concentrations found in non-neoplastic diseases, this fact limits severely the use of CEA assays in diagnosis and differential diagnosis. It is possible that sequential assays may be of greater diagnostic value, rising concentrations suggesting the presence of neoplasia and steady or falling concentrations suggesting an active or resolving inflammatory process. On the other hand, serial measurements of CEA in patients with ulcerative colitis showed that the test is unlikely to be of value as a screening test for the detection of carcinoma in this condition (Booth *et al.*, 1974); normal values were found in patients with pre-malignant histological changes or who developed a carcinoma during the period of study.

A recent application of CEA assays in distinguishing cancerous from congestive or inflammatory effusions appears promising. Although serum CEA concentrations were found to discriminate poorly between cancer and non-cancerous disease in patients with either ascites or pleural effusions, measurement of the CEA concentration in the *ascitic fluid* separated 60 per cent of the cancer patients from the non-malignant group (Booth *et al.*, 1977). Whenever the CEA concentration in the fluid was increased in association with cancer it was always several times as high as in the serum; in the cirrhotic fluids, on the other hand, CEA concentrations were always lower than in serum. A similar though less striking situation was seen in the group with pleural effusions. Combining CEA estimation with cytological examination of the fluid increased the diagnostic rate to 75 per cent.

At present the most important clinical rôle for plasma CEA assays is in surveillance to facilitate the earlier detection of recurrent or metastatic tumours known to be associated with the production and release of CEA (Neville and Cooper, 1976). A number of studies have indicated also a potential rôle of such assays in monitoring the efficacy of anti-tumour therapy (see Neville and Cooper, 1976), rising or stationary but raised concentrations suggesting the need for additional or modified therapy. Finally, plasma CEA assays may help in selecting patients who might benefit from adjuvant therapy; and monitoring the plasma concentrations of CEA after therapy might help in the detection of developing and progressive disease and the institution of further measures. For a discussion of all these aspects of CEA assays the reader is referred to the recent review by Neville and Cooper (1976).

'CCEA-2'

Glycoproteins referred to variously as non-specific cross-reacting antigen (NCA) (von Kleist *et al.*, 1972), 'normal glycoprotein' (NGP) (Mach and Pusztaszeri, 1972), CEX (Darcy *et al.*, 1973), colonic carcinoembryonic antigen 2 (CCEA-2) (Turberville *et al.*, 1973), and breast cancer glycoprotein (BCGP) (Kuo *et al.*, 1973) have been found both in normal and in neoplastic human colonic tissue. It is probable that these are all identical. Assay of this glycoprotein appears to offer no advantage over that of CEA in monitoring and diagnosing various types of tumour (Neville and Cooper, 1976). Since it shares common antigenic determinants with carcinoembryonic antigen, no antiserum to the latter should be considered as specific until it has been absorbed with normal tissues (Mach and Pusztaszeri, 1972). The glycoprotein is reported to be produced by circulating mononuclear cells (Martin, 1974).

α-Fetoprotein

In 1944 Pederson reported the discovery of a protein with α-globulin mobility in fetal calf serum. This protein, which he called *fetuin*, was absent from adult bovine serum.

Bergstrand and Czar in 1956 described an analogous protein, present in serum from human fetuses, which had an electrophoretic mobility between that of albumin and α_1-globulin. The concentration of this protein (α-fetoprotein) rises to a maximum of about 2.8 g/l at about 13 weeks, and then declines to less than 2 per cent of the maximum by 34 weeks' gestation (Gitlin and Boesman, 1966). After birth, the concentration in the infant's blood decreases rapidly, suggesting a sharp curtailment of α-fetoprotein synthesis either at birth or during the few weeks before birth.

The appearance of a fetal globulin in *adult* mammalian blood serum was first noted by Abelev (Abelev, 1963; Abelev *et al.*, 1963), who reported the presence of such a protein in the serum of adult mice and rats bearing a primary hepatoma.

Although—as judged by the screening tests in general use—α-fetoprotein is almost absent from the serum in the normal, healthy human adult, it was detected in the serum of 4 patients with primary carcinoma of the liver (Tatarinov, 1963, 1964, 1965). The value of a positive finding in confirming this diagnosis has since been amply confirmed (Uriel *et al.*, 1967; Abelev, 1968; Alpert *et al.*, 1968; Masopust *et al.*, 1968; Purves *et al.*, 1968; Sankalé *et al.*, 1968; Smith and Todd, 1968); however, it should be noted that positive results have also been found in patients with malignant neoplasms at other sites, as well as in certain non-cancerous diseases (see Chapter 3).

An important collaborative study was initiated in 1966 by the International Agency for Research on Cancer (Lyons, France) to evaluate and compare the specificity and sensitivity of the α-fetoprotein test in primary carcinoma of the liver. Serum samples were collected at centres in Kenya, Uganda, the Republic of Congo, Nigeria, Senegal, Singapore, and Jamaica, and tested by a modified Ouchterlony double-diffusion test at institutes in Villejuif (France) and Moscow and Astrakhan (USSR). Sera from a total of 813 patients were examined. Of 247 patients who were diagnosed on clinical and/or histological grounds as having primary carcinoma of the liver, 151 (61.1 per cent) had positive tests in all three test laboratories; 80 (32.4 per cent) gave negative tests; and in 16 (6.5 per cent) there was disagreement. Of the 566 control patients, with hepatic cirrhosis, hepatitis, carcinoma of the bile duct, other lesions of the liver, primary carcinoma at extrahepatic sites, and a variety of infectious, nutritional, and metabolic diseases, only 12 (2.1 per cent) were found to give a positive test in all three laboratories, and 11 (1.9 per cent) were subject to disagreement; the remaining 543 gave a negative test in all three laboratories (O'Conor *et al.*, 1970). Of the 12 patients with a positive test, two were found to have teratocarcinomas of the testicle. This is the only type of tumour, apart from primary carcinoma of the liver, with a substantial incidence of positive α-fetoprotein tests (Abelev *et al.*, 1967).

In the collaborative study referred to above, it was noted that, if only those cases with histological confirmation of primary carcinoma of the liver were considered, the number of positive cases increased to about 75 per cent. This is in agreement with the findings of Purves and his colleagues (1968), who reported a 75 per cent incidence of positive tests in this condition.

The highest frequency of raised serum α-fetoprotein concentration in primary hepatocarcinoma is apparently found in areas where the condition is endemic, such as South Africa (Purves *et al.*, 1970), Indonesia (Kresno *et al.*,

1970), and Senegal (Uriel *et al.*, 1967). On the other hand, in most parts of Europe (Abelev *et al.*, 1967; Foli *et al.*, 1969) and in the USA (Smith, 1970; Hull *et al.*, 1970) the proportion of positive tests is lower.

Application of the more sensitive method of radioimmunoassay has shown that sera from patients with primary hepatocarcinoma giving negative results by the double-diffusion method are positive by radioimmunoassay (Ruoslahti *et al.*, 1972). In 12 of 14 patients with primary carcinoma of the liver, α-fetoprotein concentrations ranged from 100 μg/l to 840 mg/l, and most were more than a thousand times the upper (non-pregnancy) normal level of 25 μg/l. In 14 of 17 patients with secondary carcinoma of the liver, the serum concentrations were less than 25 μg/l, and in the remaining three they ranged from 60 to 400 μg/l.

The presence of abnormally high concentrations of α-fetoprotein in the serum tends to be associated with poorly differentiated tumours; well-differentiated tumours (i.e. those most closely resembling normal liver tissue) tend to be associated less frequently with the production of α-fetoprotein (Glazer *et al.*, 1974).

In patients who undergo surgical operation for removal of the primary hepatocarcinoma the serum concentration of α-fetoprotein falls sharply, to rise again if growth of the tumour recurs. The determination of α-fetoprotein in the serum may be used to indicate growth of the tumour or its regression on treatment (McIntire *et al.*, 1972); raised concentrations after surgical operation or chemotherapy indicate incomplete removal of the tumour, or its spread, or the presence of metastases (Kohn and Weaver, 1974).

As mentioned in Chapter 3, rises in the serum concentration of α-fetoprotein sometimes occur in diseases other than primary carcinoma of the liver. Mention has been made above of the occurrence of high serum concentrations of α-fetoprotein in patients with testicular teratoma. Frequent sequential estimation of serum α-fetoprotein has been found of value in the diagnosis, prognosis, and management of the condition (Kohn, 1976; Kohn *et al.*, 1976). According to Newlands and his colleagues (1976), both α-fetoprotein and human chorionic gonadotrophin should be measured in patients with testicular tumours. Rises also occur in pregnancy (see Chapter 11).

The site of α-fetoprotein synthesis appears to be the parenchymal cells of the liver (Abelev, 1968). The localization of α-fetoprotein in hepatoma tissues has been studied by means of immunofluorescence staining (Engelhardt *et al.*, 1971; Nishioka *et al.*, 1972).

Function of α-fetoprotein

There have been several theories as to the rôle of α-fetoprotein in the mammalian fetus. It is possible that the protein protects the fetus from immunological attack from its mother. The evidence for this and other theories has recently been reviewed (*Lancet*, 1976).

Other oncofetal and tumour-associated antigens

Some of these are listed in Table 9.4. It is possible that further work will show that several of these, in addition to carcinoembryonic antigen and α-fetoprotein, may usefully be assayed for clinical purposes.

Table 9.4. Human tumour-associated macromolecules

	Present in	Raised serum values in
Carcinoembryonic antigen	Alimentary tract, liver and pancreas of fetuses between 2nd and 6th months, and in smaller amounts in normal adult tissues	Patients with various types of tumours (see text)
α-Fetoprotein	Fetal tissues and blood	Highest values in primary hepatoma and malignant teratoma. Elevated values in other conditions also (see text)
α_2H-Fetoprotein	Fetal liver, serum; serum up to end of second post-natal month (Buffe *et al.*, 1970)	Various tumours, including hepatoma, cholangiocarcinoma, and lymphoma, as well as certain non-neoplastic diseases (Rimbaut, 1973)
βS-Fetoprotein	Fetal serum and tissues (Takahashi *et al.*, 1967)	Hepatocarcinoma (10/23), cholangiocarcinoma (1/5), gastric carcinoma (2/7), leukaemia (1/4), lymphoma (1/3) (Wada *et al.*, 1971)
γ-Fetoprotein	Serum and some tissues of normal fetus	Detected in 75 per cent of a wide variety of benign and malignant tumours, and in serum of 23/210 patients with cancer (Edynak *et al.*, 1970, 1972)
Leukaemia-associated antigens (LAA)	Embryonic tissues and serum	Approx. one third of patients with various types of leukaemia (Harris *et al.*, 1971)
Fetal sulpho-glycoprotein antigen	Fetal alimentary canal (Häkkinen *et al.*, 1968)	Present in gastric juice of most patients with gastric carcinoma (Häkkinen and Viikari, 1969); and in gastric juice of some patients with peptic ulceration and some with non-epithelial neoplasms. See also Häkkinen (1974)
Pancreatic oncofetal antigen	Fetal pancreas	Carcinoma of pancreas (Banwo *et al.*, 1974)
'T-globulin'	Serum in cancer and in pregnancy (Tal and Halperin, 1970)	
Bronchial-tumour-associated antigens	Lung cancers (Yachi *et al.*, 1968; Sega *et al.*, 1974; McIntire and Sizaret, 1974; Bagshawe *et al.*, 1976)	

Calcitonin

Mention has been made above of the so-called *ectopic hormones* secreted by some non-endocrine tumours. One of these, *calcitonin*, is released by a variety of tumours, especially mammary and bronchial (Coombes *et al.*, 1974). *In vitro* tissue-culture studies have demonstrated its production and release by mammary and lung cancer cells (Ellison *et al.*, 1975).

Measurement of plasma concentrations of calcitonin in patients with breast diseases helps in the discrimination of local from disseminated disease; most patients with benign disease, or localized carcinoma, have plasma concentrations below 0.1 μg/l, whereas most patients with metastases have plasma concentrations above this value (Neville and Cooper, 1976). The finding of a raised plasma concentration in patients with apparently localized disease, or with no evidence of disease after operation, carries a poor prognosis.

Recent work has been concerned with the chemical nature of calcitonin produced by non-endocrine tumours. Preliminary data suggest that in breast carcinomas and some bronchial carcinomas the 'ectopic' calcitonin has a similar molecular size to calcitonin derived from human medullary carcinoma; however, material of a larger molecular weight, and also having biological and immunological activity, has been found in a lung carcinoma (Neville and Cooper, 1976).

Milk proteins

Two milk proteins, *casein* and *lactoferrin*, have been investigated in relation to the diagnosis and monitoring of cancer of the breast.

Casein, which consists of a mixture of phosphoproteins, can be estimated by a radioimmunoassay (Hendrick and Franchimont, 1974). In the majority of healthy men and non-pregnant women the protein is undetectable in the plasma, but in lactating women high concentrations are found. Hendrick and Franchimont reported that most patients with breast cancer had detectable concentrations before therapy; so did most patients after therapy, when there was local recurrence or the formation of distant metastases. According to the same authors, casein may be an 'ectopic' product of some bronchial and gastrointestinal carcinomas.

Lactoferrin is present in circulating neutrophil leucocytes, and precautions must be taken to prevent leakage if the serum concentration is to be measured (Rümke *et al.*, 1971). This iron-binding protein, which is also known as *lactotransferrin* and *lactosiderophilin*, migrates as an α_2-globulin on electrophoresis.

Reaction of various antigens with lymphocytes

In recent years interest has been focused on the interaction of various antigenic materials with peripheral lymphocytes from patients with cancer. The reaction *in vitro* of several structurally related basic proteins with lymphocytes isolated from patients with cancer has been studied, and forms the basis of a diagnostic test, the *macrophage electrophoretic mobility* (MEM) test, for all forms of cancer (Field and Caspary, 1970; Field *et al.*, 1973). According to the originators of the test, such sensitized lymphocytes react specifically with a common tumour antigen, releasing some material that slows the electrophoretic migration of normal lymphocytes; this slowing is taken as an indicator of such an interaction.

A modification of the MEM test having increased sensitivity was introduced by Pritchard and his colleagues in 1973 (Pritchard *et al.*, 1973a). Although they have concluded that the modified MEM test can be used with confidence for the exclusion of cancer, the false-negative rate being as low as 0.2 per cent (Pritchard *et al.*, 1976), an earlier report by Field (1973) indicated that of 30 patients with histologically proved localized prostatic carcinoma no less than 6 had a negative MEM test. Clearly, further work is necessary to evaluate the reliability, reproducibility, and clinical value of these tests.

According to Fish (1975), the MEM test is unlikely to have an immunological basis, a non-specific mechanism being involved.

Although the test is not specific for cancer (Field *et al.*, 1973; Pritchard *et al.*, 1973b), it apparently has the ability to detect primary malignant tumours while they are localized. Recent work by Pritchard and his colleagues, using their modification of the MEM test, is consistent with this assessment (Pritchard *et al.*, 1976). Other workers, however, have been unable to show that the test, either in its original form or modified, reliably discriminates between patients with benign disorders and patients with cancer (Lewkonia *et al.*, 1974; Crozier *et al.*, 1976).

Another test using lymphocytes is the '*structuredness of the cytoplasmic matrix*' (SCM) test (Cercek *et al.*, 1974). The term 'structuredness' refers to the physical state of organization of the cytoplasmic matrix at the molecular level (Cercek and Cercek, 1973), and the test is based upon measurement of physicochemical changes that occur in the cytoplasm of lymphocytes after interaction of the cell preparations with the common tumour antigen used in the MEM test. The tumour extract is allowed to react with lymphocyte preparations isolated from both normal subjects and patients with cancer, and fluorescein diacetate is then added to the cell suspensions. Enzymic hydrolysis of the fluorescein diacetate, which is non-fluorescent, occurs in the cytoplasm of the cells from both sources, with formation of the fluorescing molecule, fluorescein. The polarization of the emitted light ('P-value') from the cells is measured by means of a fluorescence spectrophotometer fitted with a polarization accessory. When the tumour extract is interacted with lymphocyte preparations from patients with cancer a decrease in the P-value is found, whereas no change occurs with lymphocyte preparations from healthy donors or from patients with non-malignant diseases. In the series of patients investigated by Cercek and his colleagues, exceptions to this clear-cut separation were found to be rare, but no doubt larger numbers of patients will have to be studied before the true value of the test can be assessed.

Finally, in the *histone agglutination test* (Sabolović *et al.*, 1975) blood lymphocytes are incubated with a histone fraction prepared from calf thymus glands: a positive reaction, shown by massive agglutination of the lymphocytes, was given by most of the patients studied; the test was positive in many non-malignant diseases as well as in many types of cancer.

ENZYME CHANGES IN CANCER

A comprehensive account of the enzyme changes that have been reported in cancer would fill many volumes, and only the briefest outline is possible here. It will be convenient to deal with the enzymes in three groups, *viz.* (a) those involved in glycolysis; (b) the phosphohydrolases; and (c) a miscellaneous group including amylase, leucine aminopeptidase, arylamidase, the aminotransferases, and a few others. For a fuller account of the subject the reader is referred to the reviews of Schwartz (1973, 1977) and Bodansky (1975).

Enzymes involved in glycolysis

The classic studies by Warburg and his colleagues (Warburg, 1930) showed that, in general, the rate of both aerobic and anaerobic glycolysis is greater in tumours than in normal tissues. Warburg's observations, which were made on both human and animal tumours, have been confirmed by subsequent investigators (e.g. Macbeth and Bekesi, 1962a), though exceptions to his generalization have been noted (Dickens and Weil-Malherbe, 1936, 1941). In general, Warburg's *in vitro* findings are consistent with a number of biochemical observations made *in vivo*; for example, the old observations that venous blood draining tumour-bearing organs contains considerably more lactic acid and less glucose than that from comparable tumour-free organs (Cori and Cori, 1925), and that arteriovenous differences for glucose and lactate are greater for tumour-containing tissues than for the corresponding normal tissues (Warburg *et al.*, 1926). A number of investigators have studied the activities of the individual glycolytic enzymes in normal and neoplastic tissues.

Aldolase

The finding of an increased glycolytic activity in tumours led Warburg and Christian to investigate glycolytic enzymes in the general circulation, and they showed that serum aldolase activity was increased in rats bearing the Jensen sarcoma (Warburg and Christian, 1943). These observations were confirmed by Sibley and Lehninger (1948); they extended the studies to human beings and found that about 20 per cent of a series of 102 patients with various types of cancer had increased serum aldolase activity. The serum activity of this enzyme is raised in patients with advanced carcinoma of the prostate and usually returns to normal after oestrogen therapy or orchidectomy (Baker and Govan, 1953). Later studies have extended these observations and have shown that serum aldolase activity is frequently raised in carcinoma of the gastrointestinal

Table 9.5. Distribution of types of aldolase in normal human tissues based on ratio of rate of hydrolysis of fructose 1,6-diphosphate to that of fructose 1-phosphate (FDP/F-1-P ratio)*. (Reproduced from O. Bodansky, *Biochemistry of Human Cancer*, Academic Press, New York, 1975, by permission of Academic Press, Inc.)

	Average values for FDP/F-1-P ratio		
Normal tissue	data of Tsunematsu and Shiraishi (1969)	data of Dikow (1969)	data of Lebherz and Rutter (1969)
Skeletal muscle	54.0	25.5	44
Liver	1.0	1.2	1.2
Kidney	1.7	2.9	4.0
Lung	5.6		
Spleen	5.5	19.5	
Brain†	7.1		
Heart	9.0	13.1	
Stomach, mucosa	10.0		
Stomach muscle layer	42.0		
Erythrocytes	10.3		
Serum	2.8		

*Each value is the mean of determinations on 5 specimens, with the exception of that for serum, which is based on determinations on 14 specimens.

†This value for brain is distinctly lower than that, 48.9, obtained by Sato *et al.* (1971).

tract (Schwartz *et al.*, 1962a), head, neck, or oesophagus (Schwartz *et al.*, 1962b), lung (West *et al.*, 1962), and breast (Rose *et al.*, 1961), and metastatic carcinoma of the liver (Tan *et al.*, 1963). However, the fact that normal activity is often found in all these conditions, and the finding of increases in non-neoplastic diseases (Bruns and Jacob, 1954), limits the diagnostic value of this estimation.

The demonstration that aldolase exists in the form of isoenzymes, and that the enzymes from various tissues can be differentiated in a number of ways (see Bodansky, 1975), has resulted in a potential diagnostic aid. Measurement of the ratio of the activity of the enzyme on fructose 1,6-diphosphate to that on fructose 1-phosphate (the 'FDP/F-1-P ratio') has shown that aldolase derived from different tissues is characterized by different ratios (Table 9.5). Table 9.6 shows the increase in FDP/F-1-P ratio in carcinoma of the stomach, hepatoma and carcinoma of the lung. These increases are reflected in the serum (Table 9.7); as Bodansky (1975) points out, this is in agreement with the older work in which fructose 1,6-diphosphate was the substrate employed for the determination of aldolase activity.

From Table 9.7 it is evident that the serum FDP/F-1-P ratio is increased in cancer patients generally, and especially in patients with primary hepatoma. Presumably there is an increase in the serum concentration of the isoenzyme *aldolase A*, which is characteristic of tumour tissue. In acute hepatitis, on the

Table 9.6. Comparison of FDP/F-1-P ratios in normal and neoplastic human tissues.* (Reproduced from O. Bodansky, *Biochemistry of Human Cancer*, Academic Press, New York, 1975, by permission of Academic Press, Inc.)

Normal tissue	No. of speci-mens	Ratio (mean + S.E.M.)	Types of neoplasm	No. of speci-mens	Ratio (mean + S.E.M.)
Gastric mucosa	5	10.0 ±0.85	Carcinoma of stomach	8	40.7 ±4.1†
Liver	5	1.0 ±0.0058	Hepatoma	5	7.9 ±1.4†
Lung	5	5.3 ±0.30	Carcinoma of lung	5	26.8 ±3.8†

*Data of Tsunematsu and Shiraishi (1969).
†Significantly higher ($p < 0.005$) than the corresponding normal tissue.

Table 9.7. Serum aldolase activities and FDP/F-1-P ratios in normal individuals, patients with cancer, and patients with hepatitis.* (Reproduced from O. Bodansky, *Biochemistry of Human Cancer*, Academic Press, New York, 1975, by permission of Academic Press, Inc.)

Group	Num-ber	Mean value for activity of FDP-aldolase†	Mean value for activity of F-1-P aldolase†	FDP/F-1-P ratio
Normals	14	5.44	2.50	2.8
Cancer without liver metastases	20	8.68‡	0.78‡	12.3‡
Cancer with liver metastases	6	16.4‡	2.88	7.1‡
Primary hepatoma	7	16.7‡	1.50	18.2‡
Acute hepatitis	10	18.7‡	14.55‡	1.3‡

*Based on data of Tsunematsu and Shiraishi (1969). Values for standard error (S.E.M.) have been omitted from present tabulation.
†Values for serum. Activity expressed as units, with one unit defined as cleavage of 1 μmol of substrate per minute.
‡Statistically significant ($P < 0.005$) with respect to values for normal serum.

other hand, the serum FDP/F-1-P ratio is subnormal, the ratio approaching that characteristic of liver tissue itself.

Phosphohexose isomerase (glucose phosphate isomerase)

Elevation of serum phosphohexose isomerase activity was first studied in metastatic carcinoma of the breat in patients who were receiving various forms of palliative treatment. In such patients the activity could be 10 or 20 times the normal level, and the degree of elevation was found to correlate with the growth of metastatic tumour in bone, as assessed clinically and by biochemical methods. In patients with metastatic carcinoma of the prostate, also, a good degree of correlation was found, in general, between the rise in the serum activity of the enzyme and growth of the tumour (Bodansky, 1955).

Other workers have confirmed and extended these observations, and rises have been reported in carcinoma of the gastrointestinal tract (Schwartz *et al.*, 1962a), head, neck, and oesophagus (Schwartz *et al.*, 1962b), and lung (West *et al.*, 1962), and in metastatic carcinoma of the liver (Tan *et al.*, 1963). As with aldolase, rises have also been reported in conditions other than cancer; these include tuberculosis (Bodansky, 1954a), infectious hepatitis (Bodansky *et al.*, 1959; Bruns and Jacob, 1954), various myopathies (Schapira *et al.*, 1955), myocardial infarction (Bing *et al.*, 1957), cardiac failure (West *et al.*, 1961), and myelocytic leukaemia (Israels and Delory, 1956; Blanchaer *et al.*, 1958).

Although, as emphasized above, a raised phosphohexose isomerase activity in the serum is not specific for the presence of cancer, the extent of the rise is stated to be a fairly good indicator of the progress of neoplastic disease and to afford a more sensitive indicator than other serum enzymes in revealing changes in the clinical state of the cancer patient (Bodansky, 1975).

Lactate dehydrogenase

Before the recognition that lactate dehydrogenase exists in several isoenzyme forms, rises in its serum activity in a wide variety of diseases had been reported: cancer of various types (Hill and Levi, 1954; Rose *et al.*, 1961; Schwartz *et al.*, 1962a,b; West *et al.*, 1962; Tan *et al.*, 1963), and myocardial infarction, hepatitis, infectious mononucleosis, infections, anaemia, and other diseases (Bodansky, 1961).

Kaplan and his coworkers in 1962 suggested that the electrophoretically slow lactate dehydrogenase isoenzymes are associated with anaerobic glycolysis and that the fast components predominate in tissues in which the metabolism is predominantly oxidative (Cahn *et al.*, 1962). Although there are exceptions to this generalization, there is a good deal of evidence to support it, and several investigators have demonstrated a shift towards the slow isoenzyme pattern in a variety of malignant tumours (Pfleiderer and Wachsmuth, 1961; Richterich and Burger, 1963; Goldman *et al.*, 1964; Poznanska-Linde *et al.*, 1966; Starkweather *et al.*, 1966; Stagg and Whyley, 1968; Okabe *et al.*, 1968). A similar change has been reported in pre-invasive carcinoma of the cervix, even in instances where the microscopic evidence indicated no abnormality (Latner *et al.*, 1966). Okabe and his coworkers (1968) studied the lactate dehydrogenase isoenzymes of the uterus and showed that the same relationship holds, namely, an increase in the proportion of the cathodic components and a decrease in that of the anionic components in tumour tissue.

Estimation of LD_5/LD_1 ratios has been proposed as an aid to the differentiation of benign from malignant tissue (Elhilali *et al.*, 1967; Oliver *et al.*, 1970; Bredin *et al.*, 1975). According to Clark and Srinivasan (1973), however, determination of this ratio in patients with prostatism does not aid in diagnosis.

Table 9.8. Incidence of raised serum activity of ubiquitous enzymes in cancer.*† (Reproduced from O. Bodansky, *Biochemistry of Human Cancer*, Academic Press, New York, 1975, by permission of Academic Press, Inc.)

Group	No. of patients	Percent elevations of GPI	ALS	LD	ASP	ICD	MD	GTD	ALT
Gastrointestinal carcinoma (stomach, colon, pancreas)	119	74	70	53	35	40	37	30	19
Carcinoma of head, neck, and oesophagus	88	51	45	21	16	21	10	15	9
Cancer of lung	126	72	62	53	15	24	25	28	7
Carcinoma of breast	57	70	45	60		40	40	35	
Metastatic car cinoma of liver	284	84	75	69	51	53	62	47	44

*From summary of literature by Bodansky (1965).

†The abbreviations used here have been recommended by several official bodies in Great Britain (Baron *et al.*, 1971). These abbreviations together with the Enzyme Commission number of the IUB and recommended trivial names are as follows: GPI, glucosephosphate isomerase (EC 5.3.1.9); ALS, fructosediphosphate aldolase (EC 4.1.2.13); LD, lactate dehydrogenase (EC 1.1.1.27); ASP, aspartate aminotransferase (EC 2.6.1.1); ICD, isocitrate dehydrogenase (EC 1.1.1.42); MD, malate dehydrogenase (1.1.1.37); GTD, glutathione reductase (EC 1.6.4.2); and ALT, alanine aminotransferase (EC 2.6.1.8).

Recent reports have suggested that the difference between the isoenzyme patterns of tumours and normal tissues might be significant in carcinogenesis. Thus a shift towards the cathodic (slow) isoenzymes has been demonstrated not only in tumours of the colon but also in surrounding morphologically normal tissues (Langvad, 1968a), and similar findings were reported in cancer of the lung (Langvad, 1968b). Diffusion from the tumour was not considered to be the cause of the change in the isoenzyme pattern. Langvad has suggested that a tumour develops in tissue that has already undergone a change to a more anaerobic glycolytic type of metabolism and that such a change in enzyme synthesis might be an indication of a pre-cancerous state.

These changes tend to be reflected in the serum of patients with malignant neoplasms, especially if metastases are present (Starkweather *et al.*, 1966).

'Ubiquitous enzymes'

The glycolytic enzymes and enzymes involved in other metabolic sequences have been referred to as the 'ubiquitous enzymes' (Bodansky, 1965), since they are present in almost every tissue of the body and, consequently, may pass into the blood when tissues are damaged. Table 9.8 shows the incidence of increases in the serum activity of eight of these enzymes in several types of neoplastic disease. It will be noted that the serum enzyme showing the highest incidence of elevated values in each group of diseases is phosphohexose isomerase, so that, of these particular enzymes, the determination of phosphohexose isomerase activity would be the enzyme determination of choice in following the growth or regression of a tumour and in monitoring the effectiveness of certain types of therapy (Bodansky, 1954b, 1955, 1965).

The phosphohydrolases

Measurements of these enzymes have been widely used in the evaluation of cancer patients. The three enzymes in this group of greatest importance in the investigation of cancer are acid phosphatase, alkaline phosphatase, and 5′-nucleotidase.

Acid phosphatase

The finding that this enzyme is present especially in the tissues of the human genital system (Kutscher and Wörner, 1936) was soon followed by the demonstration that increases in its activity in the serum could indicate the presence of carcinoma of the prostate (Gutman and Gutman, 1938a,b). Subsequent investigations showed that increases occur in the majority of patients with carcinoma of the prostate metastatic to bone but in only a minority of patients without metastases (Bodansky, 1960), the determination serving as a confirmatory test for metastatic disease rather than a primary diagnostic tool. The observation by Abul-Fadl and King (1949) that L-tartrate inhibits the prostatic enzyme, but not that originating in other tissues, stimulated a number of studies. Fishman and his colleagues reported that determination of the 'prostatic' enzyme (i.e. the enzyme sensitive to L-tartrate) is helpful in the diagnosis of carcinoma of the prostate before the occurrence of metastases (Fishman and Lerner, 1953; Fishman *et al.*, 1953, 1956). Green and his colleagues found that the 'prostatic' enzyme was raised in 44 of 45 patients with proven cancer of the prostate at a time when the total acid phosphatase was raised in only 24 of these patients (Green *et al.*, 1967). However, other workers have not found the L-tartrate–labile acid phosphatase assay useful (Day *et al.*, 1956; Whitmore *et al.*, 1956); this group of workers found unexplained, temporary rises in prostatic acid phosphatase in some patients, and, in contrast to the findings of Fishman and his colleagues, an apparently lower incidence of raised prostatic acid phosphatase with normal total acid phosphatase values in proved cases of carcinoma of the prostate.

There have been a number of reports that the level of serum acid phosphatase activity is not always clearly related to the apparent clinical progress of the disease or the extent of metastases (Bodansky, 1955), and undoubtedly it may be influenced by a number of factors (Bodansky, 1972). It is important to remember that palpation of a non-malignant prostate may result in elevation of the serum enzyme activity (Hock and Tessier, 1949; Daniel and Van Zyl, 1952; Bonner *et al.*, 1954); small, transient increases may even be produced by impacted faeces or by a distended bladder (Cameron, 1971).

An increase in serum acid phosphatase activity has been noted in other types of carcinoma with metastases in the liver or bones, and in a number of non-neoplastic diseases, such as Gaucher's disease (Tuchman *et al.*, 1956), Paget's disease and hyperparathyroidism (Sullivan *et al.*, 1942), and thrombocytosis (Zucker and Woodard, 1962). The incidence of elevations in these conditions is greater when phenyl phosphate rather than β-glycerophosphate is used as substrate in the assay; hence, use of the latter substrate is to be preferred for the diagnosis of prostatic carcinoma. (Other substrates have been proposed, and α-naphthyl phosphate is stated to be specific for the prostatic enzyme (Babson *et al.*, 1959).)

In investigations involving large groups of patients with a variety of infectious, metabolic or neoplastic disorders, Woodard and Dean (1947) and Woodard (1952), using the Bodansky procedure with β-glycerophosphate as substrate, were unable to find any raised acid phosphatase values in diseases other than prostatic carcinoma. However, with the same substrate, increases have since been reported to occur also in myeloproliferative disorders (Bases, 1962).

Determination of the acid phosphatase in *bone marrow* has been advocated as a sensitive indicator of the presence of bone metastasis in patients with prostatic cancer (Chua *et al.*, 1970; Reynolds *et al.*, 1973; Gursel *et al.*, 1974; Yarrison *et al.*, 1976). According to Gursel and his coworkers, an increase of acid phosphatase in the marrow is the first sign of bone metastasis and seems to contraindicate radical therapy. Combining the test with X-ray examination, isotope (^{18}F) bone scans, and bone marrow biopsy was of great value in staging the disease (Reynolds *et al.*, 1973). Increases in acid phosphatase in bone marrow were also found in leukaemia, myeloma, anaemia, and metastatic oat cell carcinoma (Yarrison *et al.*, 1976).

Alkaline phosphatase

Increases in serum alkaline phosphatase activity are found in two classes of neoplastic disease, *viz.* those affecting the skeletal system and those affecting the liver. Metastases in the bones or in the liver frequently arise from primary tumours in other tissues. In common with other 'space-occupying' lesions of the liver (see p. 59), hepatic metastases are associated with a raised serum alkaline phosphatase activity, which has been found of value for their early detection (Mendelsohn and Bodansky, 1952; Shay and Siplet, 1954). Rises occur also in many patients with primary hepatoma (Galluzzi *et al.*, 1953).

About 75 per cent of carcinomas of the breast and about 65 per cent of carcinomas of the prostate metastasize to bone (Bodansky, 1961). Since the majority of metastases from breast cancers are osteolytic, with little osteoblastic activity, serum alkaline phosphatase activity in these patients is only slightly raised. On the other hand, most metastatic bone lesions associated with carcinoma of the prostate appear to be osteoblastic, and consequently many patients with such bone metastases have much higher levels of serum alkaline phosphatase. Treatment that produces a favourable clinical effect is often associated with an initial rise in serum alkaline phosphatase activity, followed by a steady fall towards normal levels (Bodansky, 1961).

Serum alkaline phosphatase is also raised in various non-neoplastic liver diseases, such as viral hepatitis, cirrhosis, and drug-induced liver damage. Similarly, high levels are also found in non-neoplastic diseases of the skeleton, such as infantile rickets and advanced Paget's disease (Gutman, 1959).

Isoenzymes of alkaline phosphatase

Although it has been known for some forty years that alkaline phosphatases derived from different tissues are not identical (Bodansky, 1937), it is only recently that the isoenzymes of alkaline phosphatase have been studied in more detail and their assay used to define the tissues of their origin in patients. Figure 9.2 shows the patterns of alkaline phosphatase isoenzymes, obtained by starch-gel electrophoresis, in extracts of various tissues.

In 1968 Fishman and his colleagues (Fishman *et al.*, 1968a) reported finding a placental-like alkaline phosphatase isoenzyme in the serum of a patient with bronchogenic carcinoma; this isoenzyme was also found at autopsy in high concentrations in the tumour and its metastases. The enzyme, which they called the 'Regan isoenzyme' (after the patient) was found in a number of other cancer patients (Fishman *et al.*, 1968b), and was subsequently shown to be very similar to or identical with the heat-stable, L-phenylalanine-sensitive alkaline phosphatase found in the human placenta. Further studies have confirmed the presence of this enzyme in a minority of patients with various types of cancer (Stolbach *et al.*, 1969; Nathanson and Fishman, 1971). On account of the similarity of the Regan isoenzyme to the alkaline phosphatase from normal placenta, Fishman has called it a *carcinoplacental antigen*, as distinct from the carcinoembryonic and fetal antigens described earlier in this chapter (Fishman *et al.*, 1971). The Regan isoenzyme may be regarded as an example of ectopic isoenzyme production (Fishman, 1969).

Nathanson and Fishman (1971) suggested that assay of the Regan isoenzyme might be useful in monitoring the efficacy of anti-tumour therapy in some patients.

A variant of alkaline phosphatase that differs from the Regan isoenzyme in its electrophoretic properties, but has similar heat stability and sensitivity to L-phenylalanine, has been found in extracts of tumour from patients with hepatocellular carcinoma (Warnock and Reisman, 1969). A leucine-sensitive, heat-stable alkaline phosphatase has been observed in a patient with pleural carcinoma (Nakayama *et al.*, 1970).

The production of such placental-like phosphatase isoenzymes by tumours is thought to be due to derepression of the genome of the cancer cells (Fishman *et al.*, 1968b).

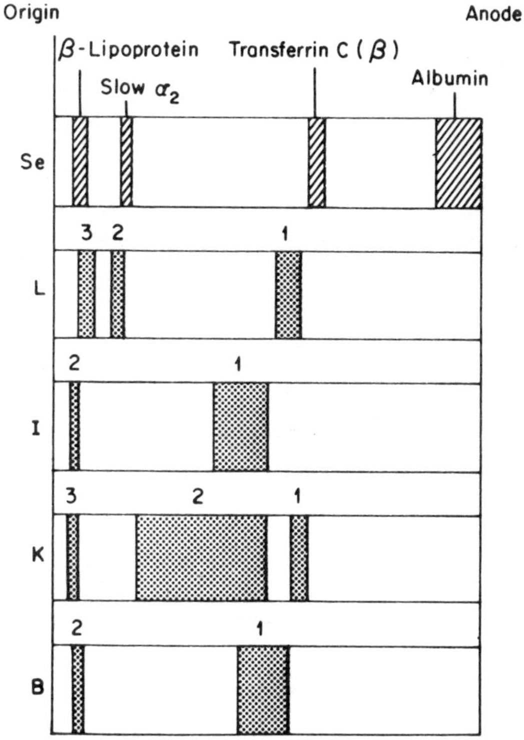

Figure 9.2. Location of alkaline phosphatase isoenzyme fractions after starch-gel electrophoresis of concentrated butan-1-ol extracts of bone (B), liver (L), kidney (K) and small intestine (I), compared with those of principal protein fractions of normal blood serum (Se). (Reproduced, with permission, from D. W. Moss and E. J. King, *Biochem. J.*, 1962, **84**, 192.)

5′-Nucleotidase

Most studies have indicated that serum 5′-nucleotidase activity is raised in patients with hepatic disease but not in those with bone disease (Dixon and Purdom, 1954; Kowlessar *et al.*, 1961). Slight increases have been reported to occur, very rarely, in Paget's disease (Schwartz and Bodansky, 1965), after bone fracture and in patients with cardiovascular, gastrointestinal, endocrine, pulmonary, and other diseases (Eschar *et al.*, 1967); however, as Bodansky (1975) points out, these increases may well reflect slight and unrecognized hepatic involvement. It would seem that assay of serum 5′-nucleotidase is a fairly specific indicator of hepatic disease and that in neoplastic hepatic disease, in the absence of skeletal lesions, it is frequently a more sensitive indicator than serum alkaline phosphatase (Bodansky, 1975). However, Eschar and his coworkers (1967) found 5′-nucleotidase to be a less sensitive measure than alkaline phosphatase in the study of hepatobiliary disease and felt that it added little specificity.

5′-Nucleotide phosphodiesterase

A study of the isoenzymes of 5′-nucleotide phosphodiesterase showed the appearance of a fast-moving component ('Band V isoenzyme') in the serum of 38 of 43 patients with primary hepatoma, of whom only 6 gave a positive reaction for α-fetoprotein by the immunodiffusion test (Tsou *et al.*, 1974); in 55 patients having liver involvement with primary cancer of other organs, 44 sera showed the Band V isoenzyme. There appeared to be no relationship between the occurrence of the isoenzyme and that of α-fetoprotein, the two proteins being independent markers for hepatoma.

The Band V isoenzyme could not be detected in cord serum with the methods available.

Aryl sulphatase

The aryl sulphatases are a group of enzymes that hydrolyse aryl sulphates. Three isoenzymes exist (A, B, and C), which are distinguished by their substrate specificity, response to inorganic inhibitors, pH optima, and subcellular localization (Barrett, 1972). Aryl sulphatases A and B are localized mainly in lysosomes (Sellinger and Hiatt, 1968), and aryl sulphatase C is found in the microsomal, nuclear, and mitochondrial fractions of various tissues (Milsom *et al.*, 1968; Perumal and Robins, 1973). In a series of 243 patients with colorectal cancer investigated by Morgan and his coworkers (1975), increased urinary aryl sulphatase B activity was found in 172 patients, the activity being related to the state of the disease. It was suggested that measurement of the urinary enzyme, when raised, might be used to monitor response to therapy, since in those patients with raised urine enzyme activity a favourable response to therapy was associated with a return or approach to normal values. In contrast to the urinary findings, aryl sulphatase B activity in tumour tissue was increased in only 24 per cent of the patients examined.

Miscellaneous enzymes

Amylase

The principal use of serum amylase assays in the clinical laboratory is in the diagnosis of acute pancreatitis, though substantial increases can occur also in chronic recurrent pancreatitis. Liver disease and renal impairment may also be associated with high values. Changes in serum amylase activity in cancer, unassociated with any of these conditions, do occur, as in some patients with carcinoma of the pancreas (Heifetz *et al.*, 1941; Comfort *et al.*, 1943). In a case of acinar cell carcinoma of the pancreas described by the latter group of authors, the serum amylase activity was many times greater than that usually encountered in carcinoma of the pancreas, and it was suggested that this was due to functioning carcinomatous cells (Comfort *et al.*, 1943). Unexplained increases to extremely high values have been found in patients with bronchogenic carcinoma (Weiss *et al.*, 1951; and others).

Leucine aminopeptidase

Measurement of the activity of this enzyme in serum and urine was found by Rutenberg and his associates (1958) to be an aid to the diagnosis of cancer of the pancreas; the finding of normal serum and urine values was especially useful in ruling out this condition. Other causes of hepatic obstruction, and liver diseases such as hepatitis, cirrhosis, and cholecystitis, were associated with lesser increases. Although some workers have obtained similar results, others have questioned the value of the estimation in routine diagnosis on account of the overlapping of results in various intra- and extrahepatic diseases (Batsakis and Briere, 1967). Rises in serum activities occur in a variety of hepatobiliary diseases (Fleisher *et al.*, 1957; Arst *et al.*, 1959; Bressler *et al.*, 1960; Kowlessar *et al.*, 1961). Measurement of the serum enzyme does not permit differentiation between malignant and benign obstruction.

In liver disease, measurement of leucine aminopeptidase is reported to have the sensitivity and diagnostic significance of that of alkaline phosphatase; it is not raised in bone disease and hence its measurement—like that of 5′-nucleotidase—may be useful in establishing the tissue of origin of elevated alkaline phosphatase. Rises are seen in pregnancy, especially in the later stages and at the time of delivery (Arst *et al.*, 1959); they do not seem to occur in any extrahepatic disease, with the exception of carcinoma of the head of the pancreas and leukaemia—in both of which a degree of involvement of the liver might, according to Bodansky (1975), account for the reported rises.

γ-Glutamyl transferase

The serum activity of this enzyme is raised in patients with carcinoma metastatic to the liver, but rises also occur in various non-malignant types of liver damage (Szewczuk and Orłowski, 1960; Szczeklik *et al.*, 1961; Orłowski, 1963; Rutenberg *et al.*, 1963; Zein and Discombe, 1970). It is also raised in many alcoholics (Spencer-Peet *et al.*, 1972), and in such diverse conditions as myocardial infarction (Ewen and Griffiths, 1971a), and certain neurological diseases (Ewen and Griffiths, 1971b) as well as in patients receiving long-term anticonvulsant therapy (Rosalki *et al.*, 1971); in this last case, the rise in serum γ-glutamyl transferase activity may be due either to microsomal injury or to enzyme induction by the drug.

Simultaneous assay of γ-glutamyl transferase and carcinoembryonic antigen is stated to be of value in the early detection of hepatic metastases in patients with colorectal cancer (Steele *et al.*, 1974; Cooper *et al.*, 1975b).

Lysozyme (muramidase)

Lysozyme activity is raised in the urine and serum of patients with certain types of leukaemia (Osserman and Lawlor, 1966; Perillie *et al.*, 1968; Wiernik and Serpick, 1969), the greatest increases, both in serum and in urine, being found in the acute myelomonocytic and the acute monocytic forms. The source of the serum enzyme in these cases appears to be the proliferating circulating monocytic leukaemic cells (Osserman and Lawlor, 1966). The increase in serum lysozyme activity is not specific for leukaemias, and increased whole-blood lysozyme has been found in patients with various types of neoplasms (Fogelson and Lobstein, 1954).

Low plasma lysozyme activity is found in acute lymphocytic leukaemia, probably mainly because of the low lysozyme content of mature neutrophilic granulocytes and the fact that lymphoblasts do not contain lysozyme (Hansen, 1974).

The value of plasma lysozyme assays in the differential diagnosis of monocytic or myelomonocytic leukaemia as against other haematological diseases is limited to very high plasma levels. In the differential diagnosis of the various acute leukaemias, again only high plasma levels are of value. Although mean plasma lysozyme levels in most types of leukaemia are somewhat different, there is so much overlapping between the various groups that difficulties of interpretation arise in the individual case (Hansen, 1974). Plasma lysozyme assays may be of value in monitoring chronic myelocytic leukaemia, particularly for giving advance warning of the onset of malignant transformation (Hansen, 1974).

Serum lysozyme assays have been found of value in identifying those patients who are unlikely to respond to certain types of intensive chemotherapy; this allows them to receive alternative forms of treatment without first being subjected to highly toxic but ineffective drug combinations (Currie, 1976).

As mentioned in Chapter 4, the post-γ-globulin of Butler and Flynn (1961) appears to consist largely of lysozyme. It has been found to be present in the urine in a number of non-neoplastic conditions, including the Fanconi syndrome, renal tubular acidosis, and an organic-aciduria syndrome (Butler and Flynn, 1961), and sometimes in cadmium poisoning (Piscator, 1966b). In the latter condition increases in serum lysozyme activity have also been found (Piscator, 1966a).

Proline hydroxylase

The serum activity of this enzyme, which is essential for the biosynthesis of collagen, is elevated in some 50 to 70 per cent of patients with hepatocellular carcinoma (Keiser *et al.*, 1972; Glazer *et al.*, 1974). According to McGee and his colleagues (1975), the assay of both proline hydroxylase activity and α-fetoprotein in serum enables all patients with the condition to be identified. The observation that the activity of the enzyme rises early in the premalignant phase of the disease makes the assay of potential value in detecting such tumours in high-risk populations (Baillie *et al.*, 1975).

Other enzymes

Increases in serum *aspartate aminotransferase*, *adenosine deaminase*, *ornithine carbamoyltransferase*, *cholinesterase*, and *isocitrate dehydrogenase* have been reported in patients with various forms of cancer, but the estimation of these enzymes for the diagnosis of cancer appears to be of little value. *Sialytransferase* activity is raised in human mammary and colonic carcinomas as compared with the normal tissues (Bossmann and Hall, 1974), and plasma activity of the enzyme is found to be raised in patients with a variety of neoplasms (Kessel and Allen, 1975); the plasma activity declined after removal of a tumour. Although increases in plasma sialyltransferase activity are not specific for cancer, having been noted, for example, in rheumatoid arthritis, it is nevertheless possible that assay of the enzyme may be useful in cancer monitoring.

Enzymes in miscellaneous body fluids

Cerebrospinal fluid

In 21 of 33 patients with primary or secondary tumours of the central nervous system, *phosphohexose isomerase* activity in the cerebrospinal fluid was found to be raised, whereas in all but one of seven patients with benign tumours the activity was within normal limits (Thompson *et al.*, 1959). Increases were also observed in half the patients with meningitis and meningoencephalitis caused by pyogenic, viral, or yeast organisms, as well as in acute infections and in some patients with cerebral thrombosis. In the series of patients studied by Hulanicka and his colleagues (1963), however, patients with primary or secondary tumours of the central nervous system usually had cerebrospinal fluid phosphohexose isomerase activity within the normal range.

Pleural and ascitic effusions

Brauer and his colleagues (1963) investigated the activity of a number of enzymes in pleural and ascitic effusions in patients with neoplastic and non-neoplastic conditions. High effusion/serum ratios were common in the case of certain enzymes, but the authors concluded that the diagnostic usefulness of such ratios is limited.

Vaginal fluid

The finding by Fishman (1956) that in invasive cancer of the uterus the *β-glucuronidase* activity of the neoplastic tissue is substantially higher than that of normal cervical tissue suggested the possibility of leakage of enzyme into the vaginal fluid; and increased β-glucuronidase activity in this fluid was indeed found in a proportion of cases (Kasdon, 1956; Lawson, 1969). However, high values may be found in conditions unrelated to cervical cancer; and this fact, together with certain technical difficulties associated with the assay (Lawson, 1969), limits severely the diagnostic value of such assays.

Another enzyme investigated as a possible aid to the diagnosis of cancer of the uterus is *6-phosphogluconate dehydrogenase*. Bonham and Gibbs (1962) found that whereas all but 3 of 93 patients without uterine malignancy had vaginal enzyme levels within the normal range, 46 patients with uterine malignancies all had levels above the upper limit of normal. Subsequent reports, however, failed to confirm this clear-cut distinction (Nerdrum, 1964; Longnecker and White, 1965; Cameron and Husain, 1965; Hoffman and Merritt, 1965).

In order to express vaginal enzyme activity in such a way as to accentuate the differences between normal subjects and patients with uterine neoplasms, Lawson and Watkins (1965) related enzyme activity to the amount of protein in the fluid rather than to its dry weight. They found β-glucuronidase activity to be high in two out of five women without cancer and low in two out of nine women with invasive cervical cancer; for 6-phosphogluconate dehydrogenase the false negative rate (10 per cent of 49 cases) was somewhat better and the false positive rate (47 per cent of 64 cases) rather worse than for β-glucuronidase.

Expression of 6-phosphogluconate dehydrogenase activity as the enzyme/potassium ratio (Gibbs *et al.*, 1968) rather than in terms of units per gram dry weight appeared to have little or no advantage in detecting uterine carcinoma in premenopausal women, but was more successful with postmenopausal women.

Many patients with trichomonas vaginitis (Bell and Egerton, 1965), moniliasis, and non-specific vaginitis (Batsakis and Briere, 1967) have raised 6-phosphogluconate dehydrogenase activity in the vaginal fluid. It seems likely that the disappointing results of estimations of vaginal enzyme activity are due, partly, to this ability of infection to produce increased enzyme activity in the vaginal secretions. Altered hormonal states can also produce increases in 6-phosphogluconate dehydrogenase activity: thus no less than 56 per cent of a group of patients with menopausal vaginitis resulting from oestrogen deficiency had increased enzyme activity (Hoffman and Merritt, 1965); and high values were found in women taking contraceptive pills (Bell and Egerton, 1965).

LABORATORY INVESTIGATION OF PROTEINS IN CANCER

It is evident that, in spite of the vast amount of research undertaken over many years, there is still no specific biochemical test for cancer. However, within a particular clinical context certain tests may be helpful, taken in conjunction with the clinical history of the patient; for example, a markedly raised serum α-fetoprotein concentration in a patient suspected of having a primary hepatoma, or a high serum acid phosphatase activity in a patient with an enlarged prostate. The non-specificity of the tests in use, and the possibility of 'false' positives, must always be borne in mind; however, the limitations imposed by non-specificity should not be over-emphasized, since in practice many non-malignant conditions associated with positive tests can often be excluded.

Perhaps the most important application of the tests at present available is in *monitoring*. This has four objects:

1. to allow the early detection of recurrences or metastases by giving a 'lead time' over other methods of tumour detection;
2. to help in the assessment of the rate of progression of established metastases;
3. to indicate the response to treatment; and
4. as a guide to prognosis.

The choice of test(s) will depend on the circumstances: no one test is applicable in all cases, and indeed much investigative work is in progress with various potential 'markers'. The measurement of two or more such markers rather than only one is often of significant value. An example is the measurement of both α-fetoprotein and prolyl hydroxylase in the diagnosis of hepatoma. Similarly, the detection rate of bronchial carcinoma is enhanced by the measurement of several markers, *viz*. human chorionic gonadotrophin (and its subunits), human placental lactogen, and placental alkaline phosphatase (Charles *et al.*, 1973; Sussman *et al.*, 1974; Rosen *et al.*, 1975); the presence of each of these has been found to be independent of the other two, and when more than one of them are present their concentrations are independent of each other. Again, simultaneous assay of carcinoembryonic antigen and γ-glutamyl

Table 9.9. A few selected publications on the monitoring of various types of cancer

Cancer	Substances measured	Reference
Breast	CEA and ferritin	Wang, 1976
	CEA, α-fetoprotein, HCG, β subunit of HCG, and kappa-casein	Franchimont *et al.*, 1976
Colorectal	CEA, γ-glutamyl transferase and routine liver function tests	Cooper *et al.*, 1975b
	α-Globulins	Cooper *et al.*, 1976a
	CEA, γ-glutamyl transferase haptoglobin, α_1-antitrypsin, α_1-acid glycoprotein, prealbumin	Cooper *et al.*, 1976b
Bladder	Haptoglobin, α_1-antitrypsin, α_1-acid glycoprotein, prealbumin	Cooper *et al.*, 1976b
Prostate	Sex-hormone-binding globulin	Cooper *et al.*, 1976b
Testicular teratoma	α-Fetoprotein	Kohn, 1976

transferase is a valuable aid to the early detection of hepatic metastases from colorectal cancer. In the case of breast cancer it would seem from the work of Tormey and his collaborators (1975), and others, that a combination of tumour markers, rather than a single one, may offer the best chance of predicting the course of the disease and of monitoring its progress. Other examples of this use of 'multiparametric' studies are discussed by Neville and Cooper (1976).

'Longitudinal' or serial studies can be very useful, since they can enable a mean or baseline value, applicable to a particular patient, to be established; changes from this mean over a period of time may be of greater significance than the finding of an isolated value that is elevated with respect to an arbitrarily established upper limit of normal for a group of people. Examples of such studies have been given in the section on carcinoembryonic antigen.

Table 9.9 lists a few selected recent publications on the biochemical monitoring of various types of cancer.

REFERENCES

Abelev, G. I. (1963), *Acta. Unio Intern. Cancer*, **19**, 80.
Abelev, G. I. (1968), *Cancer Res.*, **18**, 1344.
Abelev, G., S. Perova, N. Khramkova, Z. Postnikova, and I. Irlin (1963), *Biokhimiya*, **28**, 625.
Abelev, G. I., I. V. Assecritova, N. A. Kraevsky, S. D. Perova, and N. I. Perevodchikova (1967), *Int. J. Cancer*, **2**, 551.
Ablin, R. J. (1972), *Lancet*, **ii**, 874.
Abul-Fadl, M. A. M., and E. J. King (1949), *Biochem. J.*, **45**, 51.
Almquist, P. O., and E. Lausing (1957), *Scand. J. Clin. Lab. Invest.*, **9**, 179.
Alpert, M. E., J. Uriel, and B. de Nechaud (1968), *New Engl. J. Med.*, **278**, 984.
Anderson, G. (1973), *Paramalignant Syndromes in Lung Cancer*, Heinemann, London.
Anderson, J. M., W. H. Stimson, and F. Kelly (1976), *Brit. J. Surg.*, **63**, 819.
Arst, H. E., R. T. Manning, and D. Delp (1959), *Amer. J. Med. Sci.*, **238**, 598.
Babson, A. L., P. A. Read, and G. E. Phillips (1959), *Amer. J. Clin. Path.*, **32**, 83.
Bagshawe, K. D., M. J. Frost, G. T. Rogers, and F. Searle (1976), *Protides of the Biological Fluids: Proceedings of 24th Colloquium, Bruges, 1976* (Ed. H. Peeters), Pergamon Press, Oxford, p. 535.
Baillie, J., M. S. Al Adnani, R. S. Patrick, J. A. Kirrane, and J. McGee (1975), *Proc. Path. Soc. G. B. and Ireland* (July), p. 21. (Cited by Neville and Cooper, 1976.)
Baker, R., and E. Govan (1953), *Cancer Res.*, **13**, 141.
Banwo, O., J. Versey, and J. R. Hobbs (1974), *Lancet*, **i**, 643.
Barlow, J. J., and P. H. Dillard (1972), *Obstet. Gynec.*, **39**, 727.
Baron, D. N., D. W. Moss, P. G. Walker, and J. H. Wilkinson (1971), *J. Clin. Path.*, **24**, 656.
Barrelet, V., and J.-P. Mach (1975), *Amer. J. Obstet. Gynec.*, **121**, 164.
Barrett, A. J. (1972), in *Lysosomes* (Ed. J. T. Dingle), Elsevier, New York, pp. 68, 114.
Bases, R. (1962), *New Engl. J. Med.*, **266**, 538.
Batsakis, J. G., and R. O. Briere (1967), *Interpretive Enzymology*, Thomas, Springfield, Ill.
Bell, J. L., and M. E. Egerton (1965), *J. Obstet. Gynaec. Brit. Commonw.*, **72**, 603.
Bergstrand, C. G., and B. Czar (1956), *Scand. J. Clin. Lab. Invest.*, **8**, 174.
Berne, B. H., H. Bohn, R. Hofmann, B. Klausch, W. Straube, C. H. W. Horne, R. Kasukawa, Ch. Rittner, W. H. Stimson, and G. N. Than (1975), *Lancet*, **ii**, 367.
Bing, R. J., A. Castellanos, and A. Siegel (1957), *J. Amer. Med. Assoc.*, **164**, 647.
Blanchaer, M. C., P. T. Green, J. P. Maclean, and M. J. Hollenberg (1958), *Blood*, **13**, 245.

Bodansky, O. (1937), *J. Biol. Chem.*, **118**, 341.
Bodansky, O. (1945a), *Cancer*, **7**, 1191.
Bodansky, O. (1954b), *Cancer*, **7**, 1200.
Bodansky, O. (1955), *Cancer*, **8**, 1087.
Bodansky, O. (1960), in *Enzymes in Health and Disease* (Eds. D. M. Greenberg and H. M. Harper), Thomas, Springfield, Ill., p. 269.
Bodansky, O. (1961), *Adv. Cancer Res.*, **6**, 1.
Bodansky, O. (1965), *Proc. 5th Natl. Cancer Conference*, Philadelphia, Lippincott, Philadelphia, p. 687. (Cited by Bodansky, 1975.)
Bodansky, O. (1972), *Adv. Clin. Chem.*, **15**, 43.
Bodansky, O. (1975), *Biochemistry of Human Cancer*, Academic Press, New York.
Bodansky, O., S. Krugman, R. Ward, M. K. Schwartz, J. P. Giles, and A. M. Jacobs (1959), *Amer. J. Dis. Child.*, **98**, 166.
Bolker, N. (1953), *Amer. J. Roentgenol., Radium Ther. Nucl. Med.*, **69**, 839.
Bonham, D. G., and D. F. Gibbs (1962), *Brit. Med. J.*, **ii**, 823.
Bonner, C. D., F. Homburger, and W. H. Fishman (1954), *Surg. Gynec. Obstet.*, **99**, 179.
Booth, S. N., J. P. G. King, J. C. Leonard, and P. W. Dykes (1974), *Scand. J. Gastroent.*, **9**, 651.
Booth, S. N., G. Lakin, P. W. Dykes, D. Burnett, and A. R. Bradwell (1977), *J. Clin. Path.*, **30**, 537.
Bossmann, H. B., and T. C. Hall (1974), *Proc. Nat. Acad. Sci.*, **71**, 1833.
Brauer, M. J., M. West, and H. J. Zimmerman (1963), *Cancer*, **16**, 533.
Bredin, H. C., J. J. Daly, and G. R. Prout (1975), *J. Urol.*, **113**, 487.
Bressler, R., B. R. Forsyth, and G. Klatskin (1960), *J. Lab. Clin. Med.*, **56**, 417.
Bruns, H. F., and W. Jacob (1954), *Klin. Woch.*, **32**, 1041.
Buffe, D., C. Rimbaut, J. Lemerle, O. Schweisguth, and P. Burtin (1970), *Int. J. Cancer*, **5**, 85.
Butler, E. A., and F. V. Flynn (1961), *J. Clin. Path.*, **14**, 172.
Cahn, R. D., N. O. Kaplan, L. Levene, and E. Zwilling (1962), *Science*, **136**, 962.
Cameron, C. B. (1971), *J. Clin. Path.*, **24**, Suppl. (Assoc. Clin. Path.) 4, 80.
Cameron, C. B., and O. A. N. Husain (1965), *Brit. Med. J.*, **i**, 1529.
Cameron, E., A. Campbell, and W. Plenderleith (1961), *Scot. Med. J.*, **6**, 301.
Cercek, L., and B. Cercek (1973), *Biophysik*, **9**, 105.
Cercek, L., B. Cercek, and C. I. V. Franklin (1974), *Brit. J. Cancer*, **29**, 345.
Charles, M. A., R. Claypool, M. Schaaf, S. W. Rosen, and B. D. Weintraub (1973), *Arch. Int. Med.*, **132**, 427.
Chua, D. T., R. J. Veenema, F. Muggia, and A. Graff (1970), *J. Urol.*, **103**, 462.
Clark, S. S., and V. Srinivasan (1973), *J. Urol.*, **109**, 444.
Comfort, M. W., H. R. Butt, A. H. Baggenstoss, A. E. Osterberg, and J. T. Priestly (1943), *Ann. Int. Med.*, **19**, 808.
Coombes, R. C., C. Hillyard, P. B. Greenberg, and I. McIntyre (1974), *Lancet*, **ii**, 1080.
Cooper, E. H., R. Turner, A. Geake, and A. M. Neville (1975a), cited by Neville and Cooper, 1976.
Cooper, E. H., R. Turner, L. Steele, A. M. Neville, and A. M. Mackay (1975b), *Brit. J. Cancer*, **31**, 111.
Cooper, E. H., R. Turner, A. Geekie, A. M. Neville, J. C. Goligher, N. G. Graham, G.-R. Giles, R. Hall, and W. A. F. Macadam (1976a), *Biomedicine*, **24**, 171.
Cooper, E. H., R. Turner, A. M. Ward, and A. M. Neville (1976b), in *Cancer Related Antigens* (Ed. P. Franchimont), Elsevier/North-Holland, Amsterdam, p. 179.
Cori, C. F., and G. T. Cori (1925), *J. Biol. Chem.*, **65**, 397.
Crozier, E. H., M. E. Hollinger, B. E. Woodend, and J. H. Robertson (1976), *J. Clin. Path.*, **29**, 608.
Currie, G. (1976), *Lancet*, **i**, 835.
Daniel, O., and J. J. Van Zyl (1952), *Lancet*, **i**, 998.

Darcy, D. A., C. Turberville, and R. James (1973), *Brit. J. Cancer*, **28**, 147.

Day, E., S. H. Ying, M. K. Schwartz, W. F. Whitmore, Jr., and O. Bodansky (1956), *Cancer*, **9**, 222.

Dickens, F., and H. Weil-Malherbe (1936), *Biochem. J.*, **30**, 659.

Dickens, F., and H. Weil-Malherbe (1941), *Biochem. J.*, **35**, 7.

Dikow, A. L. (1969), *Z. klin. Chem.*, **7**, 278.

DiSaia, P. J., B. J. Haverback, B. J. Dyce, and C. P. Morrow (1975), *Amer. J. Obstet. Gynec.*, **121**, 159.

Dixon, T. F., and M. Purdom (1954), *J. Clin. Path.*, **7**, 341.

Edynak, E. M., L. J. Old, M. Vrana, and M. Lardis (1970), *Proc. Amer. Assoc. Cancer Res.*, **11**, 22.

Edynak, E. M., L. J. Old, M. Vrana, and M. P. Lardis (1972), *New Engl. J. Med.*, **286**, 1178.

Elhilali, M. M., J. A. Oliver, A. L. Sherwin, and K. J. MacKinnon (1967), *J. Urol.*, **98**, 686.

Ellison, M. L., D. Woodhouse, C. Hillyard, M. Dowsett, R. C. Coombes, E. D. Gilby, P. B. Greenberg, and A. M. Neville (1975), cited by Neville and Cooper (1976).

Engelhardt, N. V., A. I. Goussev, L. J. Shipova, and G. I. Abelev (1971) *Int. J. Cancer*, **7**, 198.

Eschar, J., C. Rudzki, and H. J. Zimmerman (1967), *Amer. J. Clin. Path.*, **47**, 598.

Evans, A. S., M. F. Dolan, P. Z. Sobocinski, and F. A. Quinn (1974), *Cancer Res.*, **34**, 538.

Ewen, L. M., and J. Griffiths (1971a), *Amer J. Clin. Path.*, **56**, 614.

Ewen, L. M., and J. Griffiths (1971b), *Clin. Chem.*, **17**, 642.

Field, E. J. (1973), in *Immunological Techniques for Detection of Cancer* (Ed. B. Björklund), Bonniers, Sollentuna, p. 79.

Field, E. J., and E. A. Caspary (1970), *Lancet*, **ii**, 1337.

Field, E. J., E. A. Caspary, and K. S. Smith (1973), *Brit. J. Cancer*, **28**, Suppl. 1, p. 208.

Fish, R. G. (1975), *Med. Hypotheses*, **1**, 144.

Fishman, W. H. (1956), in *The Laboratory Diagnosis of Cancer of the Cervix* (Eds. F. Homburger and W. H. Fishman), Karger, Basel, p. 46.

Fishman, W. H. (1969), *Ann. N. Y. Acad. Sci.*, **166**, 745.

Fishman, W. H., and F. Lerner (1953), *J. Biol. Chem.*, **200**, 89.

Fishman, W. H., R. M. Dart, C. D. Bonner, W. F. Leadbetter, F. Lerner, and F. Homburger (1953), *J. Clin. Invest.*, **32**, 1034.

Fishman, W. H., C. D. Bonner, and F. Homburger (1956), *New Engl. J. Med.*, **255**, 925.

Fishman, W. H., N. R. Inglis, L. L. Stolbach, and M. J. Krant (1968a), *Cancer Res.*, **28**, 150.

Fishman, W. H., N. R. Inglis, S. Green, C. L. Anstiss, N. K. Ghosh, A. E. Reif, R. Rustigian, M. J. Krant, and L. L. Stolbach (1968b), *Nature*, **219**, 697.

Fishman, W. H., N. R. Inglis, and S. Green (1971), *Cancer Res.*, **31**, 1054.

Fleisher, G. A., H. R. Butt, and K. A. Huizenga (1957), *Proc. Staff Meet. Mayo Clin.*, **32**, 410.

Fogelson, S. J., and O. E. Lobstein (1954), *Amer. J. Dig. Dis.*, **21**, 324.

Foli, A. K., S. Sherlock, and M. Adinolfi (1969), *Lancet*, **ii**, 1267.

Franchimont, P., P. F. Zangerle, J. Nogarede, J. Bury, F. Molter, A. Reuter, J. C. Hendrick, and J. Colette (1976), in *Protides of the Biological Fluids: Proceedings of 24th Colloquium, Bruges, 1976* (Ed. H. Peeters), Pergamon Press, Oxford, p. 571.

Galluzzi, N. J., W. Weingarten, F. D. Regan, and A. A. Doerner (1953), *J. Amer. Med. Assoc.*, **152**, 15.

Gibbs, D. F., A. H. Labrum, and B. H. Stagg (1968), *Amer. J. Obstet. Gynec.*, **102**, 982.

Gitlin, D., and M. Boesman (1966), *J. Clin. Invest.*, **45**, 1826.

Glazer, R. I., C. L. Vogel, I. R. Patel, and P. P. Anthony (1974), *Cancer Res.*, **34**, 2975.

Gold, P., and S. O. Freedman (1965a), *J. Exp. Med.*, **121**, 439.

Gold, P., and S. O. Freedman (1965b), *J. Exp. Med.*, **122**, 467.
Goldman, R. D., N. O. Kaplan, and T. C. Hall (1964), *Cancer Res.*, **24**, 389.
Green, S., T. J. Giovanniello, and W. H. Fishman (1967), in *Automation in Analytical Chemistry* (Technicon Symposium I. 1966) (Eds. N. B. Scova *et al.*), Mediad, White Plains, N. Y., p. 480.
Greenspan, E. M. (1954), *A. M. A. Arch. Int. Med.*, **93**, 863.
Greenspan, E. M. (1955), *Adv. Int. Med.*, **7**, 101.
Greenspan, E. M., and D. A. Dreiling (1953), *A. M. A. Arch. Int. Med.*, **91**, 494.
Greenspan, E. M., B. Tepper, L. L. Terry, and E. B. Schoenbach (1952), *J. Lab. Clin. Med.*, **39**, 44.
Gursel, E. O., M. Rezvan, F. A. Sy, and R. J. Veenema (1974), *J. Urol.*, **111**, 53.
Gutman, A. B. (1959), *Amer. J. Med.*, **27**, 875.
Gutman, A. B., and E. B. Gutman (1938a), *Proc. Soc. Exp. Biol. Med.*, **38**, 470.
Gutman, A. B., and E. B. Gutman (1938b), *J. Clin. Invest.*, **17**, 473.
Häkkinen, I. P. T. (1974), *Transplant. Rev.*, **20**, 61.
Häkkinen, I., and S. Viikari (1969), *Ann. Surg.*, **169**, 277.
Häkkinen, I., K. Korhonen, and L. Saxén (1968), *Int. J. Cancer*, **3**, 582.
Hansen, N. E. (1974), *Ser. Haematol.*, **7**, 87.
Harris, R., D. Viza, R. Todd, J. Phillips, R. Sugar, R. F. Jennison, G. Marriott, and M. H. Gleeson (1971), *Nature*, **233**, 556.
Harshman, S., P. T. Patikas, K. Dayani, and V. H. Reynolds (1967), *Cancer Res.*, **27**, 1286.
Harshman, S., V. H. Reynolds, T. Neumaster, T. Patikas, and T. Worrall (1974), *Cancer*, **34**, 291.
Heifetz, C. J., J. G. Probstein, and S. H. Gray (1941), *Arch. Int. Med.*, **67**, 819.
Hendrick, J. C., and P. Franchimont (1974), *Europ. J. Cancer*, **10**, 725.
Henry, R. J., S. Berkman, M. S. Little, and R. J. Winzler (1951), *J. Amer. Med. Assoc.*, **147**, 37.
Hill, B. R., and C. Levi (1954), *Cancer Res.*, **14**, 513.
Hirszfeld, L., W. Halber, and J. Rosenblat (1932), *Z. Immunitätsforsch.*, **75**, 209.
Hock, E., and R. N. Tessier (1949), *J. Urol.*, **62**, 488.
Hoffman, R. L., and J. W. Merritt (1965), *Amer. J. Obstet. Gynec.*, **92**, 650.
Horne, C. H. W., H. Bohn, A. L. C. McLay, E. H. Wood, and W. D. Thompson (1975), *Behring Inst. Mitt.*, **58**, 50.
Horne, C. H. W., I. N. Reid, and G. D. Milne (1976), *Lancet*, **ii**, 279.
Hulanicka, K., R. Arend, and M. Orlowski (1963), *Arch. Neurol.*, **8**, 194.
Hull, E. P., P. P. Carbone, C. G. Moertel, and G. T. O'Conor (1970), *Lancet*, **i**, 779.
Israels, L. G., and G. E. Delory (1956), *Brit. J. Cancer*, **10**, 318.
Kasdon, S. C. (1956), in *The Laboratory Diagnosis of Cancer of the Cervix* (Eds. F. Homburger and W. H. Fishman), Karger, Basel, p. 59.
Keiser, H. R., C. L. Vogel, and F. Sadikali (1972), *J. Nat. Cancer. Inst.*, **49**, 1251.
Kelley, V. C., R. A. Good, and I. M'Quarrie (1950), *Pediatrics*, **5**, 824.
Kelley, V. C., F. H. Adams, and R. A. Good (1953), *Pediatrics*, **12**, 607.
Kessel, D., and J. Allen (1975), *Cancer Res.*, **35**, 670.
Keyser, J. W. (1952), *J. Clin. Path.*, **5**, 194.
Keyser, J. W. (1954), *Brit. J. Cancer*, **8**, 238.
Keyser, J. W., and A. M. Ward (1977), *Lancet*, **i**, 258.
Keyser, J. W., R. B. Payne, and B. T. Stephens (1962), *Clin. Chem.*, **8**, 270.
Kohn, J. (1976), in *Protides of the Biological Fluids: Proceedings of 24th Colloquium, Bruges, 1976* (Ed. H. Peeters), Pergamon Press, Oxford, p. 377.
Kohn, J., and P. C. Weaver (1974), *Lancet*, **ii**, 334.
Kohn, J., A. H. Orr, T. J. McElwain, M. Bentall, and M. J. Peckham (1976), *Lancet*, **ii**, 433.
Kowlessar, O. D., L. J. Haeffner, E. M. Riley, and M. H. Sleisenger (1961), *Amer. J. Med.*, **31**, 231.
Kresno, S. B., R. Gandasoebrata, and P. Rümke (1970), *Lancet*, **i**, 1178.

Kuo, T. T., J. Rosai, and T. W. Tillack (1973), *Int. J. Cancer*, **12**, 532.
Kutscher, W., and A. Wörner (1936), *Z. physiol. Chem.*, **239**, 109.
Lancet (1976), **i**, 522.
Langvad, E. (1968a), *Int. J. Cancer*, **3**, 17.
Langvad, E. (1968b), *Europ. J. Cancer*, **4**, 107.
Latner, A. L., D. M. Turner, and S. A. Way (1966), *Lancet*, **ii**, 814.
Laurence, D. J. R., and A. M. Neville (1972), *Brit. J. Cancer*, **26**, 335.
Laurence, D. J. R., U. Stevens, R. Bettelheim, D. Darcy, C. Leese, C. Turberville, P Alexander, E. W. Johns, and A. M. Neville (1972), *Brit. Med. J.*, **iii**, 605.
Lawson, J. G. (1969), in *Proceedings of World Conference on Cancer of the Uterus*, Amer. Cancer Soc., New Orleans, p. 116.
Lawson, J. G., and D. K. Watkins (1965), *J. Obstet. Gynaec. Brit. Commonw.*, **72**, 1.
Lebherz, H. G., and W. J. Rutter (1969), *Biochemistry*, **8**, 109.
Lewkonia, R. M., E. J. L. Kerr, and W. J. Irvine (1974), *Brit. J. Cancer*, **30**, 532.
Liddle, G. W., W. E. Nicholson, D. P. Island, D. N. Orth, K. Abe, and S. C. Lowder (1969), *Rec. Progr. Hormone Res.*, **25**, 283.
Lipsett, M. B. (1968), *Adv. Metab. Disorders*, **3**, 111.
Lockey, E., A. J. Anderson, and N. F. Maclagan (1956), *Brit. J. Cancer*, **10**, 209.
Longnecker, D. S., and C. A. White (1965), *Amer. J. Obstet. Gynec.*, **93**, 1088.
Lustig, B., and A. Langer (1931), *Biochem. Z.*, **272**, 320.
Macbeth, R. A. L., and J. G. Bekesi (1962a), *Cancer Res.*, **22**, 244.
Macbeth, R. A. L., and J. G. Bekesi (1972b), *Cancer Res.*, **22**, 1170.
Mach, J.-P., and G. Pusztaszeri (1972), *Immunochemistry*, **9**, 1031.
Martin, F. (1974), cited by Neville and Cooper (1976).
Masopust, J., K. Kithier, J. Rádl, J. Koutecký, and L. Kotál (1968), *Int. J. Cancer*, **3**, 364.
McGee, J. O'D., J. Baillie, M. S. Al Adnani, and R. S. Patrick (1975), *Proc. Path. Soc. G. B. and Ireland* (July), p. 20. (Cited by Neville and Cooper, 1976.)
McIntire, K. R., and P. P. Sizaret (1974), *Abstr. 11th Int. Cancer Congress*, **1**, 295.
McIntire, K. R., C. L. Vogel, G. L. Princler, and I. R. Patel (1972), *Cancer Res.*, **32**, 1941.
Mendelsohn, M. L., and O. Bodansky (1952), *Cancer*, **5**, 1.
Mider, G. B. (1951), *Cancer Res.*, **11**, 821.
Mider, G. B., E. L. Alling, and J. J. Morton (1950), *Cancer*, **3**, 56.
Milsom, D. W., F. A. Rose, and K. S. Dodgson (1968), *Biochem. J.*, **109**, 40P.
Morgan, L. R., M. S. Samuels, W. Thomas, E. T. Krementz, and W. Meeker (1975), *Cancer*, **36**, 2337.
Mueller, J. (1889), *Z. klin. Med.*, **16**, 496.
Mueller, W. K., R. Handschumacher, and M. E. Wade (1971), *Obstet. Gynec.*, **38**, 427.
Nakayama, T., M. Yoshida, and M. Kitamura (1970), *Clin. Chim. Acta*, **30**, 546.
Nathanson, L., and W. H. Fishman (1971), *Cancer*, **27**, 1388.
Nerdrum, H. J. (1964), *Scandinav. J. Clin. Lab. Invest.*, **16**, 565.
Neville, A. M., and E. C. Cooper (1976), *Ann. Clin. Biochem.*, **13**, 283.
Newlands, E. S., J. Dent, A. Kardana, F. Searle, and K. D. Bagshawe (1976), *Lancet*, **ii**, 744.
Nishioka, M., T. Ibata, K. Okita, T. Harada, and T. Fujita (1972), *Cancer Res.*, **32**, 162.
O'Conor, G. T., Y. S. Tatarinov, G. I. Abelev, and J. Uriel (1970), *Cancer*, **25**, 1091.
Ogryzlo, M. A., M. Maclachlan, J. A. Dauphinee, and A. A. Fletcher (1960), *Med. Serv. J., Can.*, **16**, 208.
Okabe, K., T. Hayakawa, M. Hamada, and M. Koike (1968), *Biochemistry*, **7**, 79.
Oliver, J. A., M. M. Elhilali, P. Belitsky, and K. J. MacKinnon (1970), *Cancer*, **25**, 863.
Orłowski, M. (1963), *Arch. Immunol. Ther. Exp.*, **11**, 1.
Osserman, E. F., and D. P. Lawlor (1966), *J. Exp. Med.*, **124**, 921.
Pareira, M. D., E. J. Conrad, W. Hicks, and R. Elman (1955), *Cancer*, **8**, 803.
Pederson, K. O. (1944), *Nature*, **154**, 575.

Perillie, P. E., S. S. Kaplan, E. Lefkowitz, W. Rogaway, and S. C. Finch (1968), *J. Amer. Med. Assoc.*, **203**, 317.
Perumal, A. S., and E. Robins (1973), *Brain Res.*, **59**, 349.
Petermann, M. L., D. A. Karnofsky, and K. R. Hogness (1948), *Cancer*, **1**, 109.
Pfleiderer, G., and E. D. Wachsmuth (1961), *Biochem. Z.*, **334**, 185.
Piscator, M. (1966a), *Arch. Environ. Health*, **12**, 335.
Piscator, M. (1966b), *Arch. Environ. Health*, **12**, 345.
Poznanska-Linde, H., J. H. Wilkinson, and W. A. Withycombe (1966), *Nature*, **209**, 727.
Pritchard, J. A. V., J. L. Moore, W. H. Sutherland, and C. A. Joslin (1973a), *Brit. J. Cancer*, **28**, Suppl. 1., p. 229.
Pritchard, J. A. V., J. L. Moore, W. H. Sutherland, and C. A. F. Joslin (1973b), *Brit. J. Cancer*, **27**, 1.
Pritchard, J. A. V., W. H. Sutherland, and T. J. Deeley (1976), *Lancet*, **i**, 637.
Purves, L. R., M. MacNab, E. W. Geddes, and I. Bersohn (1968), *Lancet*, **i**, 921.
Purves, L. R., I. Bersohn, and E. W. Geddes (1970), *Cancer*, **25**, 1261.
Ratcliffe, J. G., and L. H. Rees (1974), *Brit. J. Hosp. Med.*, 685.
Rees, L. H. (1975), *J. Endocrin.*, **67**, 143.
Rees, L. H., and J. G. Ratcliffe (1974), *Clin. Endocrin.*, **3**, 263.
Reynolds, R. D., B. R. Greenberg, N. D. Martin, R. N. Lucas, C. N. Gaffney, and L. Hawn (1973), *Cancer*, **32**, 181.
Rhees, M. C., L. D. Ellerbrook, and S. W. Lippincott (1954), *Amer. J. Clin. Path.*, **24**, 774.
Richterich, R., and A. Burger (1963), *Enzym. biol. clin.*, **3**, 65.
Rimbaut, C. (1973), *Bull. Cancer*, **60**, 411.
Roberts, J., J. W. Keyser, and M. Baum (1975), *Brit. J. Surg.*, **62**, 816.
Rosalki, S. B., P. Tarlow, and D. Raw (1971), *Lancet*, **ii**, 376.
Rosato, F. E., M. Seltzer, J. Mullen, and E. F. Rosato (1971), *Cancer*, **28**, 1575.
Rose, A., M. West, and H. J. Zimmerman (1961), *Cancer*, **14**, 726.
Rosen, S. W., B. D. Weintraub, J. L. Vaitukaitis, H. H. Sussman, J. M. Hershman, and F. M. Muggia (1975), *Ann. Int. Med.*, **82**, 71.
Rümke, Ph., D. Visser, H. G. Kwa, and A. A. M. Hart (1971), *Folia Med. Neerl.*, **14**, 156.
Ruoslahti, E., M. Seppälä, P. Vuopio, E. Saksela, and P. Peltokallio (1972), *J. Nat. Cancer Inst.*, **49**, 623.
Rutenberg, A. M., J. A. Goldbarg, and E. P. Pineda (1958), *New Engl. J. Med.*, **259**, 469.
Rutenberg, A. M., J. A. Goldbarg, and E. Pineda (1963), *Gastroenterology*, **45**, 43.
Sabolović, D., N. Sabolović, A. Moutte, S. Leibovici, B. Sauvezie, P. Chollet, and R. Plagne (1975), *Brit. J. Cancer*, **32**, 28.
Sankalé, M., R. Masseyeff, R. Camain, C. Quénum, J.-P. Ancelle, and L. LeBlanc (1968), *Presse méd.*, **76**, 2047.
Sato, S., T. Sugimura, T. C. Chien, and K. Takakura (1971), *Cancer*, **27**, 223.
Schapira, G., J. C. Dreyfus, F. Schapira, and J. Kruh (1955), *Amer. J. Phys. Med.*, **34**, 313.
Schwartz, M. A., M. West, W. S. Walsh, and H. J. Zimmerman (1962a), *Cancer*, **15**, 346.
Schwartz, M. A., W. S. Walsh, N. M. West, and H. J. Zimmerman (1962b), *Cancer*, **15**, 927.
Schwartz, M. K. (1973), *Clin. Chem.*, **19**, 10.
Schwartz, M. K. (1977), *Ann. Clin. Lab. Sci.*, **7**, 99.
Schwartz, M. K., and O. Bodansky (1965), *Cancer*, **18**, 886.
Searle, F., B. A. Leake, K. D. Bagshawe, and J. Dent (1978), *Lancet*, **i**, 579.
Sega, E., P. G. Natali, C. Ricci, C. T. Mineo, and G. Citro (1974), *IRCS (Research on: Cancer; Immunology and Allergy; Respiratory System; Surgery and Transplantation)*, **2**, 1278.
Seibert, F. B., M. V. Seibert, A. J. Atno, and H. W. Campbell (1947), *J. Clin. Invest.*, **26**, 90.
Sellinger, O., and R. A. Hiatt (1968), *Brain Res.*, **7**, 191.

Seppälä, M., E.-M. Rutanen, M. Heikinheimo, H. Jalanko, and E. Engvall (1978), *Int. J. Cancer*, **21**, 265.
Shay, H., and H. Siplet (1954), *J. Lab. Clin. Med.*, **43**, 741.
Shetlar, M. R., J. V. Foster, K. H. Kelley, C. L. Shetlar, R. S. Bryan, and M. R. Everett (1949), *Cancer Res.*, **9**, 515.
Shetlar, M. R., R. W. Payne, J. A. Bullock, D. R. Patrick, A. A. Hellbaum, and W. K. Ishmael (1953), *J. Clin. Invest.*, **32**, 1208.
Sibley, J. A., and A. L. Lehninger (1948), *J. Nat. Cancer Inst.*, **9**, 303.
Simkin, B., H. C. Bergman, and M. Prinzmetal (1949), *Amer. J. Med.*, **6**, 734.
Smith, J. B. (1970), *Med. Clin. N. America*, **54**, 797.
Smith, J. B., and D. Todd (1968), *Lancet*, **ii**, 833.
Snyder, S., and G. Ashwell (1971), *Clin. Chim. Acta*, **34**, 449.
Spencer-Peet, J., D. Wood, and M. M. Glatt (1972), *Lancet*, **i**, 1122.
Stagg, B. H., and G. A. Whyley (1968), *Clin. Chim. Acta*, **22**, 521.
Starkweather, W. H., R. A. Green, H. H. Spencer, and H. K. Schoch (1966), *J. Lab. Clin. Med.*, **68**, 314.
Steele, L., E. H. Cooper, A. M. Mackay, M. S. Losowsky, and J. C. Goligher (1974), *Brit. J. Cancer*, **30**, 319.
Stimson, W. H. (1972), *Lancet*, **i**, 684.
Stimson, W. H. (1975a), *Lancet*, **i**, 777.
Stimson, W. H. (1975b), *J. Clin. Path.*, **28**, 868.
Stolbach, L. L., M. J. Krant, and W. H. Fishman (1969), *New Engl. J. Med.*, **281**, 757.
Stonehill, E. H., and A. Bendich (1970), *Nature*, **228**, 370.
Suga, S., and Z. Tamura (1972), *Cancer Res.*, **32**, 426.
Sullivan, T. J., E. B. Gutman, and A. B. Gutman (1942), *J. Urol.*, **48**, 426.
Sussman, H. H., B. D. Weintraub, and S. W. Rosen (1974), *Cancer*, **33**, 820.
Szczeklik, E., M. Orłowski, and A. Szewczuk (1961), *Gastroenterology*, **41**, 353.
Szewczuk, A., and M. Orłowski (1960), *Clin. Chim. Acta*, **5**, 680.
Takahashi, A., A. Yachi, T. Anzai, and T. Wada (1967), *Clin. Chim. Acta*, **17**, 5.
Tal, C., and M. Halperin (1970), *Israel J. Med. Sci.*, **6**, 708.
Tan, C. O., J. Cohen, M. West, and H. J. Zimmerman (1963), *Cancer*, **16**, 1373.
Tatarinov, Y. S. (1963), in *Proceedings of the 45th Scientific Session, Astrakhan Medical Institute*, p. 31.
Tatarinov, Y. S. (1964), *Vopros. Med. Khim.*, **1**, 90.
Tatarinov, Y. S. (1965), *Vopros. Med. Khim.* **11**, 20 (see *Fed. Proc.*, 1966, **25**, T344).
Tatarinov, Y. S., D. M. Falalleva, and V. V. Kalashnikov (1976), *Int. J. Cancer*, **17**, 626.
Terepka, A. R., and C. Waterhouse (1956), *Amer. J. Med.*, **20**, 225.
Thompson, H. G., Jr., E. Hirschberg, M. Osnos, and A. Gellhorn (1959), *Neurology*, **9**, 545.
Thomson, D. M. P., J. Krupey, S. O. Freedman, and P. Gold (1969), *Proc. Nat. Acad. Sci.* **64**, 161.
Tormey, D. C., T. P. Waalkes, D. Ahmann, C. W. Gehrke, R. W. Zumwatt, J. Snyder, and H. Hansen (1975), *Cancer*, **35**, 1095.
Tsou, K. C., M. G. McCoy, and K. W. Lo (1974), *Cancer Res.*, **34**, 2459.
Tsunematsu, K., and T. Shiraishi (1969), *Cancer*, **24**, 637.
Tuchman, L. R., H. Suna, and J. J. Carr (1956), *J. Mt. Sinai Hosp., New York*, **23**, 227.
Turberville, C., D. A. Darcy, D. J. R. Laurence, E. W. Johns, and A. M. Neville (1973), *Immunochemistry*, **10**, 841.
Turner, G. C., F. Schaffner, D. E. Eshbaugh, and J. de la Huerga (1953), *Dis. Chest*, **23**, 154.
Uriel, J., B. de Nechaud, M. S. Birencwajg, R. Masseyeff, L. Leblanc, C. Quenum, F. Loisillier, and P. Grabar (1967), *Compt. rend. Acad. Sci.*, Series D, **265**, 75.
von Kleist, S., G. Chavanel, and P. Burtin (1972), *Proc. Nat. Acad. Sci.*, **69**, 2492.
Wada, T., T. Anzai, A. Yachi, A. Takahashi, and S. Sakamoto (1971), in *Protides of the*

Biological Fluids: Proceedings of 18th Colloquium, Bruges, 1970 (Ed. H. Peeters), Pergamon Press, Oxford, p. 221.
Wallersteiner, E. (1914), *Deut. Arch. klin. Med.*, **116**, 145.
Wang, D. Y. (1976), *Protides of the Biological Fluids: Proceedings of 24th Colloquium, Bruges, 1976* (Ed. H. Peeters), Pergamon Press, Oxford, p. 481.
Warburg, O. (1930), *The Metabolism of Tumours*, Constable, London.
Warburg, O., and W. Christian (1943), *Biochem. Z.*, **314**, 399.
Warburg, O., F. Wind, and E. Negelein (1926), *Klin. Woch.*, **5**, 829.
Warnock, M. L., and R. Reisman (1969), *Clin. Chim. Acta*, **24**, 5.
Waterhouse, C., L. D. Fenninger, and E. H. Keutmann (1951), *Cancer*, **4**, 500.
Weiss, M. J., H. A. Edmondson, and M. Wertman (1951), *Amer. J. Clin. Path.*, **21**, 1057.
West, M., D. Gelb, C. G. Pilz, and H. J. Zimmerman (1961), *Amer. J. Med. Sci.*, **241**, 350.
West, M., M. A. Schwartz, W. S. Walsh, and H. J. Zimmerman (1962), *Cancer*, **15**, 931.
Whitmore, W. F., Jr., O. Bodansky, M. K. Schwartz, S. H. Ying, and E. Day (1956), *Cancer*, **9**, 228.
Wiernik, P. H., and A. A. Serpick (1969), *Amer. J. Med.*, **46**, 330.
Winzler, R. J., and I. M. Smyth (1948), *J. Clin. Invest.*, **27**, 617.
Woodard, H. Q. (1952), *Cancer*, **5**, 236.
Woodard, H. Q., and A. L. Dean (1947), *J. Urol.*, **57**, 158.
Yachi, A., Y. Matsuura, C. M. Carpenter, and L. Hyde (1968), *J. Nat. Cancer Inst.*, **40**, 663.
Yarrison, G., B. F. Mertens, and J. C. Mathues (1976), *Amer. J. Clin. Path.*, **66**, 667.
Yoshioka, N., K. Takahashi, T. Oshima, and T. Watanabe (1977), *Tohoku J. Exp. Med.*, **122**, 383.
Zein, M., and G. Discombe (1970), *Lancet*, **ii**, 748.
Zucker, M. B., and H. Q. Woodard (1962), *J. Lab. Clin. Med.*, **59**, 760.

CHAPTER 10

Neurological diseases

Many groups of workers have studied the proteins of the cerebrospinal fluid in a search for abnormalities that would help in the differential diagnosis of neurological disorders. For some years a simple estimation of the total protein concentration, together with a test for excess of globulin and perhaps a Lange colloidal gold test*, were the only available investigations of the protein constituents of the fluid. More recently electrophoretic and immunoelectrophoretic techniques have made possible a more refined analysis of the composition of the cerebrospinal fluid protein, and have made a limited contribution to diagnosis.

Total protein

Most investigations of the cerebrospinal fluid have been made on specimens obtained by lumbar puncture. Reported normal ranges for total protein have varied quite considerably, not only according to the method of estimation used but also between different laboratories using the same method. Laterre (1965) and Lumsden (1972) have reviewed many of the available methods.

Increases in the protein concentration occur if the fluid stagnates as a result of a blockage in the spinal subarachnoid space, and very high concentrations, up to 20 or 30 g/l, may be attained in these circumstances. This may happen in cases of spinal tumour, fractures of the vertebrae, spinal tuberculosis, chronic meningitis, and other less common conditions. Intracranial tumours and acute infections of the meninges or central nervous system, whether due to bacteria, rickettsia, or viruses, are also associated with increased concentrations of protein. Probably more than half the patients with multiple sclerosis, irrespective of the stage and severity of the disease, have a slightly elevated concentration of protein in the cerebrospinal fluid (Lumsden, 1972).

Lower concentrations of protein are normally found in cisternal fluid, and still lower concentrations in ventricular fluid.

COMPOSITION OF CEREBROSPINAL FLUID PROTEIN

Electrophoretic analysis of normal lumbar cerebrospinal fluid, using agar gel or cellulose acetate, shows an overall resemblance to serum, except for

*The well-known Lange collodial gold test depends on an increase in the γ-globulin concentration in the cerebrospinal fluid. Typical patterns of precipitation of the gold sol have been thought to be associated with particular neurological diseases. However, opinion is divided as to the value of the test in clinical diagnosis, and it is being increasingly replaced by specific immunochemical determinations of the immunoglobulins.

certain differences, notably a more conspicuous prealbumin fraction, a fraction ('tau') moving between the β- and γ-globulins, and a proportionately lower γ-globulin content. These and other differences are discussed by Schultze and Heremans (1966).

By the use of antisera raised against normal human plasma proteins it has been demonstrated that many of the proteins in the cerebrospinal fluid are immunologically identical with those in plasma. Plasma proteins of high molecular weight are normally absent or almost absent from the cerebrospinal fluid. A number of proteins that are apparently specific for cerebrospinal fluid have been reported (Clausen, 1961; MacPherson and Cosgrove, 1961; Hochwald and Thorbecke, 1962; Link, 1965; and others); however, for the demonstration of such trace proteins it is necessary to concentrate the fluid to an extent which cannot be achieved with plasma, and it may well be that these trace proteins are present in plasma and indeed throughout the extracellular fluids (Schultze and Heremans, 1966).

PATTERNS OF CEREBROSPINAL FLUID PROTEINS IN DISEASE

A variety of protein patterns are seen in the cerebrospinal fluid in disease. According to Schultze and Heremans (1966) these can be classified in four groups:

1. the pattern of increased admixture of plasma proteins;
2. patterns reflecting changes in the plasma proteins;
3. the pattern of local production of immunoglobulin; and
4. degenerative patterns.

Increased admixture of plasma proteins

This is found in conditions associated with inflammatory changes or processes, such as meningitis and chronic meningoencephalitis, as well as in the presence of intracranial malignancies and in cerebrovascular diseases. This pattern, together with the next, would appear to correspond with the 'transudative' type described by Laterre (1965).

Changes in the plasma proteins

The protein pattern of the cerebrospinal fluid is affected by changes in the plasma proteins, even if no increased admixture of the latter occurs. The most striking example is found in the paraproteinaemias, in which numerous investigators have reported the presence, in the cerebrospinal fluid, of paraprotein bands similar to those in the blood serum. In cirrhosis and in the nephrotic syndrome, also, changes in the plasma proteins are reflected in the cerebrospinal fluid. Since such changes in the cerebrospinal fluid occur even in the absence of neurological disease, it is important not to interpret an electrophoretic pattern of the cerebrospinal fluid proteins without first comparing it with the patient's serum protein pattern.

Local immunoglobulin production

A more or less isolated increase in the γ-globulin fraction of the cerebrospinal fluid has been reported in a variety of conditions, including chronic and subacute infections of the central nervous system, multiple sclerosis, subacute panencephalitis, and a number of other neurological diseases. The abnormalities of the γ-globulin fraction are both quantitative and qualitative, the increased γ-globulin usually being found to differ in composition from the normal. For example, the presence of IgM has frequently been recorded; and, secondly, there often appears to be a selective increase in the faster-moving 7S γ-globulins (Dencker, 1964). The local production of immunoglobulins is discussed below (see p. 200).

A number of investigators have shown that the essential feature of the electrophoretic γ-globulin pattern of the cerebrospinal fluid of patients with multiple sclerosis and other inflammatory diseases of the central nervous system is a 'restricted heterogeneity distribution', shown by the appearance of striations and discrete bands within the diffuse γ-globulin area (Lowenthal *et al.*, 1960; Laterre *et al.*, 1962; Lowenthal, 1965; Laterre, 1965, 1966; Link, 1967). In a series of more than 2000 cases, Laterre and his colleagues (1970) found this electrophoretic pattern in some 75 to 87 per cent of multiple sclerosis patients, depending upon the diagnostic category ('possible', 'probable', or 'definite'). Link and Müller (1971) found agar-gel electrophoresis to be the most valuable cerebrospinal fluid investigation for establishing the diagnosis of multiple sclerosis, oligoclonal IgG bands being found in 94 per cent of their cases.

It is not to be inferred that the pattern of discrete bands of oligoclonal IgG is found only in multiple sclerosis: it was noted in 39 per cent of patients with infections of the central nervous system and in 3 per cent of patients with other neurological disorders (Link and Müller, 1971). This last group excluded patients with the Guillain–Barré syndrome, in which a separate study demonstrated the presence of two such bands in five of 12 patients (Link, 1973). In subacute sclerosing panencephalitis these bands were found in all of the eight cases investigated (Link *et al.*, 1973).

More recently the use of isoelectric focusing has confirmed the presence of these bands in more than 90 per cent of patients with multiple sclerosis (Delmotte and Gonsette, 1977; Trotter *et al.*, 1977).

'Degenerative' patterns

Certain proteins of the cerebrospinal fluid, notably transferrin and haemopexin, may occur in more than one electrophoretic position. For example, part of the transferrin (the so called 'tau' fraction) may have an abnormally slow electrophoretic mobility and migrate behind the β_1-position; and haemopexin, which normally migrates slightly faster than transferrin, may be retarded to an even greater extent. The result of these changes is to leave the β_1-globulin area of the electrophoretic pattern largely depleted of proteins. Patterns of this sort are found, in a proportion of patients, in a variety of degenerative disorders of the central nervous system involving progressive damage to nervous tissue—cerebral and cerebellar atrophy, spasmodic paraplegia, motor-neurone disease, syringomyelia, and the neurological syndromes associated with chronic anaemias, etc. Such degenerative patterns are, however, rarely seen in multiple sclerosis (Laterre *et al.*, 1962).

The changes in electrophoretic mobility are apparently consistent with the occurrence of enzymic breakdown of normal cerebrospinal fluid proteins (Laterre, 1965), though the possibility of a dual origin for the transferrin has been suggested (Frick and Scheid-Seydel, 1960, 1963; Parker and Bearn, 1962; Frick, 1963), whereby the β_1-transferrin could be derived from the plasma and the tau transferrin synthesized locally in the central nervous system.

GLOBULINS OF THE CEREBROSPINAL FLUID

Interest in the protein fractions of the cerebrospinal fluid was stimulated by the work of Kabat and his coworkers (1942). By the use of the Tiselius electrophoresis method they found that the γ-globulin concentration was increased in some patients with multiple sclerosis or neurosyphilis. Their findings have largely been confirmed by many workers—including Kabat's own group—using varied techniques: paper and gel electrophoresis, immunoelectrophoresis, chemical precipitation, immunoprecipitation, and electroimmunodiffusion (see Riddoch and Thompson (1970) for references).

In addition to neurosyphilis and multiple sclerosis, most investigators have found that some patients with other neurological diseases have a raised concentration of γ-globulin in the cerebrospinal fluid. From the work of Kabat and his associates (1948), Schneck and Claman (1969), and others, it would seem that while many conditions may be associated with larger increases in the γ-globulin concentration, in multiple sclerosis increases usually occur in this fraction even when the total protein concentration is within the normal range (Table 10.1). Although Riddoch and Thompson (1970) found higher than usual values of IgG in a variety of disorders, the rise tended to be small and was more common when the concentration of total protein exceeded 1 g/l. In their experience, conditions likely to be confused clinically with multiple sclerosis showed uniformly normal concentrations of IgG.

IgM was not detected in 'normal' cerebrospinal fluid, even (in some cases) after tenfold concentration, by several groups of workers (Dencker, 1964; Bauer and Gottesleben, 1969; Riddoch and Thompson, 1970; Smith *et al.*, 1973), but it has been shown to occur in cerebrospinal fluid from some patients with multiple sclerosis (Bauer and Gottesleben, 1969; Schneck and Claman, 1969; Riddoch and Thompson, 1970; Schuller *et al.*, 1972); however, it is also found in infections and in the presence of cerebrovascular disease. Its presence or absence appears to be of no diagnostic value (Laterre *et al.*, 1962; Schneck and Claman, 1969; Riddoch and Thompson, 1970).

IgA in the cerebrospinal fluid has been measured in many neurological conditions. Riddoch and Thompson (1970) could detect it only when the total

Table 10.1. Elevation in c.s.f. IgG concentration in various diseases. (After S. A. Schneck and H. N. Claman, *Arch. Neurol.*, 1969, **20**, 132, with permission. Copyright 1969, American Medical Association.)

	Multiple sclerosis		Other demyelinating diseases		Optic and retrobulbar neuritis	
	no. of fluids	no. with ↑ IgG	no. of fluids	no. with ↑ IgG	no. of fluids	no. with ↑ IgG
Entire group	54	30 (55.6%)	8	1 (12.5%)	5	1 (20%)
With normal total protein	35	25 (71.4%)	5	1 (20%)	3	1 (33.3%)
With raised total protein	19	5 (26.3%)	0	0	0	0
	Landry–Guillain–Barré syndrome		Neurosyphilis		Miscellaneous	
	no. of fluids	no. with ↑ IgG	no. of fluids	no. with ↑ IgG	no. of fluids	no. with ↑ IgG
Entire group	4	2 (50%)	5	3 (60%)	118	15 (12.7%)
With normal total protein	0	0	3	2 (66.7%)	85	12 (14.1%)
With raised total protein	4	2 (50%)	2	1 (50%)	33	3 (9%)

protein concentration was 400 mg/l or higher; in agreement with Laterre and his coworkers (1962) and Schneck and Claman (1969), its presence or absence was not found to be of any diagnostic value.

Although Riddoch and Thompson were unable to detect *IgD* in the cerebrospinal fluid of patients with various neurological disorders, its presence has been reported by Tavolato and De Zanche (1968) in many patients with neurological disease, whereas in normal subjects it was either undetectable or present only in trace amounts.

Synthesis of IgG and IgA within the central nervous system

The finding that the γ-globulin: albumin ratio of cerebrospinal fluid is, on average, more increased than that of serum in a number of neurological diseases (including neurosyphilis, multiple sclerosis, and subacute sclerosing panencephalitis) suggests that some formation of γ-globulin can occur within the tissues of the central nervous system, since it seems unlikely that an alteration in the permeability of the blood–central nervous system barrier that would allow an increase in the concentration of γ-globulin would not also allow a similar or even greater increase in that of albumin. Speculations that γ-globulin can be synthesized in the central nervous system have been supported by experiments in which radioactively-labelled albumin and IgG have been used to trace the exchange between blood, cerebrospinal fluid, and the central nervous system (Frick and Scheid-Seydel, 1958; Lippincott *et al.*, 1965; Hochwald and Wallenstein, 1967a,b; Cutler *et al.*, 1970). This work is too extensive to be described here, and the reader is referred to the review by Tourtellotte (1970).

In addition to the dynamic studies referred to above, evidence of the synthesis of IgG and IgA by the leucocytes of the cerebrospinal fluid has been presented. Experiments in which mononuclear cells of the cerebrospinal fluid from a patient with multiple sclerosis were incubated *in vitro* with ^{3}H-L-leucine, and the immunoglobulins isolated by specific immune precipitation, have demonstrated that these cells can synthesize IgG and IgA, but not IgM (Cohen and Bannister, 1967). Serial studies of a patient with multiple sclerosis have confirmed the synthesis of IgG by mononuclear cells of the cerebrospinal fluid and have shown that the rate of synthesis was significantly higher during a relapse than during remissions (Sandberg-Wollheim *et al.*, 1969).

In spite of these observations, it is clear that in a small percentage of multiple sclerosis patients there is no significant increase in the concentration of IgG in the cerebrospinal fluid. Although, clinically, there appear to be no consistent differences between multiple sclerosis patients with and without an elevated concentration of IgG, the suggestion has been made that further studies might indicate that not all cases of multiple sclerosis have the same aetiology (Lamoureux *et al.*, 1975). In this connexion it may be significant that treatment of multiple sclerosis with adrenocorticotrophic hormone and antilymphocytic serum was reported to be effective only in those patients who had a raised cerebrospinal fluid γ-globulin/total protein ratio (Seland *et al.*, 1974).

To return to the question of local production of IgM within the central nervous system, it is interesting to note that a case has been described of a late-onset type of immunodeficiency with chronic progressive encephalopathy, in which IgM was not detected in the patient's serum but was nevertheless demonstrable in the cerebrospinal fluid. Other high molecular weight serum proteins, such as α_2-macroglobulin and fibrinogen, were absent from the cerebrospinal fluid, and it appears that the IgM may have been produced by lymphoid cells in the brain (Lord *et al.*, 1973). The IgM present in the cerebrospinal fluid appeared to be similar to the normally occurring polymeric form.

Immunoglobulin production within the central nervous system may be indirectly assessed by measuring the concentration in the cerebrospinal fluid, and applying a correction to allow for the permeability of the blood–cerebrospinal fluid barrier in order to account for immunoglobulin derived from the plasma in the normal way. Since it has been shown that the permeability of this barrier is reflected by the cerebrospinal fluid total protein or albumin concentration (Tourtellotte, 1970; and others), most investigators have related the actual concentration of immunoglobulin to the total protein or albumin: if the derived relative concentration of immunoglobulin ('immunoglobulin quotient') is raised, this is taken to indicate local synthesis within the central nervous system.

To allow for the influence of the plasma proteins several workers (Delpech and Lichtblau, 1972; Laterre, 1975) proposed expressing the concentration of IgG in the spinal fluid as a ratio or index that takes account also of the concentration of IgG in the plasma and of that of albumin in both fluids, *viz.*

$$\frac{\text{spinal fluid IgG/albumin}}{\text{plasma IgG/albumin}}.$$

The superiority of this index over the other IgG ratios proposed, both for demonstrating an increase of IgG concentration in the spinal fluid due to synthesis within the central nervous system and for distinguishing patients with multiple sclerosis from those with other neurological disorders, has been confirmed by other workers (Roberts-Thomson *et al.*, 1976; Link and Tibbling, 1977).

Tourtellotte (1970) has devised a means of calculating the quantity of IgG synthesized per day by the central nervous system in patients with multiple sclerosis. The principle of the method is that an excess of albumin in the cerebrospinal fluid is a quantitative marker of a damaged blood–central nervous system–cerebrospinal fluid barrier; it is assumed that for each milligram of excess albumin that passes the damaged barrier from the blood, a proportional amount of IgG accompanies it. After determining the excess of IgG in the cerebrospinal fluid and correcting it for the amount derived from the blood, one arrives at a value which, if it exceeds zero, reflects the synthesis of IgG in the central nervous system. On the assumption that 500 ml of fluid is formed and absorbed each day, the amount of IgG synthesized can be calculated. Tourtellotte obtained figures of 0–100 mg (average 16 mg) for the daily synthesis of IgG by the central nervous system in a series of 55 patients with multiple sclerosis.

Another approach is that of Felgenhauer and his colleagues (1976), who utilize the serum/cerebrospinal fluid concentration ratios of three proteins of widely differing size—*viz.* albumin, caeruloplasmin, and α_2-macroglobulin—for evaluating the permeability of the blood–cerebrospinal fluid barrier.

Local synthesis of other proteins

There is evidence that certain other proteins (prealbumin, transferrin, β-trace protein and γ-trace protein) may be synthesized within the central nervous system, since their concentration in the cerebrospinal fluid is considerably greater than would be expected on the basis of their molecular weights and concentration in the serum (Link *et al.*, 1972).

Other protein ratios

The finding of an increased concentration of γ-globulin in the cerebrospinal fluid in some patients in conditions other than multiple sclerosis, and the fact that it is not shown by all patients with this disease, has led to attempts to find other diagnostically useful measurements. Of these, one of the most promising appears to be the ratio of the β- and γ-globulins of the cerebrospinal fluid as determined by agar-gel electrophoresis. This ratio (i.e. β-/γ-globulin) was found to be decreased in 93 per cent of a series of 153 patients with multiple sclerosis, and the decrease seemed to parallel the severity, progression, and acuteness of the disease process (Cosgrove and Agius, 1966). The decrease in the ratio was found more frequently, in multiple sclerosis, than either elevation of the γ-globulin fraction alone or an abnormal Lange colloidal gold curve. Little overlap of values was found with other neurological or non-neurological diseases. In the majority of cases the decrease in the ratio was due to an increase in the γ-globulin fraction, the β-globulin remaining in the low–normal range.

Studies with cerebrospinal fluid in the writer's laboratory, in which a number of specific proteins were measured and the ratios of their concentrations to one another and to the total protein were calculated, revealed only a few measurements of possible diagnostic value (J.M. Fuller *et al.*, unpublished). One ratio (haptoglobin/IgG) showed complete separation of multiple sclerosis from the Guillain–Barré syndrome (ratios 0–1.1 and 2.9–7.0 respectively). Ratios for other pairs of proteins showed greater or less degrees of overlap, but they might occasionally be of diagnostic use.

Kappa/lambda ratio

Abnormal kappa/lambda ratios—usually due to preferential increase in the kappa light-chain subclass—were reported for cerebrospinal fluid (but not serum) in some patients with multiple sclerosis (Link and Zettervall, 1970; Zettervall and Link, 1970). Increases in the ratio in multiple sclerosis have been confirmed by other workers (Bauer *et al.*, 1975; Roberts-Thomson *et al.*, 1976), and have been reported also in neurosyphilis, cysticercosis, subacute sclerosing panencephalitis, and other chronic inflammatory conditions with a high total protein and a pronounced increase in IgG concentration in the cerebrospinal fluid (Bauer *et al.*, 1975). According to Link and Müller (1971), determination of the kappa/lambda ratio may allow differentiation between multiple sclerosis and viral infections of the central nervous system, the ratio being normal in infections.

A further diagnostic aid may be found in the formation of double rings when cerebrospinal fluid from many patients with multiple sclerosis, or subacute sclerosing panencephalitis, is subjected to radial immunodiffusion against antiserum to chains of type kappa (Iwashita *et al.*, 1974). Bollengier and his coworkers (1975) found double ring formation also with lambda light chains in some cases, though these double rings did not appear so clearly as with type kappa. They found that in multiple sclerosis kappa chains predominate, whereas lambda chains predominate in subcute sclerosing panencephalitis.

In more recent investigations Bollengier and his associates (1978) have shown that disturbed kappa/lambda light-chain ratios may be found in a number of neurological conditions, including multiple sclerosis. They conclude that free light chains are an index of 'either hyperimmunization, or strong immunological processes in the central nervous system.'

In short, it would seem that the presence of free light chains in the cerebrospinal fluid is not as strong an indication of multiple sclerosis as was originally thought; it is rather an indication of any chronic form of antigenic stimulation, of which multiple sclerosis is the most common example.

CHANGES IN PROTEIN CONCENTRATIONS DURING THE COURSE OF MULTIPLE SCLEROSIS

Studies have been made of the proteins of the cerebrospinal fluid in patients with multiple sclerosis of the intermittent and chronic types, and in various stages of the disease (Schwartz *et al.*, 1970; Lamoureux *et al.*, 1975). Lamoureux and his coworkers found that in patients in acute relapse there was a significant increase in total protein, γ-globulin, IgG, IgA, IgM, caeruloplasmin and 7S-γ_1-globulin (a fast-moving IgG component), and a significant decrease in prealbumin, α_1-globulin, and α_2-globulin and of the β-/γ-globulin ratio. The concentrations of IgG, IgA, and IgM were often reduced while patients were on steroid treatment or in remission, though they remained significantly higher than in control subjects. During remission, or during treatment with adrenocorticotrophic hormone and/or steroids, the concentrations of caeruloplasmin and 7S-γ_1-globulin were significantly reduced, while the prealbumin, α_1-globulin, α_2-globulin and β-/γ-globulin ratio showed a tendency to return to normal.

POLYACRYLAMIDE-GEL ELECTROPHORESIS OF CEREBROSPINAL FLUID PROTEINS

A number of investigators have examined the proteins of the cerebrospinal fluid by polyacrylamide-gel electrophoresis (Cunningham, 1964; Nakamura, 1964; Weiss *et al.*, 1965; Monseu and Cumings, 1965; Cumings *et al.*, 1970; Takeoka *et al.*, 1976). Takeoka and his coworkers applied disc electrophoresis to a large number of specimens from patients with and without diseases of the nervous system. In all the diseases studied, the percentage of the prealbumin zone (Figure 10.1) was found to be decreased and those of the A_1- and G-zones increased, under the experimental conditions employed, when the total protein concentration was above normal. In general, the disc electrophoretic patterns of the cerebrospinal fluid tended to resemble those of the plasma proteins in proportion to the increase in the concentration of cerebrospinal fluid total protein. In patients with brain tumours, when the total protein averaged about 1.3 g/l, the mean percentages of the A_2- and B-zones were lowered. In spite of a normal total protein concentration the mean value of the G-zone was found to be increased in patients with multiple sclerosis, brain tumours, or intervertebral disc protrusion. In the latter two disorders there was also an increase in the percentage of the A_1-zone. In the diseases studied, the relative concentration of the Alb- and B_1-zones did not show any significant increase or decrease.

It seems likely that refined electrophoretic analysis of this sort will play an increasing part in diagnosis. However, the high resolution achieved in polyacrylamide-gel electrophoresis reveals genetic differences between healthy subjects, and allowance must be made for these differences when interpreting the patterns obtained in disease.

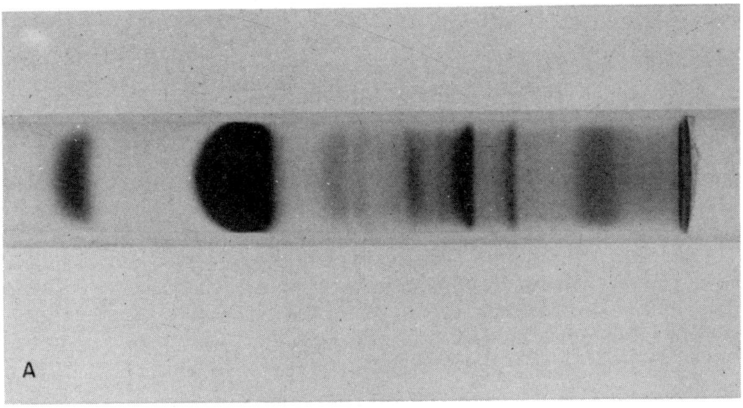

Figure 10.1(A). Normal protein pattern of native cerebrospinal fluid. Disc electrophoresis was performed at 4 °C for approx. 3 h in polyacrylamide gel with 5mM Tris–0.038 M glycine buffer (pH 8.3). The anode is at the left and the cathode at the right. Approx. 200 μg of protein was employed; 2.5 mA per tube was applied. The gel was stained with Amidoschwartz 10B. (Reproduced from T. Takeoka *et al.*, *J. Neurol. Sciences*, 1976, **29**, 213, by permission of Elsevier Scientific Publishing Co., Amsterdam, and the authors.)

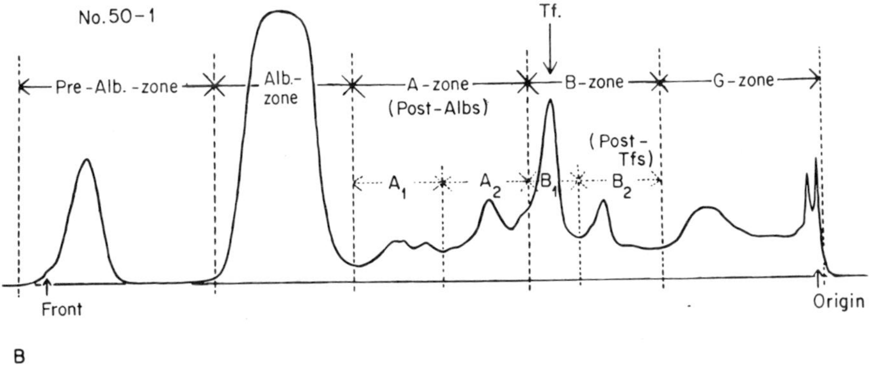

Figure 10.1(B). Densitometric recording of the gel pattern of normal cerebrospinal fluid. Pre-alb = prealbumin; Alb = albumin; Post-albs = post-albumins; Tf = transferrin; Post-Tfs = post-transferrins. (Reproduced from T. Takeoka *et al.*, *J. Neurol. Sciences*, 1976, **29**, 213, by permission of Elsevier Scientific Publishing Co., Amsterdam, and the authors.)

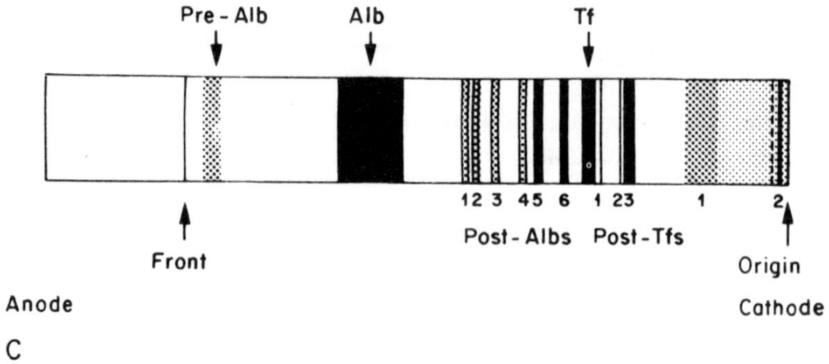

Figure 10.1(C). Schematic representation of the pattern obtained with normal cerebrospinal fluid when subjected to disc acrylamide-gel electrophoresis. For abbreviations see above (B). The globulin zones are not designated as α-, β-, etc., since the positions taken up by the various proteins do not for the most part correspond exactly to those found in conventional paper or cellulose acetate electrophoresis. (Reproduced from T. Takeoka *et al.*, *J. Neurol. Sciences*, 1976, **29**, 213, by permission of Elsevier Scientific Publishing Co., Amsterdam, and the authors.)

ENZYME MEASUREMENTS IN NEUROLOGICAL DISEASES

Owing to the presence of the 'blood–brain barrier', the majority of diseases involving lesions in the central nervous system are not associated with an alteration in serum enzyme activity, and studies of enzymes in neurological diseases have mostly been confined to the cerebrospinal fluid. Of the many enzymes known to be present in the body, only a few have been investigated for their possible value as aids to the diagnosis of neurological disorders, and such observations as have been made do not appear to have proved useful in clinical medicine. Table 10.2 shows some of the enzyme changes that have been report-

Table 10.2. Some of the reported changes in enzyme activity in the cerebrospinal fluid in neurological disorders.

Enzyme	Condition	References
Phosphohexose isomerase	Malignant tumours in brain	Thompson *et al.* (1959); see also p. 185.
Aldolase	Amaurotic family idiocy; Niemann-Pick disease	Aronson *et al.* (1958)
Creatine phosphokinase	Active multiple sclerosis	Culebras and Richards (1969)
Aspartate transaminase	Cerebral infarcts and haemorrhages	Several authors—see Lumsden (1972)

ed. For a detailed discussion of the enzymes and cofactors in the cerebrospinal fluid the reader is referred to the review by Lumsden (1972).

'BRAIN-SPECIFIC (S-100) PROTEIN'

A highly soluble, acidic protein of low molecular weight was first isolated by Moore (1965) from bovine and rabbit brain. The protein, designated S-100 on account of its solubility in saturated ammonium sulphate solution, was detected, by immunological techniques, solely in the nervous system of many species of mammals. It appears to be not a single species but a class of proteins (Stewart, 1972). Haglid and Carlsson (1971) have reported that a protein immunologically identical with the S-100 protein is present in tumours of glial origin but not in tumours originating from non-glial structures.

Williams (1975) isolated an acidic brain-specific protein (S-100) from adult human brain and, by means of a sensitive immunoradiometric assay, showed that it is present in brain tissue at a concentration some thousand times as great as in other organs of the body. The analysis of cerebrospinal fluid and sera from a few patients with various neurological diseases showed that some had raised concentrations of S-100 proteins in the spinal fluid, but further studies will be necessary to establish whether the test is likely to be useful in diagnosis.

OTHER CEREBROSPINAL FLUID PROTEINS IN DIAGNOSIS

Lysozyme is normally absent from the cerebrospinal fluid, but appreciable amounts have been found in fluid from patients with primary and secondary tumours of the central nervous system (Newman *et al.*, 1974). It is also present in the fluid in children with bacterial meningitis, and in many with cerebral convulsions, but is not found in viral meningitis, so determination of this protein would appear to offer an important aid to the differential diagnosis between viral and bacterial meningitis (Gekle *et al.*, 1977).

Children with viral meningitis were found to have, on the average, about twice the concentration of β_2-*microglobulin* in the cerebrospinal fluid as healthy children, but there was considerable overlapping; those with bacterial meningitis usually had even higher concentrations, but these overlapped the range for viral meningitis (Gekle *et al.*, 1977).

An additional aid to the differential diagnosis of meningitis might be found in the high concentration of IgM in the cerebrospinal fluid in the acute phase of purulent meningitis, the mean concentration in acute viral meningitis being much lower (Smith *et al.*, 1973).

LABORATORY EXAMINATION OF CEREBROSPINAL FLUID

Cerebrospinal fluid for protein investigations should, ideally, be collected in three tubes. If the lumbar puncture produced tissue trauma, with rupture of blood vessels, this will be shown by a progressive clearing of the fluid from tubes 1 to 3. Protein tests should be done using the specimen that is least contaminated with red blood cells. It is desirable also to use a specimen taken *before* an air encephalogram, since this procedure leads to considerable variation (perhaps as much as 300–400 mg/l) in the protein concentration, and the variation is not consistently in one direction (Thompson *et al.*, 1975).

A number of methods are available for the estimation of total protein. These are discussed in Appendix 2. Whichever method is used, allowance must be made, in interpreting the result, for the slightly lower range of values found in children and the slightly higher values found in the elderly and in people who have been recumbent for long periods (Thompson *et al.*, 1975).

As indicated above, determination of the cerebrospinal fluid IgG concentration, expressed as a quotient, or of the kappa/lambda ratio, will often be helpful in differential diagnosis. The value of agar-gel electrophoresis has been emphasized by several authors.

PROTEINS IN CEREBRAL-CYST FLUID

The protein electrophoretic pattern of cerebral-cyst fluids has been investigated by several groups of workers. Cumings (1953) found no correlation between the electrophoretic pattern of the serum proteins and those of cerebrospinal and cerebral-cyst fluids, except in the case of cyst fluids associated with cerebellar haemangioblastoma, and cerebrospinal fluids from patients with meningitis and post-operative conditions in which blood had become mixed with the fluid. An excess of globulin migrating in the same position on electrophoresis as serum β-globulin was found in cyst and cerebrospinal fluids from patients with malignant tumours.

Gardner and his coworkers (1963) examined fluid from a number of cystic brain tumours by free-moving-boundary (Tiselius) electrophoresis, supplemented in some cases by starch-gel and immunoelectrophoresis. They found that the proteins of the cyst fluids and sera were composed of a similar number of fractions, usually with similar electrophoretic mobilities and relative concentrations. Ultracentrifugal analysis showed the presence of fractions with flotation rates similar to those of α- and β-lipoproteins of serum. These and other analytical observations, such as the similarity in the electrolyte composition of the two fluids, suggested that the fluid forms in cystic brain tumours by diffusion of plasma from the capillaries of the tumour.

de Rougement and his coworkers (1962), on the other hand, distinguished three categories of cystic fluids:

1. those identical with serum;
2. those similar to cerebrospinal fluid; and
3. fluids different from both serum and cerebrospinal fluid.

Most fluids were of the third type, and it was concluded that they were formed not by simple exudation of plasma but rather by an active secretory process.

Szliwowski and Cumings (1961) examined cyst fluids for total protein, electrophoretic protein fractions, enzymes, and cholesterol. They found raised lactate dehydrogenase and phosphohexose isomerase activities in malignant tumours. They also reported that after tapping cysts which have previously been evacuated, the results do not parallel those obtained on the first examination.

Although biochemical studies of cerebral-cyst fluids in association with tumours may be of diagnostic value, there is evidence that in some cases the accumulation of fluid may result from a breakdown of barrier permeability, since the more malignant the tumour, the higher is the protein content of the fluid and the greater the resemblance of its lactate dehydrogenase isoenzyme pattern to that of serum (Cumings *et al.*, 1970).

Electrophoretic studies, including acrylamide-gel electrophoresis (Cumings *et al.*, 1970), do not appear as yet to have revealed any abnormal proteins in cerebral-cyst fluids.

A detailed account of the biochemical changes associated with brain tumours, with particular attention to isoenzyme patterns, has been given by Wollemann (1974).

REFERENCES

Aronson, S. M., A. Saifer, G. Perle, and B. W. Volk (1958), *Proc. Soc. Exp. Biol. Med.*, **97**, 331.

Bauer, H., and A. Gottesleben (1969), *Int. Arch. Allergy*, **36**, Suppl., 643.

Bauer, H., D. Grunwald, and J. V. Drach (1975), in *Immunopathologie du système nerveux* (Ed. E. Schuller), Editions INSERM, Paris, p. 155.

Bollengier, F., A. Lowenthal, and W. Henrotin (1975), *Z. Klin. Chem. Klin. Biochem.*, **13**, 305.

Bollengier, F., N. Rabinovitch, and A. Lowenthal (1978), *J. Clin. Chem. Clin. Biochem.*, **16**, 165.

Clausen, J. (1961), *Proc. Soc. Exp. Biol. Med.*, **107**, 170.

Cohen, S., and R. Bannister (1967), *Lancet*, **i**, 366.

Cosgrove, J. B. R., and P. Agius (1966), *Neurology*, **16**, 197.

Culebras, A., and N. G. Richards (1969), *Cleveland Clin. Quart.*, **36**, 47.

Cumings, J. N. (1953), *J. Neurol. Neurosurg. Psychiat.*, **16**, 152.

Cumings, J. N., R. C. Shortman, and M. Tooley (1970), *Clin. Chim. Acta*, **27**, 29.

Cunningham, V. R. (1964), *J. Clin. Path.*, **17**, 143.

Cutler, R. W. P., G. V. Watters, and J. P. Hammerstad (1970), *J. Neurol. Sci.*, **10**, 259.

Delmotte, P., and G. Gonsette (1977), *J. Neurol.*, **215**, 27.

Delpech, B., and E. Lichtblau (1972), *Clin. Chim. Acta*, **37**, 15.

Dencker, S. J. (1964), *Acta neurol. scand.*, **40**, Suppl. 10, 57.

de Rougemont, J., Y. Manuel, and M. Jeannin (1962), *Compt. rend. Soc. Biol.*, **156**, 1862.

Felgenhauer, K., G. Schliep, and N. Rapic (1976), *J. Neurol. Sci.*, **30**, 113.

Frick, E. (1963), *Klin. Woch.*, **41**, 75.

Frick, E., and L. Scheid-Seydel (1958), *Klin. Woch.*, **36**, 857.

Frick, E., and L. Scheid-Seydel (1960), *Klin. Woch.*, **38**, 1240.

Frick, E., and L. Scheid-Seydel (1963), *Klin. Woch.*, **41**, 589.

Gardner, W. J., J. S. Collis, Jr., and L.A. Lewis (1963), *Arch. Neurol.*, **8**, 291.

Gekle, D., J. Kult, and R. Roth (1977), *Klin. Woch.*, **55**, 189.

Haglid, K. G., and C.-A. Carlsson (1971), *Neurochirurgia*, **14**, 24.

Hochwald, G. M., and G. J. Thorbecke (1962), *Proc. Soc. Exp. Biol. Med.*, **109**, 91.
Hochwald, G. M., and M. C. Wallenstein (1967a), *Exp. Neurol.*, **19**, 115.
Hochwald, G. M., and M. Wallenstein (1967b), *Amer. J. Physiol.*, **212**, 1199.
Iwashita, H., F. Grunwald, and H. Bauer (1974), *J. Neurol.*, **207**, 45.
Kabat, E. A., D. H. Moore, and H. Landow (1942), *J. Clin. Invest.*, **21**, 571.
Kabat, E. A., M. Glusman, and V. Knaub (1948), *Amer. J. Med.*, **4**, 653.
Lamoureux, G., R. Jolicoeur, N. Giard, M. St-Hilaire, and F. Duplantis (1975), *Neurology*, **25**, 537.
Laterre, E. C. (1965), *Les Protéines du Liquide céphalo-rachidien à l'Etat normal et pathologique*, Editions Arscia, Brussels, p. 17.
Laterre, E. C. (1966), *Acta neurol. belg.*, **66**, 305.
Laterre, E. C. (1975), in *Immunopathologie du système nerveux* (Ed. E. Schuller), Editions INSERM, Paris, p. 211.
Laterre, E. C., J.-F. Heremans, and G. Demanet (1962), *Rev. Neurol.*, **107**, 500.
Laterre, E. C., A. Callewaert, J. F. Heremans, and Z. Sfaello (1970), *Neurology*, **20**, 982.
Link, H. (1965), *J. Neurol. Neurosurg. Psychiat.*, **28**, 552.
Link, H. (1967), *Acta neurol. scand.*, **43**, Suppl. 28, 1.
Link, H. (1973), *J. Neurol. Sci.*, **18**, 11.
Link, H., and R. Müller (1971), *Arch. Neurol.*, **25**, 326.
Link, H., and G. Tibbling (1977), *Scand. J. Clin. Lab. Invest.*, **37**, 397.
Link, H., and O. Zettervall (1970), *Clin. Exp. Immunol.*, **6**, 435.
Link, H., O. Zettervall, and G. Blennow (1972), *Z. Neurol.*, **203**, 119.
Link, H., M. Panelius, and A. A. Salmi (1973), *Arch. Neurol.*, **28**, 23.
Lippincott, S. W., S. Korman, L. C. Lax, and C. Corcoran (1965), *J. Nucl. Med.*, **6**, 632.
Lord, R. A., E. Dupree, R. M. Goldblum, W. D. Storey, P. M. Forman, and A. S. Goldman (1973), *Lancet*, **ii**, 528.
Lowenthal, A. (1965), *Agar Gel Electrophoresis in Neurology*, Elsevier, Amsterdam. (Cited by Laterre *et al.*, 1970.)
Lowenthal, A., M. Van Sande, and D. Karcher (1960), *J. Neurochem.*, **6**, 51.
Lumsden, C. E. (1972), in *Multiple Sclerosis: a Reappraisal* (by D. McAlpine, C. E. Lumsden, and E. D. Acheson), Churchill Livingstone, Edinburgh and London, p. 368.
MacPherson, C. F. C., and J. B. R. Cosgrove (1961), *Can. J. Biochem.*, **39**, 1567.
Monseu, G., and J. N. Cumings (1965), *J. Neurol. Neurosurg. Psychiat.*, **28**, 56.
Moore, B. W. (1965), *Biochem. Biophys. Res. Comm.*, **19**, 739.
Nakamura, S. (1964), *Saishin-igaku (Tokyo)*, **19**, 827. (Cited by Takeoka *et al.*, 1976.)
Newman, J., A. S. Josephson, A. Cacatian, and A. Tsang (1974), *Lancet*, **ii**, 756.
Parker, W. C., and A. G. Bearn (1962), *J. Exp. Med.*, **115**, 84.
Riddoch, D., and R. A. Thompson (1970), *Brit. Med. J.*, **i**, 396.
Roberts-Thomson, P. J., M. M. Esiri, A. C. Young, and I. C. M. MacLennan (1976), *J. Clin. Path.*, **29**, 1105.
Sandberg-Wollheim, M., O. Zettervall, and R. Müller (1969), *Clin. Exp. Immunol.*, **4**, 401.
Schneck, S. A., and H. N. Claman (1969), *Arch. Neurol.*, **20**, 132.
Schuller, E., M. Lefèvre, and L. Tömpe (1972), *Clin. Chim. Acta*, **42**, 5.
Schultze, H. E., and J. F. Heremans (1966), *Molecular Biology of Human Proteins*, Vol. 1, Elsevier, Amsterdam, p. 732.
Schwartz, S., H. P. Rieder, and R. Wüthrich (1970), *Europ. Neurol.*, **4**, 267.
Seland, T. P., T. A. McPherson, M. Grace, G. Lamoureux, and J. G. Blain (1974), *Neurology*, **24**, 34.
Smith, H., B. Bannister, and M. J. O'Shea (1973), *Lancet*, **ii**, 591.
Stewart, J. A. (1972), *Biochim. Biophys. Acta*, **263**, 178.
Szliwowski, H. B., and J. N. Cumings (1961), *Brain*, **84**, 204.
Takeoka, T., F. Gotoh, K. Furumi, and K. Mori (1976), *J. Neurol. Sci.*, **29**, 213.
Tavolato, B., and L. De Zanche (1968), *Acta Neurol. Scand.*, **44**, 384.
Thompson, E. J., P. M. Norman, and J. MacDermot (1975), *Brit. J. Hosp. Med.*, **14**, 645.

Thompson, H. G., E. Hirschberg, M. Osnos, and A. Gellhorn (1959), *Neurology*, **9**, 545.
Tourtellotte, W. (1970), *J. Neurol. Sci.*, **10**, 279.
Trotter, J. L., G. Banks, and P. Wang (1977), *Clin. Chem.*, **23**, 2213.
Weiss, A. H., E. Smith, N. Christoff, and S. Kochwa (1965), *J. Lab. Clin. Med.*, **66**, 280.
Williams, E. J. (1975), *An Immunological Study of Brain Proteins*, Ph.D. Thesis, University of Wales.
Wollemann, M. (1974), *Biochemistry of Brain Tumours*, Macmillan, London.
Zettervall, O., and H. Link (1970), *Clin. Exp. Immunol.*, **7**, 365.

CHAPTER 11

Fetal and neonatal monitoring

In this chapter the contribution of specific protein determinations to three types of clinical situation will be discussed: firstly, the detection of intrauterine infection; secondly, the assessment of fetal well-being in pregnancy; and finally, the detection of neural-tube defects in the fetus.

FETAL INFECTION*

The clinical diagnosis of chronic intrauterine or acute perinatal infections has long been a problem, and the laboratory diagnosis also is not always straightforward. Although the causative maternal infections are often asymptomatic, or are so mild as to escape notice, severe damage to the developing embryo can be caused (Sever and London, 1969).

Current evidence indicates that the human fetus, far from being immunologically incompetent, as was once thought, can mount an immune response when appropriately stimulated (Silverstein, 1964). Koch and his coworkers (1956) appear to have been the first to demonstrate that a *raised concentration of IgM* in cord blood serum could indicate the presence of intrauterine infection, such as congenital syphilis. Their findings have been fully confirmed, in a variety of infections. At least part of the antibody produced by the fetus can be distinguished from the large pool of maternally transferred antibodies. This can be done in two ways. The first is the detection of fetal antibody of the IgM class, specific for a given pathogen, mainly by the use of fluorescence microscopy (Cohen *et al.*, 1968; Hanshaw *et al.*, 1968; Remington *et al.*, 1968; Alford *et al.*, 1969b). The second method involves the demonstration of raised serum IgM concentrations as a non-specific monitor to detect newborn infants who are at high risk (Stiehm *et al.*, 1966; Alford *et al.*, 1967, 1968, 1969a; and others).

Estimation of the serum IgM concentration is of value in the investigation of sickness in newborn infants, with symptoms due to chronic congenital infections. In those with raised values the aetiologic organism must be identified by other means, and here the specific IgM fluorescent antibody procedures have proved of great value for rapid diagnosis.

In acute intrauterine infections that are acquired shorly before or during birth, the demonstration of increases in IgM concentration is of lesser value than in the chronic group; this is because of the considerable variations in the

*This section is based largely on the review by Alford (1971).

period that must elapse before IgM elevations can be demonstrated (Alford *et al.*, 1967; Blankenship *et al.*, 1969; Sever, 1969). Nevertheless, serial estimations of IgM can be of value, especially in aseptic meningitis, bacterial infections of the urinary tract, viral conjunctivitis, and various diarrhoeal states (Blankenship *et al.*, 1969; Sever, 1969); they are also helpful in diagnosing acute systemic viral infections caused by Coxsackie B, herpes virus, or other viral agents, in which conditions the concentrations of IgM increase more rapidly and reach higher values (Blankenship *et al.*, 1969).

Estimation of IgM has also been used as a screening procedure to detect subclinical congenital infections in the newborn (Alford *et al.*, 1969a; Alford, 1970).

It is important to note that a raised cord serum concentration of IgM is not always due to infection, since other stimuli, such as maternal allotypic proteins or intrauterine transfusion (Hobbs *et al.*, 1968), can also cause elevations. Conversely, a normal value does not exclude infection: for example, McCracken and his coworkers (1969) found a significant elevation in the IgM concentration in only 16 of 88 infants with congenital rubella.

Laboratory investigation of intrauterine infection

In interpreting a serum IgM value it is important to remember that there is an overlap of values for uninfected and infected infants, and also that (as mentioned above) raised IgM values can sometimes be found in the absence of infection. Although it is desirable to define a level of elevation that would select as many infected babies as possible, this level should not result in an inordinate number of false positives. Most investigators have chosen 18–20 mg/100 ml (180–200 mg/l) as the cut-off region for raised values of IgM in cord sera (Sever, 1969); this is between one and two standard deviations above the (geometric) mean of normal cord IgM concentrations found in most studies.

If the blood specimen is not taken within a few days of birth, allowance must be made, in interpreting the result, for the changing concentration of IgM with age (Figure 11.1). The upper limit represented by the mean plus two standard deviations is relatively so low up to 6 weeks of age that elevations due to infection readily stand out; after that time the distinction can be lost (Hobbs, 1971).

Finally, it must be emphasized that the IgM estimation affords only a non-specific indicator of infection and that the finding of a raised concentration must always be supplemented with tests for specific pathogens (Alford, 1971).

FETAL WELL-BEING IN PREGNANCY

The causes of fetal mortality and morbidity are complex and little understood. Many tests have been proposed for assessing the function and development of the fetus and placenta, most of which give information mainly about either one or other of these components. The fetal component is often monitored by

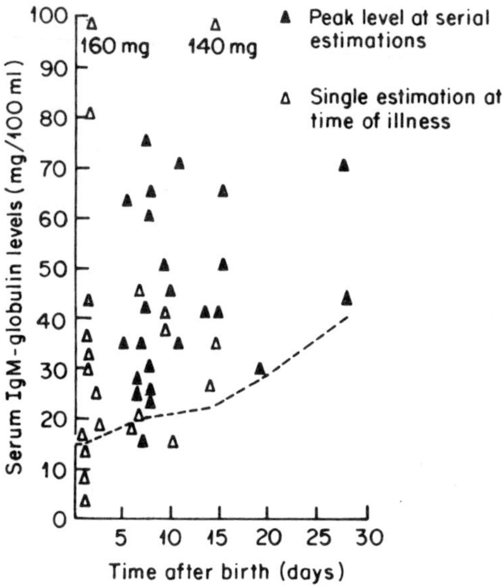

Figure 11.1. Serum IgM concentrations in 45 consecutive neonates in whom proof of infection was obtained. The broken line indicates the 2SD (logarithmic) upper limit for uninfected controls in the same unit. (C. Y. Yeung and J. R. Hobbs). (Reproduced from J. R. Hobbs, *Brit. J. Hosp. Med.*, 1970, **3**, 669, by permission of Hospital Medical Publications Ltd. and Prof. Hobbs.)

measurement of *α-fetoprotein* (p. 218), *lecithin-containing surfactants* secreted by the fetal lung, *bilirubin* as an index of Rhesus sensitization, and so on. In many cases poor nutrition of the fetus due to placental failure is an important factor. Substances measured to assess placental development and function include: *progesterone and its metabolites*; the maternal serum peptide hormones *human chorionic gonadotrophin* (HCG) and *human placental lactogen* (HPL); and the maternal serum enzymes *heat-stable alkaline phosphatase*, *diamine oxidase*, and *cystine aminopeptidase* (oxytocinase). The function of the whole fetoplacental unit may be assessed by measurement of the production or excretion of *oestriol*.

In this section a brief account is given of the use of HPL and HCG determinations in monitoring fetal well-being in pregnancy. Some mention is also made of the possible applications of *pregnancy-specific β_1-glycoprotein* determinations.

Human placental lactogen (HPL)

This is a protein hormone produced exclusively by the placenta. During uncomplicated pregnancies it progressively increases in concentration in the maternal blood plasma until the 36th or 37th week, after which concentrations are fairly stable (Keller *et al.*, 1971b; Lindberg *et al.*, 1972). Typical mean concentrations are: 0.2 mg/l at 10 weeks, 1 mg/l at 15 weeks, 3 mg/l at 25 weeks, 4.5 mg/l at 30 weeks, and 6.5 mg/l at 40 weeks. Although its concentration in maternal plasma reflects only placental function, of which it appears to be a sensitive indicator (Saxena *et al.*, 1969), its estimation is nevertheless a valuable guide to fetal well-being (Spellacy *et al.*, 1971; Keller *et al.*, 1971a,b). HPL is usually determined by radioimmunoassay, though radial immunodiffusion offers a simple and reliable alternative (Keller, 1976).

The usefulness of plasma HPL (and other) determinations has been reviewed by Chard (1975a) and by Wilde and Oakey (1975). During the first and second trimesters of pregnancy, the determination is useful in assessing the outcome of threatened abortion: in most reported cases, low concentrations have been associated with abortion (Genazzani *et al.*, 1969, 1971; Saxena *et al.*, 1969; Singer *et al.*, 1970; Spona and Janisch, 1971; Niven *et al.*, 1972; Gartside and Tindall, 1975), and determination of plasma HPL can be a valuable aid to prognosis. In late pregnancy, however, there appears to be little correlation between plasma HPL concentrations and impending fetal death.

According to most reports, plasma HPL concentrations tend to be low in pregnancies that result in 'small-for-dates' babies (Seppälä and Ruoslahti, 1970; Letchworth *et al.*, 1971; Spellacy *et al.*, 1971), at least when the determination is carried out late in pregnancy. These findings presumably reflect the smaller placental mass in such cases.

In toxaemia of pregnancy, most investigators have found a tendency for mean plasma concentrations of HPL to be lower than in normal subjects (Josimovich *et al.*, 1970; Spona and Janisch, 1971; Genazzani *et al.*, 1971; Spellacy *et al.*, 1971; Letchworth and Chard, 1972a). This is probably due to the reduction in placental volume which is common in patients with pre-eclampsia (Aherne and Dunnill, 1966). The relationship to severity or to increased risk to the fetus is uncertain.

In diabetic pregnancies that progress normally, it is now well established that there is a higher range of plasma HPL concentrations than in normal pregnancies, with significantly lower concentrations in the presence of placental insufficiency (Ursell *et al.*, 1973). Ursell and his coworkers concluded that the interpretation of results in diabetic pregnancies depends on knowledge of the HPL concentrations normally associated with this particular complication; on account of the considerable overlap between groups of patients with and without placental dysfunction they emphasize the need for serial measurements at frequent intervals.

In Rhesus isoimmunization, if the child is severely affected, values are raised. This is probably a reflection of the increase in placental size associated with this condition (Ward *et al.*, 1974). A value more than two standard deviations above the normal mean before the 26th week of gestation suggests a 90 per cent probability that the child is severely affected (Chard, 1975a). The test provides an index of fetal outcome at a stage when other measurements—such as that of the liquor bilirubin concentration—may be unreliable.

In prolonged pregnancy, HPL concentrations fall if fetal distress occurs (Genazzani *et al.*, 1971).

An important application of HPL estimations is in the screening of pregnancies that appear clinically quite normal; the development of complications during or immediately after labour can be predicted by serial estimations of circulating HPL, falling concentrations between the 35th and 40th weeks of pregnancy indicating a risk of fetal distress in labour or neonatal asphyxia (Letchworth and Chard, 1972b).

Persistently low maternal serum HPL concentrations associated with gross fetal abnormality have been reported (Gau and Cadle, 1974, 1977).

An investigation of the efficacy of five different biochemical tests for the early detection of fetoplacental distress led Keller and his associates (1971a) to conclude that the most effective monitoring is obtained by the simultaneous use of at least two tests—preferably urinary oestriol and serum HPL estimations.

For further information on the monitoring of the fetoplacental unit the reader is referred to the reviews by Chard (1975a) (placenta), Klopper (1975) (fetus), and Wilde and Oakey (1975).

Human chorionic gonadotrophin (HCG)

Maternal plasma and urine concentrations of HCG rise rapidly during pregnancy to reach a peak between the 50th and 70th days of gestation, and appear to fall during the second trimester with a small secondary peak between 30 and 36 weeks (Wilde and Oakey, 1975). The normal ranges for both blood and urine are very wide at all stages of pregnancy. The hormone is produced by the placenta, and its measurement in maternal urine has been extensively used as a test for pregnancy. Bioassay methods have been used for its determination, but radioimmunoassay is now usually preferred.

From the work of a number of investigators (summarized by Wilde and Oakey, 1975) it is clear that measurement of HCG in maternal serum or urine is not helpful in the management of pregnancy in the second half of gestation. In threatened abortion in the first half of pregnancy, however, measurement of urinary HCG excretion may have a useful predictive rôle (Wide, 1962). In the case of plasma, Nygren and his collaborators (1973) found that the determination of HCG gave a very good prediction of the outcome in threatened abortion, low values being associated with abortion, and high values nearly always with a favourable outcome.

HCG is a glycoprotein hormone composed of two dissimilar subunits, the α- and β-subunits (Canfield *et al.*, 1971). The former is virtually identical to the α-subunit of human luteinizing hormone (HLH) physicochemically, structurally, and immunologically, while the β-subunit of HCG differs from that of HLH in containing an extra 30 amino acid residues (Bahl *et al.*, 1972). Antisera directed against the β-subunit of HCG were found not to show significant cross-reaction with physiological concentrations of intact HLH (Vaitukaitis *et al.*, 1972) or with the α-subunit of HCG (Vaitukaitis and Ross, 1972).

By the use of a radioimmunoassay specific for the β-unit, HCG was detected in the serum as early as 6 days after presumed conception, and showed a peak concentration between 56 and 68 days; no secondary rise in HCG concentration could be demonstrated, indicating that the non-specific immunoassays give spuriously high values for HCG during the last trimester of pregnancy (Braunstein *et al.*, 1976). These observations are of great interest; however, as indicated above, it is in the first half of pregnancy that measurement of this hormone may have a useful rôle.

Pregnancy-specific β_1-glycoprotein

In pregnancy certain proteins appear in the blood that are not commonly identifiable in non-pregnant subjects (MacLaren *et al.*, 1959; Afonso and de Alvarez, 1964; Studd *et al.*, 1970; Bohn, 1971; Lin *et al.*, 1974; Than *et al.*, 1974). Owing partly to the terminology employed, some confusion may arise between three pregnancy-associated proteins, *viz. pregnancy-specific β_1-glycoprotein, steroid-binding β-globulin*, and *pregnancy-associated α_2-glycoprotein*; Table 11.1 may help to clarify the position.

It is possible that measurement of the plasma concentration of pregnancy-specific β_1-glycoprotein (abbreviated to SP_1 or PSβG) may provide another useful index of fetal well-being. This protein, first described by Bohn (1971), is synthesized by the placenta and rises in concentration in the plasma throughout pregnancy until about the 34th week, thereafter tending to remain constant until term (Towler *et al.*, 1976). Plasma concentrations correlate well with placental weight (Tatra *et al.*, 1975), and appear to fall outside the normal range in many or most of the abnormal pregnancies reported (Tatra *et al.*, 1974;

Table 11.1. Some pregnancy-associated globulins

Usual and other names	Abbreviations	References
Pregnancy-specific β_1-glycoprotein	SP_1 PSβG	Bohn, 1971
Steroid-binding β-globulin	SP_2	
Pregnancy-associated α_2-glycoprotein	SP_3	Stimson and Eubank-Scott, 1972; Bohn 1972; von Schoultz and Stigbrand, 1973; Than *et al.*, 1974; etc.
Pregnancy-zone protein	PZ	
Pregnancy-associated globulin	Pa_1	
α_2-pregnoglobulin	PAG	
α_2A.P. glycoprotein	PAα_2G	
Pregnancy-associated α_2-macroglobulin	α_2PAG PAM	
Schwangerschaftsprotein$_3$		
Xh		
etc.		

Gordon *et al.*, 1977; Towler *et al.*, 1977). In about 60 or 70 per cent of women with fetal growth retardation, low concentrations of plasma SP_1 were found (Gordon *et al.*, 1977; Towler *et al.*, 1977). It has been suggested also that measurement of plasma SP_1 (or, better, both SP_1 and HPL) may help in the detection of multiple pregnancies at an early stage of gestation, since in the majority of such pregnancies higher values are found than in singleton pregnancies (Towler *et al.*, 1976).

Laboratory monitoring of fetoplacental function

The tests available for assessing fetoplacental function all yield fairly wide ranges of normal values, and there is often considerable overlap between these ranges and those found in the presence of fetoplacental dysfunction. Furthermore, the appropriate normal or reference range may not be the same in pregnancies with different complications: an example has been given on p. 215, in relation to diabetes; the range of plasma HPL concentrations in pregnant women with diabetes, or with Rhesus incompatibility, who are delivered of normal babies is higher than in uncomplicated pregnancies. Finally, results may differ from one laboratory to another, on account of the use of different methods or standards. In all these circumstances, a single result can rarely give unequivocal information on fetoplacental function. Serial determinations are preferable, and will in addition indicate any trend.

At present, the determination of urinary oestrogens appears to be the best single test available for assessing fetoplacental function, and detecting fetal distress, in late pregnancy. In very early pregnancy, the estimation of urinary *chorionic gonadotrophin* is a valuable indicator of placental development.

The situations in which plasma HPL determinations are likely to be useful have been outlined above. As already indicated, one of the most valuable applications of the test is in helping to decide which of those patients with bleeding in early pregnancy are in danger of imminent abortion.

α-Fetoprotein concentrations in maternal serum are often increased in association with fetal death during the second and third trimesters (Seppälä and Ruoslahti, 1972a,b), and the increase may occur before the death of the fetus (Seppälä and Ruoslahti, 1973b); apart from this, the value of maternal serum α-fetoprotein measurement as an additional test of fetal viability in late pregnancy has not been substantiated.

For a critical evaluation of the range of tests available for the assessment of feto-placental function the reader is referred to the extensive review by Wilde and Oakey (1975).

DETECTION OF NEURAL-TUBE DEFECTS IN THE FETUS

The occurrence of large amounts of α-fetoprotein in fetal blood, and its almost complete disappearance from the blood soon after birth, have been described in Chapter 3. The protein is found at lower concentrations in amniotic fluid than in the fetal circulation.

In 1972 Brock and Sutcliffe reported an association between neural-tube defects in the fetus and abnormally high concentrations of α-fetoprotein in the amniotic fluid. Of 31 cases of anencephaly investigated by them, all were found to have greatly increased concentrations of α-fetoprotein in amniotic fluid taken between the 25th and 35th weeks of gestation; and in one case of spina bifida the concentration was high at the 13th week. These observations have since been confirmed by many groups (Brock and Scrimgeour, 1972, 1974; Brock *et al.*, 1973; Allan *et al.*, 1973; Field *et al.*, 1973; Leek *et al.*, 1973; Nevin *et al.*, 1973, 1974; Seller *et al.*, 1973; Harris *et al.*, 1974; Milunsky and Alpert, 1974; Stewart *et al.*, 1975), and it is now generally accepted that a significantly raised concentration of α-fetoprotein in the amniotic fluid, in conjunction with radiographic and/or ultrasonographic investigations, will detect the presence of 'open' *spina bifida or anencephaly. Since the concentration of α-fetoprotein is normal in the fetus itself (Seller *et al.*, 1974a), raised concentrations in the amniotic fluid probably result from leakage of fetal cerebrospinal fluid or transudation of proteins from fetal capillaries exposed directly to the amniotic fluid, though other mechanisms may be involved in other conditions (see below). The concentrations associated with 'closed' spina bifida lesions, on the other hand, are normal or only slightly raised. Increased concentrations of α-fetoprotein in the amniotic fluid can occur in association with other congenital abnormalities and after intrauterine death of the fetus (Table 11.2). Possible mechanisms by which the concentration of α-fetoprotein in the amniotic fluid may be increased include, in addition to those mentioned above, fetal proteinuria (in nephrosis) and impaired fetal swallowing or digestion (when a congenital malformation of the orogastrointestinal tract is present) (Brock, 1976a).

The concentration of α-fetoprotein in amniotic fluid normally decreases from the 14th week of pregnancy until term (Seppälä and Ruoslahti, 1972c).

Maternal blood α-fetoprotein

The presence of α-fetoprotein in the serum of pregnant women was first demonstrated by Foy and his colleagues (1970). During pregnancy, the concentration increases (Seppälä and Ruoslahti, 1972a; Ishiguro, 1973), probably as a result of passage of the protein either across the placenta or through the membranes, peak concentrations occurring early in the third trimester (Ishiguro, 1973; Seppälä and Ruoslahti, 1972a, 1973b). Such peak concentrations may range between 100 and 550 μg/l—i.e. some 10–50 times the normal concentration in non-pregnant adults—though actual estimates may vary from one laboratory to another.

In 1973 preliminary reports (Leek *et al.*, 1973; Brock *et al.*, 1973) suggested that a raised concentration of α-fetoprotein in the amniotic fluid might some-

*Spina bifida lesions are classified as 'open' if there is completely exposed neural tissue or a lesion covered by thin transparent membrane, or 'closed' if the lesion is completely covered by skin or thick opaque membrane.

Table 11.2. Pathological conditions of the fetus, other than spina bifida and anencephaly, in which increased concentrations of α-fetoprotein may be found in amniotic fluid and/or maternal serum.

Condition	Gestation	Usual finding* maternal serum α-fetoprotein	Usual finding* amniotic fluid α-fetoprotein	Reference*
Congenital nephrosis	2nd and 3rd trimesters	↑	↑	Seppälä and Ruoslahti, 1972c; Kjessler *et al.*, 1975
Hydrocephaly	3rd trimester	Normal	↑	Seppälä and Unnérus, 1974
Death of fetus; spontaneous abortion		↑		Seppälä and Ruoslahti 1972a, b, 1973a; Guibaud *et al.*, 1973; Cohen *et al.*, 1973; Wald *et al.*, 1977a
Gastroschisis	2nd trimester	↑		Douglas, 1977; Clarke *et al.*, 1977
Omphalocele (exomphalos)	2nd and 3rd trimesters	↑	↑	Nevin and Armstrong, 1975; De Bruijn and Huisjes, 1975; Leschot and Treffers, 1975; Kunz and Schmid, 1976; Seppälä *et al.*, 1976; Clarke *et al.*, 1977
Turner's syndrome (?)*	1st trimester		↑	Seller *et al.*, 1974b
Duodenal atresia	2nd trimester		↑	Weinberg *et al.*, 1975
Oesophageal atresia	3rd trimester	Normal	↑	Seppälä, 1973
Severe Rh-iso-immunization (?)*		↑	↑	Seppälä and Ruoslahti, 1973b
Sacrococcygeal teratoma	2nd trimester		↑	Schmid and Mühlethaler, 1975
Fallot's tetralogy	3rd trimester		↑	Seppälä, 1975.

*Note:

1. Not all the references cited refer to both amniotic fluid and maternal serum.
2. In some cases (e.g. Fallot's tetralogy, oesophageal atresia) the data are obtainable only late in pregnancy and may not apply to the gestational period when diagnostic amniocentesis is performed.
3. In some conditions (e.g. exomphalos, Turner's syndrome) there is disagreement as to whether raised α-fetoprotein concentrations will be found in all cases. It has been suggested (Sutherland *et al.*, 1977) that high values obtained for amniotic fluid in Turner's syndrome may have resulted from puncture of a fetal cervical pouch at amniocentesis.
4. In the case of rhesus isoimmunization, Whyley and his colleagues (1974) found no differences between amniotic fluid α-fetoprotein concentrations in unaffected pregnancies, in pregnancies complicated by mild or moderate disease, or in severe rhesus isoimmunization when the baby survived; however, in severe rhesus isoimmunization with an unfavourable outcome a proportion of the cases showed elevations on one or more occasions.

times be reflected in the maternal serum, giving rise to concentrations even higher than those normally found in pregnancy. Leek and his coworkers described three cases of anencephaly, in two of which the maternal serum α-fetoprotein concentrations were substantially raised, and Brock and his colleagues described a further such case. These findings also have been for the most part confirmed by many workers, either in spina bifida or in anencephaly, or both (Brock *et al.*, 1974; Wald *et al.*, 1974; Seller *et al.*, 1974a; Harris *et al.*, 1974; Leek *et al.*, 1974; Higa *et al.*, 1974; Nevin, 1974; Malmqvist *et al.*, 1975; Brock *et al.*, 1975; Vince *et al.*, 1975; Leighton *et al.*, 1975; Monk and Goldie, 1976). Such abnormally high serum α-fetoprotein concentrations probably originate by absorption of amniotic fluid proteins through the membranes.

Since the collection of maternal blood, unlike that of amniotic fluid, is without risk, these observations suggested that measurement of maternal blood α-fetoprotein might offer a routine screening procedure for neural-tube defects in the fetus.

In 1974 a major collaborative study (UK Collaborative Study on Alpha-fetoprotein in Relation to Neural-tube Defects) was initiated with the object of obtaining a reliable estimate of the efficiency of maternal serum α-fetoprotein measurement in the antenatal detection of neural-tube defects. Since the distributions of maternal serum α-fetoprotein concentrations in pregnancies with and without neural-tube defects overlap, it was clear that any selection of a 'cut-off' concentration above which further investigations would be called for, and below which the pregnancy would be regarded as normal, must necessarily be a compromise. If the cut-off level were set too high, many affected pregnancies would be missed, whereas if it were too low, a large number of unaffected pregnancies would have to be investigated further.

The UK Collaborative Study (Wald *et al.*, 1977b) has established that the best time to discriminate between normal and abnormal pregnancies by examination of maternal blood is between the 16th and 18th weeks of gestation. A single cut-off point, applicable in all circumstances, is not recommended; but for many centres the report favours, at 16–18 weeks, a value 2.5 times the median value for normal pregnancies as established in individual assay laboratories. Cut-off points expressed as multiples of the normal median are preferred to those based on percentiles as the latter are more subject to large random errors, while the median can be determined accurately with relatively few values. The advantage of relating cut-off points to a statistic such as the median is that it allows results obtained by different laboratories to be more easily compared; results expressed as weight per volume may vary widely from one laboratory to another (see below, p. 222).

If a value above the cut-off point is found, a second blood sample may be obtained if necessary, and the average of the two results used. If amniocentesis is indicated, ultrasonography should first be performed in order to establish whether the pregnancy is single or multiple, since multiple pregnancy is associated with raised maternal serum α-fetoprotein concentrations (Garoff and Seppälä, 1973).

The results of the UK Collaborative Study indicated that, using the median × 2.5 cut-off point, 88 per cent of cases of anencephaly and 79 per cent of cases of open spina bifida could be detected by maternal serum α-fetoprotein screening. Three per cent of unaffected singleton pregnancies also had α-fetoprotein concentrations equal to or greater than 2.5 times the median. Amniocentesis is thought to be justified in these 3 per cent of cases, since they form part of a high-risk group in which the detection rate of neural-tube defects probably much exceeds the risk of fetal mortality resulting from amniocentesis.

Laboratory investigations

Patients involved in laboratory investigations to detect neural-tube defects fall into two categories. On the one hand are those women who have previously given birth to an infant with a neural-tube defect. Such women are recognized as being at high risk and can be offered amniocentesis, measurement of amniotic fluid α-fetoprotein and termination of pregnancy if the concentration is grossly higher than it is in normal pregnancies.

On the other hand are those women who are included in a routine screening programme but who are not thought to be at high risk. In such cases, if a high serum α-fetoprotein concentration is found this is an indication for ultrasonography and amniocentesis. In no circumstances is termination of pregnancy justified on the basis of serum α-fetoprotein concentrations alone.

It must be emphasized that each laboratory should establish its own ranges for normal pregnancies, both for amniotic fluid and for serum. The precise cut-off point above which ultrasonography and amniocentesis are indicated is a matter for arrangement with the obstetricians, since (as mentioned above) if this point is set too low an unacceptably large number of normal pregnancies will need to be investigated.

The actual values for α-fetoprotein obtained by radioimmunoassay in different laboratories vary widely. One reason for this is probably the use of different standards, often of unknown purity (cf. Keyser *et al.*, 1976). Another reason may be the variety of antisera and methods used. Purified α-fetoprotein, although homogeneous by many criteria, appears to exist in several forms (Alpert *et al.*, 1971, 1972; Purves *et al.*, 1970), one of which apparently undergoes a structural alteration, during the purification procedure, which affects the antigenic determinant (Alpert and Perencevich, 1975). The presence of similar α-fetoprotein isoproteins, with altered antigenic determinants, may be one explanation for the wide variation in standards and serum concentrations found in different laboratories.

According to a recent report (Young *et al.*, 1976), molecular aggregates form when α-fetoprotein is stored; the presence of ^{125}I-labelled aggregates affects the double antibody radioimmunoassay by increasing non-specific binding, thereby reducing assay sensitivity.

Chard (1975b) has listed the causes of 'false' positive results, i.e. the finding of an elevated maternal serum α-fetoprotein concentration in the absence of a neural tube defect. Some of these have already been mentioned above. They include:

1. overlap between the upper end of the normal range and the abnormal range;
2. technical errors in performing the estimation;
3. multiple pregnancy (Garoff and Seppälä, 1973; Wald *et al.*, 1975; Vince *et al.*, 1977);
4. intrauterine death of the fetus (Seppälä and Ruoslahti, 1972a,b; Guibaud *et al.*, 1973; Cohen *et al.*, 1973);
5. other congenital abnormalities (Table 11.2);
6. concurrent maternal liver disease;
7. collection of the blood sample after amniocentesis, which is sometimes associated with transplacental haemorrhage and elevation of maternal blood α-fetoprotein concentrations (Chard *et al.*, 1976).

Another source of error has been reported by Rimbaut and his coworkers (1975), who found extremely high serum α-fetoprotein concentrations by radioimmunoassay, but not by immunodiffusion, in some patients with liver diseases or carcinoma with metastases in the liver; all the sera were icteric and it appeared that some component of the bile had inhibited the antigen–antibody reaction in the radioimmunoassay.

The importance of collecting maternal blood before, rather than after, amniocentesis is worth re-emphasizing, since it is important to eliminate the possibility that raised concentrations of α-fetoprotein in the maternal blood might have been caused by fetomaternal haemorrhage (Horacek *et al.*, 1976; Chard *et al.*, 1976). In the case of amniotic fluid also, contamination with fetal blood constitutes a potent source of error (Brock, 1975a; Kitau *et al.*, 1975; Goldie and Monk, 1975; Campbell *et al.*, 1975b). There have been a few cases of antenatal misdiagnosis, for example the finding of raised concentrations of α-fetoprotein in the amniotic fluid although the fetus was normal (Campbell *et al.*, 1975a; Field and Kerr, 1975); and the possibility that fetal blood in the sample might account for the high values reported in such cases has been emphasized by Brock (1975a), who recommends that all blood-stained samples of amniotic fluid should be checked for fetal erythrocytes by the Kleihauer test (cf. Ward and Stewart, 1974), and indeed that all samples with raised concentrations of α-fetoprotein should be so checked even in the absence of visible contamination.

A case has also been reported in which α-fetoprotein in the amniotic fluid was not detectable by radial immunodiffusion, although the infant was born with a large open thoracolumbar meningomyelocoele (Field and Kerr, 1975). In examining more than 1000 specimens of amniotic fluid Brock (1975a) encountered this situation six times. In two cases the period of gestation had been grossly miscalculated, and in the remaining four the specimens proved to be maternal urine. A simple routine procedure to eliminate this source of error has been recommended (Duncan, 1975). Following ultrasound B-scan to localize the placenta and immediately before amniocentesis, urine is voided and tested for sugar and protein ('Uristix', Ames Company). This test is generally negative. The urine is discarded and the 'Uristix' strip kept. Amniocentesis is performed and, after the syringe has been emptied into the container, the final drops are placed on another test strip. Protein and sugar are invariably present in sufficient concentration to give an immediate reaction, and the contrast between urine and amniotic fluid is obvious.

If, however, the pregnancy is complicated by diabetes or renal disease, the maternal urine may well contain considerable amounts of glucose or protein. In this case a clear distinction can be made on the basis of the much greater concentration of urea and potassium in maternal urine as compared with amniotic fluid (Guibaud *et al.*, 1976).

Kohn (1975) has drawn attention to the possibility that maternal serum may be mistaken for amniotic fluid—either in the laboratory or by a mistake in specimen collecting—and suggests estimation of the total protein by a simple method, such as the refractometric or the copper sulphate method, to distinguish between the two fluids.

For further information on the measurement of maternal serum α-fetoprotein in antenatal screening the reader is referred to the comprehensive report of the UK Collaborative Study.

Other constituents of amniotic fluid

Measurement of a number of other protein constituents of amniotic fluid has been proposed as an aid to the pre-natal diagnosis of neural-tube defects. These constituents include *β-trace protein* (Macri *et al.*, 1974a, b; Weiss *et al.*, 1974), *fibrinogen degradation products* (Purdie *et al.*, 1975), α_2-*macroglubulin* and *β-lipoprotein* (Brock, 1975b), and *IgM* (Cantuaria and Jones, 1975). More recent work has not confirmed that the estimation of *β-trace protein* is useful for the early antenatal diagnosis of anencephaly and spina bifida (Olsson *et al.*, 1974; Adinolfi *et al.*, 1976; Brock and Olsson, 1976). Statistically significant increases in the concentration of *fibrin/fibrinogen degradation products* were found in anencephalic pregnancies in the second and third trimesters, and in spina bifida pregnancies in the second trimester, when compared with normal pregnancies (Purdie *et al.*, 1975); since the concentration of these degradation products is stated to be relatively constant throughout normal pregnancy, a raised concentration demands attention even when the degree of fetal maturity is uncertain. However, another group of workers (Gordon *et al.*, 1976), who measured fibrin(ogen) degradation fragment E, found that although the concentration of this protein in the amniotic fluid was generally raised when a neural-tube defect was present, there was considerable overlap between the normal and abnormal ranges. These findings are in agreement with those of Weiss and his colleagues (1976).

With regard to the high molecular weight proteins α_2-*macroglobulin*, *β-lipoprotein*, and *IgM*, these have certainly been found in high concentrations in the amniotic fluid when the infant had a neural-tube defect but not in normal pregnancies. Estimation of α_2-macroglobulin has two advantages over that of α-fetoprotein in the early diagnosis of neural-tube defects: in the first place, α_2-macroglobulin is virtually absent from control amniotic fluids, and secondly, comparatively high concentrations of this protein are found in some early cases of spina bifida in which the concentrations of α-fetoprotein are more marginal (Brock, 1975b). The main disadvantage of measuring amniotic fluid α_2-macroglobulin lies in the possibility of contamination of the fluid with maternal serum; since contamination with fetal blood is far less common, measurement of a 'feto-specific parameter' remains the best way of diagnosing neural-tube defects *in utero* (Brock, 1975b). According to Brock (1976b), quantitative assay of fetal macrophages among the amniotic fluid cells (Sutherland *et al.*, 1973, 1975; Nelson *et al.*, 1974; Gosden and Brock, 1977) is likely to afford the most useful 'second-line' indication of early neural-tube defects, for example in cases where α-fetoprotein concentrations are equivocal or ultrasonography fails to detect any malformation.

REFERENCES

Adinolfi, M., S. A. Haddad, S. E. Beck, I. L. Fung, and E. Osserman (1976), *Experientia*, **32**, 53.

Afonso, J. F., and R. R. de Alvarez (1964), *Amer. J. Obstet. Gynec.*, **89**, 204.

Aherne, M., and M. S. Dunnill (1966), *J. Path. Bact.*, **91**, 123.

Alford, C. A. (1970), *Hosp. Practice*, **5**, 88.

Alford, C. A. (1971), *Pediat. Clin. N. Amer.*, **18**, 99.

Alford, C. A., J. Schaefer, W. J. Blankenship, J. V. Straumfjord, and G. Cassady (1967), *New Engl. J. Med.*, **277**, 437.

Alford, C. A., W. J. Blankenship, J. V. Straumfjord, and G. Cassady (1968), *Birth Defects, Orig. Art. Series*, **4**, 3.

Alford, C. A., J. W. Foft, W. J. Blankenship, G. Cassady, and J. W. Benton (1969a), *J. Pediat.*, **75**, 1167.

Alford, C. A., S. S. Polt, G. Cassady, J. V. Straumfjord, and J. S. Remington (1969b), *New Engl. J. Med.*, **280**, 1086.

Allan, L. D., M. A. Ferguson-Smith, I. Donald, E. M. Sweet, and A. A. M. Gibson (1973), *Lancet*, **ii**, 522.

Alpert, E., and R. C. Perencevich (1975), *Ann. N. Y. Acad. Sci.*, **259**, 131.

Alpert, E., P. H. Schur, J. Drysdale, and K. J. Isselbacher (1971), *Fed. Proc.*, **30**, 246.

Alpert, E., J. W. Drysdale, K. J. Isselbacher, and P. H. Schur (1972), *J. Biol. Chem.*, **247**, 3792.

Bahl, O. P., R. Carlson, R. Bellisario, and N. Swaminathan (1972), *Biochem. Biophys. Res. Commun.*, **48**, 416.

Blankenship, W., G. Cassady, J. Schaefer, J. V. Straumfjord, and C. A. Alford (1969), *J. Pediat.*, **75**, 1271.

Bohn, H. (1971), *Arch. Gynäk.*, **210**, 440.

Bohn, H. (1972), *Arch. Gynäk.*, **213**, 54.

Braunstein, G. D., J. Rasor, D. Adler, H. Danzer, and M. E. Wade (1976), *Amer. J. Obstet. Gynec.*, **126**, 678.

Brock, D. J. H. (1975a), *Lancet*, **ii**, 495.

Brock, D. J. H. (1975b), *Clin. Genetics*, **8**, 297.

Brock, D. J. H. (1976a), *Lancet*, **ii**, 345.

Brock, D. J. H. (1976b), *J. Clin. Path.*, **29**, Suppl. (Roy. Coll. Path.) **10**, 157.
Brock, D. J. H., and J. E. Olsson (1976), *Clin. Genetics*, **9**, 385.
Brock, D. J. H., and J. B. Scrimgeour (1972), *Lancet*, **ii**, 1252.
Brock, D. J. H., and J. B. Scrimgeour (1974), *Lancet*, **i**, 569.
Brock, D. J. H., and R. G. Sutcliffe (1972), *Lancet*, **ii**, 197.
Brock, D. J. H., A. E. Bolton, and J. M. Monaghan (1973), *Lancet*, **ii**, 923.
Brock, D. J. H., A. E. Bolton, and J. B. Scrimgeour (1974), *Lancet*, **i**, 767.
Brock, D. J. H., J. B. Scrimgeour, A. E. Bolton, N. Wald, R. Peto, and S. Barker (1975), *Lancet*, **ii**, 195.
Campbell, S., J. Pryse-Davies, T. M. Coltart, M. J. Seller, and J. D. Singer (1975a), *Lancet*, **i**, 1065.
Campbell, S., J. Pryse-Davies, T. M. Coltart, M. Seller, and J. D. Singer (1975b), *Lancet*, **i**, 1336.
Canfield, R. E., F. J. Morgan, S. Kammerman, J. J. Bell, and G. M. Agosto (1971), *Rec. Progr. Hormone Res.*, **27**, 121.
Cantuaria, A. A., and A. L. Jones (1975), *Brit. J. Obstet. Gynaec.*, **82**, 262.
Chard, T. (1975a), *Postgrad. Med. J.*, **51**, 221.
Chard, T. (1975b), *Lab-Lore* (Wellcome Foundation), **6**, 361.
Chard, T. (1976), *J. Clin. Path.*, **29**, Suppl. (Roy. Coll. Path.) **10**, 18.
Chard, T., M. J. Kitau, R. Ledward, T. Coltart, S. Embury, and M. J. Seller (1976), *Brit. J. Obstet. Gynaec.*, **83**, 33.
Clarke, P. C., Y. B. Gordon, M. J. Kitau, T. Chard, and A. D. McNeal (1977), *Brit. J. Obstet. Gynaec.*, **84**, 285.
Cohen, M. S., C. P. Ducharme, C. A. Carpenter, and R. Deibel (1968), *J. Lab. Clin. Med.*, **72**, 760.
Cohen, H., H. Graham, and H. L. Lau (1973), *Amer. J. Obstet. Gynec.*, **115**, 881.
De Bruijn, H. W. A., and H. J. Huisjes (1975), *Lancet*, **i**, 525.
Douglas, D. L. (1977), *Lancet*, **i**, 42.
Duncan, S. L. B. (1975), *Lancet*, **ii**, 709.
Field, B., and C. Kerr (1975), *Lancet*, **ii**, 324.
Field, B., G. Mitchell, W. Garrett, and C. Kerr (1973), *Lancet*, **ii**, 798.
Foy, H., A. Kondi, A. M. Parker, R. Stanley, and C. D. Venning (1970), *Lancet*, **i**, 1336.
Garoff, L., and M. Seppälä (1973), *J. Obstet. Gynec. Brit. Commonw.*, **80**, 695.
Gartside, M. W., and V. R. Tindall (1975), *Brit. J. Obstet. Gynaec.*, **82**, 303.
Gau, G., and G. Cadle (1974), *Lancet*, **ii**, 775.
Gau, G. S., and G. Cadle (1977), *Obstet. Gynec.*, **49**, 243.
Genazzani, A. R., M. L. Aubert, M. Casoli, P. Fioretti, and J.-P. Felber (1969), *Lancet*, **ii**, 1385.
Genazzani, A. R., F. Cocola, M. Casoli, G. Mello, E. J. Scarselli, P. Neri, and P. Fioretti (1971), *J. Obstet. Gynaec. Brit. Commonw.*, **78**, 577.
Goldie, D. J., and A. M. Monk (1975), *Lancet*, **i**, 1336.
Gordon, Y. B., S. M. Ratky, P. C. Leighton, M. J. Kitau, and T. Chard (1976), *Brit. J. Obstet. Gynaec.*, **83**, 771.
Gordon, Y. B., J. G. Grudzinskas, D. Jeffrey, T. Chard, and A. T. Letchworth (1977), *Lancet*, **ii**, 331.
Gosden, C. M., and D. J. H. Brock (1977), *Lancet*, **i**, 919.
Guibaud, S., M. Bonnet, J. M. Thoulon, and M. Dumont (1973), *Lancet*, **i**, 1261.
Guibaud, S., M. Bonnet, A. Dury, J. M. Thoulon, and M. Dumont (1976), *Lancet*, **i**, 746.
Hanshaw, J. B., H. J. Steinfeld, and C. J. White (1968), *New Engl. J. Med.*, **279**, 566.
Harris, R., R. F. Jennison, A. J. Barson, K. M. Laurence, E. Ruoslahti, and M. Seppälä (1974), *Lancet*, **i**, 429.
Higa, Y., T. Sasazuki, H. Nakajima, M. Takayama, M. Tada, and H. Soma (1974), *Amer. J. Obstet. Gynec.*, **119**, 932.
Hobbs, J. R. (1971), *Adv. Clin. Chem.*, **14**, 219.

Hobbs, J. R., M. I. Hughes, and W. Walker (1968), *Lancet*, **i**, 1400.

Horacek, I., R. J. Pepperell, D. L. Hay, J. U. Barrie, and B. W. Buttery (1976), *Lancet*, **ii**, 200.

Ishiguro, T. (1973), *Lancet*, **i**, 1509.

Josimovich, J. B., B. Kosor, L. Boccella, D. H. Mintz, and D. L. Hutchinson (1970), *Obstet. Gynec.*, **36**, 244.

Keller, P. J. (1976), *Lancet*, **i**, 745.

Keller, P. J., U. Baertschi, P. Bader, C. Gerber, J. Schmid, R. Soltermann, and E. Kopper (1971a), *Lancet*, **ii**, 729.

Keller, P. J., C. Gerber, and R. Soltermann (1971b), *Schweiz. Z. Gynäk. Geburtsh.*, **2**, 109.

Keyser, J. W., J. Kohn, and A. M. Ward (1976), *Lancet*, **i**, 1015.

Kitau, M. J., P. Leighton, Y. B. Gordon, and T. Chard (1975), *Lancet*, **i**, 1336.

Kjessler, B., S. G. O. Johansson, M. Sherman, K.-H. Gustavson, and G. Hultquist (1975), *Lancet*, **i**, 432.

Klopper, A. (1975), *Postgrad. Med. J.*, **51**, 227.

Koch, F., K. Schlagetter, H. E. Schultze, and G. Schwick (1956), *Z. Kinderheilk.*, **78**, 283.

Kohn, J. (1975), *Lancet*, **ii**, 663.

Kunz, J., and J. Schmid (1976), *Lancet*, **i**, 47.

Leek, A. E., C. F. Ruoss, M. J. Kitau, and T. Chard (1973), *Lancet*, **ii**, 385.

Leek, A. E., P. C. Leighton, M. J. Kitau, and T. Chard (1974), *Lancet*, **ii**, 1511.

Leighton, P. C., Y. B. Gordon, M. J. Kitau, A. E. Leek, and T. Chard (1975), *Lancet*, **ii**, 1012.

Leschot, N. J., and P. E. Treffers (1975), *Lancet*, **ii**, 1141.

Letchworth, A. T., and T. Chard (1972a), *J. Obstet. Gynaec. Brit. Commonw.*, **79**, 680.

Letchworth, A. T., and T. Chard (1972b), *Lancet*, **i**, 704.

Letchworth, A. T., R. J. Boardman, C. Bristow, J. Landon, and T. Chard (1971), *J. Obstet. Gynaec. Brit. Commonw.*, **78**, 542.

Lin, T. M., S. P. Halbert, D. Kiefer, W. N. Spellacy, and S. Gall (1974), *Amer. J. Obstet. Gynec.*, **118**, 223.

Lindberg, B., B. A. Nilsson, A. Roth, and L. Ylänen (1972), *Upsala J. Med. Sci.*, **77**, 129.

MacLaren, J. A., R. D. Thornes, C. C. Roby, and D. E. Reid (1959), *Amer. J. Obstet. Gynec.*, **78**, 939.

Macri, J. N., R. R. Weiss, M. S. Joshi, and M. I. Evans (1974a), *Lancet*, **i**, 14.

Macri, J. N., R. R. Weiss, and M. S. Joshi (1974b), *Lancet*, **i**, 1109.

Malmqvist, E., J. Lindsten, B. Nørgaard-Pedersen, B. Hellström, and B. Sundberg (1975), *Clin. Genetics*, **7**, 176.

McCracken, G. H., J. B. Hardy, T. C. Chen, L. S. Hoffman, M. R. Gilkeson, and J. L. Sever (1969), *J. Pediat.*, **74**, 383.

Milunsky, A., and E. Alpert (1974), *J. Pediat.*, **84**, 889.

Monk, A. M., and D. J. Goldie (1976), *Brit. J. Obstet. Gynaec.*, **83**, 845.

Nelson, M. M., M. T. Ruttiman, and D. J. H. Brock (1974), *Lancet*, **i**, 504.

Nevin, N. C. (1974), *Dev. Med. Child. Neurol.*, **16**, Suppl. 32, p. 122.

Nevin, N. C., and M. J. Armstrong (1975), *J. Obstet. Gynaec. Brit. Commonw.*, **82**, 826.

Nevin, N. C., S. Nesbitt, and W. Thompson (1973), *Lancet*, **i**, 1383.

Nevin, N. C., W. Thompson, and S. Nesbitt (1974), *J. Obstet. Gynaec. Brit. Commonw.*, **81**, 759.

Niven, P. A. R., J. Landon, and T. Chard (1972), *Brit. Med. J.*, **iii**, 799.

Nygren, K.-G., E. D. B. Johansson, and L. Wide (1973), *Amer. J. Obstet. Gynec.*, **116**, 916.

Olsson, J. E., M. S. Sherman, and B. Kjessler (1974), *Lancet*, **ii**, 347.

Purdie, D. W., P. W. Howie, W. Edgar, C. D. Forbes, and C. R. M. Prentice (1975), *Lancet*, **i**, 1013.

Purves, L. R., E. van der Merwe, and I. Bersohn (1970), *S. Afr. Med. J.*, **44**, 1264.

Remington, J. S., M. J. Miller, and I. Brownlee (1968), *Pediatrics*, **41**, 1082.

Rimbaut, C., C. Rudant, and D. Buffe (1975), *Lancet*, **ii**, 934.

Saxena, B. N., K. Emerson, and H. A. Selenkow (1969), *New Engl. J. Med.*, **281**, 225.
Schmid, W., and J. P. Mühlethaler (1975), *Humangenetik*, **26**, 353.
Seller, M. J., S. Campbell, T. M. Coltart, and J. D. Singer (1973), *Lancet*, **ii**, 73.
Seller, M. J., J. D. Singer, T. M. Coltart, and S. Campbell (1974a), *Lancet*, **i**, 428.
Seller, M. J., M. R. Creasy, and E. D. Alberman (1974b), *Brit. Med. J.*, **ii**, 524.
Seppälä, M. (1973), *Obstet. Gynec.*, **42**, 613.
Seppälä, M. (1975), *Ann. N. Y. Acad. Sci.*, **259**, 59.
Seppälä, M., and E. Ruoslahti (1970), *Acta Obstet. Gynec. Scand.*, **49**, 143.
Seppälä, M., and E. Ruoslahti (1972a), *Lancet*, **i**, 375.
Seppälä, M., and E. Ruoslahti (1972b), *Brit. Med. J.*, **ii**, 769.
Seppälä, M., and E. Ruoslahti (1972c), *Amer. J. Obstet. Gynec.*, **114**, 595.
Seppälä, M., and E. Ruoslahti (1973a), *Amer. J. Obstet. Gynec.*, **115**, 48.
Seppälä, M., and E. Ruoslahti (1973b), *Obstet. Gynec.*, **42**, 701.
Seppälä, M., and H.-A. Unnérus (1974), *Amer. J. Obstet. Gynec.*, **119**, 270.
Seppälä, M., O. Karjalainen, J. Rapola, and J. Lindgren (1976), *Lancet*, **i**, 303.
Sever, J. L. (1969), Ed.: Immunological responses to perinatal infections (selected papers), *J. Pediat.*, **75**.
Sever, J. L., and W. T. London (1969), *Teratology*, **2**, 39.
Silverstein, A. M. (1964), *Science*, **144**, 1423.
Singer, W., P. Desjardins, and H. G. Friesen (1970), *Obstet. Gynec.*, **36**, 222.
Spellacy, W. N., E. S. Teoh, W. C. Buhi, S. A. Birk, and S. A. McCreary (1971), *Amer. J. Obstet. Gynec.*, **109**, 588.
Spona, J., and H. Janisch (1971), *Acta Endocrin.*, **68**, 401.
Stewart, C. R., A. M. Ward, and J. Lorber (1975), *Brit. J. Obstet. Gynaec.*, **82**, 257.
Stiehm, E. R., A. J. Ammann, and J. D. Cherry (1966), *New Engl. J. Med.*, **275**, 971.
Stimson, W. H., and L. Eubank-Scott (1972), *FEBS Lett.*, **23**, 298.
Studd, J. W. W., J. D. Blainey, and D. E. Bailey (1970), *J. Obstet. Gynaec. Brit. Commonw.*, **77**, 42.
Sutherland, G. R., D. J. H. Brock, and J. B. Scrimgeour (1973), *Lancet*, **ii**, 1098.
Sutherland, G. R., D. J. H. Brock, and J. B. Scrimgeour (1975), *J. Med. Genet.*, **12**, 135.
Sutherland, G. R., D. Holt, and J. G. Rogers (1977), *Lancet*, **i**, 649.
Tatra, G., G. Breitenecker, and W. Gruber (1974), *Arch. Gynäk.*, **217**, 383.
Tatra, G., P. Placheta, and G. Breitenecker (1975), *Wien. klin. Woch.*, **87**, 279.
Than, G. N., I. F. Csaba, and D. G. Szabó (1974), *Lancet*, **ii**, 1578.
Towler, C. M., C. H. W. Horne, V. Jandial, D. M. Campbell, and I. MacGillivray (1976), *Brit. J. Obstet. Gynaec.*, **83**, 775.
Towler, C. M., C. H. W. Horne, V. Jandial, D. M. Campbell, and I. MacGillivray (1977), *Brit. J. Obstet. Gynaec.*, **84**, 258.
Ursell, W., M. Brudenell, and T. Chard (1973), *Brit. Med. J.*, **ii**, 80.
Vaitukaitis, J. L., and G. T. Ross (1972), cited by Braunstein *et al.* (1976).
Vaitukaitis, J. L., G. D. Braunstein, and G. T. Ross (1972), *Amer. J. Obstet. Gynec.*, **113**, 751.
Vince, J. D., T. J. McManus, M. A. Ferguson-Smith, and J. G. Ratcliffe (1975), *Brit. J. Obstet. Gynaec.*, **82**, 718.
Vince, J. D., H. Rawlinson, H. A. Tait, T. J. McManus, M. A. Ferguson-Smith, J. O. Struthers, and J. G. Ratcliffe (1977), *Lancet*, **i**, 43.
von Schoultz, B., and T. Stigbrand (1973), *Acta Obstet. Gynec. Scand.*, **52**, 51.
Wald, N. J., D. J. H. Brock, and J. Bonnar (1974), *Lancet*, **i**, 765.
Wald, N., S. Barker, R. Peto, D. J. H. Brock, and J. Bonnar (1975), *Brit. Med. J.*, **i**, 651.
Wald, N., S. Barker, H. Cuckle, D. J. H. Brock, and G. M. Stirrat (1977a), *Brit. J. Obstet. Gynaec.*, **84**, 357.
Wald, N. J., H. Cuckle, D. J. H. Brock, R. Peto, P. E. Polani, F. P. Woodford, and 29 others (1977b), *Lancet*, **i**, 1324.
Ward, A. M., and C. R. Stewart (1974), *Lancet*, **ii**, 345.

Ward, R. H. T., A. T. Letchworth, P. A. R. Niven, and T. Chard (1974), *Brit. Med. J.*, **i**, 347.
Weinberg, A. G., A. Milunsky, and M. J. Harrod (1975), *Lancet*, **ii**, 496.
Weiss, R. R., J. N. Macri, N. Tejani, R. Tillitt, and L. I. Mann (1974), *Obstet. Gynec.*, **44**, 368.
Weiss, R. R., J. N. Macri, and C. Merskey (1976), *Lancet*, **i**, 304.
Whyley, G. A., H. Ward, and N. R. Hardy (1974), *J. Obstet. Gynaec. Brit. Commonw.*, **81**, 459.
Wide, L. (1962), *Acta Endocrin.*, **41**, Suppl. 70, 1.
Wilde, C. E., and R. E. Oakey (1975), *Ann. Clin. Biochem.*, **12**, 83.
Young, J. L., R. G. Reid, and J. W. Crawford (1976), *Clin. Chim. Acta*, **69**, 11.

CHAPTER 12

Malnutrition

The term *malnutrition* covers a multitude of deficiency diseases, as well as conditions of nutritional deficiency brought about by disease, for example malabsorption syndromes, or carcinomata that interfere with the digestion and absorption of food. The present chapter is limited to a brief discussion of plasma protein changes in infants and children resulting from a deficiency of protein, or of both protein and calories, in the diet; the literature on protein changes in malnutrition is extensive, and the present chapter can provide only a partial background to the subject.

Protein-energy malnutrition denotes a spectrum of pathological conditions ranging from kwashiorkor to marasmus. The main distinguishing feature of kwashiorkor is the presence of oedema and (as far as the plasma proteins are concerned) the main biochemical feature is a very low albumin concentration, but the degree of body wasting can vary greatly; in marasmus, on the other hand, there no oedema and the serum albumin concentration is not so much reduced (indeed, it may be normal), but the child is extremely emaciated. These and other differences in the pathophysiology of kwashiorkor and marasmus have been assumed to indicate different dietary aetiologies, kwashiorkor being thought to result from a diet that is primarily lacking in protein but provides a sufficiency of calories, and marasmus to result from a deficiency of calories in what could otherwise be a balanced diet. This is undoubtedly an over-simplification. It has been shown, for example, that in Indian children there need be no essential difference in the protein : energy ratios of the diets consumed by children who develop kwashiorkor and those who become marasmic; the two syndromes can apparently develop in children whose diets do not demonstrably differ in protein content (Gopalan, 1968). Similar conclusions have since been reported by Arroyave (1975), Scrimshaw (1975), and Waterlow (1975). A full discussion of the aetiology of these conditions is beyond the scope of this book; the reader is referred to the contributions of Coward and Whitehead and their colleagues (Coward *et al.*, 1977; Whitehead *et al.*, 1977) in addition to those mentioned above.

PLASMA PROTEINS IN MALNUTRITION

Plasma total protein and albumin

In severe protein malnutrition in man with a very low energy and protein intake the total protein concentration in the plasma may be greatly decreased, often to as little as 40 g/l (Waterlow *et al.*, 1960). This is due mainly to a decrease in the albumin fraction. However, severely wasted marasmic children can have relatively normal concentrations of plasma total protein and albumin (Coward *et al.*, 1977); indeed, it appears that in malnutrition a reduced rate of synthesis of albumin may often be partly balanced by a reduction in the rate at which it is catabolized (James and Hay, 1968).

In countries where protein–calorie malnutrition is endemic, determinations of the concentrations of plasma total protein and albumin have long been regarded as essential measures of nutritional status; and a fall in the concentration of serum albumin has been regarded as the most sensitive biochemical index of mild or impending protein deficiency (Brock, 1961).

More recent studies suggest, however, that there are mechanisms tending to maintain the total circulating mass of albumin when protein supplies are low, and that a fall in the serum albumin concentration is a relatively late event in protein depletion (Waterlow, 1969). A reduction in the rate of catabolism of albumin has been referred to above. In animal experiments it has been shown that there is a reduction in the concentration of albumin in the interstitial fluid, which protects against oedema formation (Coward and Fiorotto, 1979), and this mechanism may well be operative in children also.

These observations are consistent with those of Schendel and his colleagues (1962), who found that even with a diet of poor quality food, such as maize, the serum albumin concentration was maintained for several weeks before it began to fall. Again, in children from families with widely different levels of income (Wittmann *et al.*, 1967), only a small difference was found between the mean albumin concentrations in the lowest and highest income groups, but there was a much greater difference in body weights. All these and other findings suggest that the serum albumin concentration is not a very sensitive index of the adequacy of protein intake.

On the other hand, Olusi and his collaborators (1975) found that the serum concentration of albumin closely reflected the severity of protein–calorie malnutrition in Nigerian children with kwashiorkor or marasmus. They suggested that this finding might have been due to their use of highly sensitive immunochemical methods of analysis.

Furthermore, Whitehead and his coworkers (1973), while accepting that there are measurements that are much more sensitive than serum albumin to dietary deprivation and its immediate consequences, have nevertheless emphasized the value of measuring serum albumin as a marker for a critical 'switch' in metabolic balance during the onset of clinical kwashiorkor in a child. Their observations indicated that major biochemical changes (low insulin, high cortisol and growth hormone, low α_2- and β-globulin, low β-lipoprotein, and very low valine and alanine concentrations in the serum, and a reduced serum colloidal osmotic pressure), and associated early clinical signs, all start to develop at about the same time; and that in the type of protein malnutrition that they were studying (in Uganda) this critical phase begins after the serum albumin concentration has fallen below 30 g/l. In a more recent publication Whitehead and his coworkers (Hay *et al.*, 1975) have reaffirmed the value of serum albumin determinations as a prognostic indicator in oedematous malnutrition.

Coward and his coworkers (1977) list a number of possible reasons for the development of hypoalbuminaemia: (a) muscle-wasting may be so extensive that this tissue can no longer provide an adequate source of amino acids for the hepatic synthesis of albumin; (b) the metabolism of the liver may become so deranged that it no longer has an adequate synthetic ability; (c) since the concentration of intravascular albumin is normally 'buffered' in protein–energy malnutrition by the extravascular albumin, principally contained in muscle and skin, the reduced amounts of such tissues might limit this capacity; and (d) in children there can be an actual loss of albumin, for example as a result of an attack of measles. The profound effect that superimposed infection may have is illustrated by studies of undernourished children who suffered an attack of measles. Such an attack often precipitates overt kwashiorkor (Gans, 1961; Murphy, 1966; Ogbeide, 1971). In addition to other possible causes, faecal protein loss and malabsorption probably contribute significantly to the development of malnutrition after measles (Dossetor and Whittle, 1975; Axton, 1975). Helminth infections may disturb the digestion, metabolism, and growth of their hosts (Scrimshaw *et al.*, 1968) and in this way become a factor in the aetiology of protein–calorie malnutrition (see FAO/WHO Recommendations, 1975; Muller, 1975). In rats infected with the nematode *Nippostrongylus brasiliensis* a considerable reduction occurred in plasma albumin concentrations below those found in uninfected animals fed the same diets (Crompton *et al.*, 1978). If severe hookworm or similar parasitic infections have a similar effect in children with subclinical features of kwashiorkor, they might be expected to reduce further the already low plasma albumin concentration and might well precipitate acute kwashiorkor (Crompton *et al.*, 1978).

Transferrin and prealbumin

Several studies have demonstrated that other plasma proteins may provide a more sensitive indicator of nutritional status. Among the tests available for evaluating protein–calorie malnutrition, estimation of transferrin has been found useful (Antia *et al.*, 1968; McFarlane *et al.*, 1968; Garib *et al.*, 1971; Grant *et al.*, 1973; Masawe and Rwabwogo-Atenyi, 1973); and the estimation of thyroxine-binding prealbumin has also been proposed for a similar purpose (Ingenbleek *et al.*, 1972). In addition to transporting thyroxine, prealbumin serves as a carrier protein for retinol-binding protein (the specific carrier protein for vitamin A alcohol), and it has been demonstrated that the concentration of the prealbumin-retinol-binding protein complex falls drastically in the acute stage of kwashiorkor and returns to normal during nutritional rehabilitation (Smith *et al.*, 1973; Ingenbleek *et al.*, 1975a).

A comparative study of the concentrations of four plasma proteins in Senegalese children suffering from severe protein–calorie malnutrition showed that plasma albumin has low sensitivity, transferrin has intermediate sensitivity, and the thyroxine-binding-prealbumin-retinol-binding protein complex has the highest sensitivity to alteration in the nutritional status (Ingenbleek *et al.*, 1975b). This high sensitivity is apparently related to the rapid turnover rates of these proteins and to their high content of tryptophan, an amino acid which plays a special rôle in the regulation of polyribosome aggregation and protein synthesis in the liver (Sidransky *et al.*, 1968; Rothschild *et al.*, 1969). Measurement of either thyroxine-binding prealbumin or retinol-binding was proposed as a method for the detection of pre-kwashiorkor and early marasmus.

It is important to note that serum prealbumin is not a suitable indicator of low protein intake in patients with chronic renal failure who are being treated by dialysis (Wardle *et al.*, 1975). Many of these patients were found to have normal or raised serum prealbumin but low transferrin and near-normal albumin concentrations. Possible reasons for the maintenance of the prealbumin concentration are (Wardle *et al.*, 1975): the high binding capacity of the plasma proteins for tryptophan (of which prealbumin has a high content), as a result of which only small losses occur during haemodialysis; reduced renal filtration (i.e. assuming catabolism of prealbumin by the kidney); and, possibly, depression of thyroid function (Fankhauser *et al.*, 1967; Ramirez *et al.*, 1972). The lowering of the serum transferrin concentration, which has often been noted in patients with chronic renal failure (Young and Parsons, 1970; Kluthe *et al.*, 1971; Ooi *et al.*, 1972; Müller *et al.*, 1973), appears to reflect restricted protein intake and poor nutritional status. Loss of amino acids through the dialyser may be a contributory factor (Wardle *et al.*, 1975).

Although, as mentioned above, plasma transferrin might appear to be a more suitable index of nutritional status than albumin, it shows a wide range of individual values in patients on admission to hospital (Grant *et al.*, 1973; Ingenbleek *et al.*, 1975b), and in spite of the onset of severe kwashiorkor some patients may have values within the normal range. After the first week of dietary treatment some individuals may show a six- or eightfold increase in plasma transferrin concentration (Antia *et al.*, 1968), while others may show no change or even a fall. Moreover, plasma transferrin responds also to alterations in the supply of iron. Thus, raised plasma transferrin concentrations are found in iron-deficient patients and a progressive return to normal values may be seen on treatment with iron (Awai and Brown, 1963). Since protein malnutrition and iron deficiency usually occur in association in developing countries, the plasma transferrin concentration is subjected to opposing stimuli and thus expresses the relative predominance of one deficiency over the other; this invalidates, at least in part, the use of transferrin measurements as a dependable method for evaluating protein status alone (Ingenbleek *et al.*, 1975b). For the same reason, the plasma concentration of transferrin is not a reliable index of the severity of the iron deficit, at least until protein replenishment has been achieved. For an assessment of iron deficiency, the best available test would appear to be measurement of the serum *ferritin* concentration. In patients with iron deficiency low serum concentrations of ferritin are found (Jacobs *et al.*, 1972). An increased concentration, however, does not necessarily indicate iron overload, since inflammation, liver disease and increased red-cell turnover have been shown to raise the serum ferritin concentration to a degree disproportionate to that corresponding to the iron stores of the body (Lipschitz *et al.*, 1974).

Other serum proteins in malnutrition

Sirisinha and his colleagues (1973) investigated the serum concentrations of the *complement proteins* C1q, C1s, C3, C4, C5, C6, C8, C9, and C3 proactivator in children with protein–calorie malnutrition in Thailand. On admission the serum concentrations of all the complement proteins, except C4, were markedly lower in the malnourished children than in normal, well-nourished children, and children with kwashiorkor had lower concentrations than those with marasmus. The authors point out that most of the children were suffering from bacterial infections on admission, and that these might have been responsible for the observed reductions in complement, as a result of activation and rapid clearance from the circulation. The finding that two children who died in septic shock had serum complement concentrations appreciably lower than those in children who recovered is consistent with the report of McCabe (1973) referred to in Chapter 1.

Olusi and his collaborators (1975), in their study of Nigerian children referred to above, also found normal C4 concentrations in children with kwashiorkor, but significantly lowered concentrations of C3; the amount of lowering was greater the more severe the kwashiorkor. In marasmus the mean concentration of C3 was also lowered but not to the same extent. The reason for the different behaviour of C4 as compared with the other complement components is not known.

Immunoglobulins

Immunoglobulin concentrations have been measured in malnutrition by a number of workers, but the findings (reviewed by Garrow, 1974) have varied. Taking the data as a whole, Garrow concludes that it seems unlikely that malnourished children have any impairment of antibody production, the differences in the findings between one series and another probably being due to variations in the type and severity of infection.

Plasma lipoproteins

Plasma α_1- and β-lipoprotein concentrations have usually been found to be low in kwashiorkor, the α-lipoprotein being more severely affected than the β- (Cravioto *et al.*, 1959, in Mexico; Chatterjee and Chaudhuri, 1961, in India; Coward and Whitehead, 1972, in Uganda). Apparently the β-lipoprotein concentration does not fall significantly until the serum albumin concentration is less than a certain critical value (25 g/l) (Coward and Whitehead, 1972).

Marasmic children, however, were found to have normal serum concentrations of β-lipoprotein and of the other components measured. It was considered that, in Ugandan children with serum albumin concentrations below 25 g/l, the concentration of β-lipoprotein was probably insufficient for normal mobilization of fat from the liver and that the children were therefore more susceptible to the development of a fatty liver (a well known feature of kwashiorkor).

As noted above, the three studies mentioned were made in Mexico, India, and Uganda respectively. A significantly different finding was reported by Truswell and his coworkers (1969), who found that in South African children with kwashiorkor only the β-lipoprotein concentration was reduced, the α-lipoprotein being unaltered. It would seem—as Coward and Whitehead point out—that some of the biochemical features of kwashiorkor may well differ in different parts of the world.

The suggestion has been made that the principal mechanism for the pathogenesis of fatty liver in protein–calorie malnutrition is reduced synthesis of the apoprotein of low-density and/or very-low-density lipoproteins (Truswell and Hansen, 1969; Truswell *et al.*, 1969). According to Truswell (1975), measurement of the serum concentration of cholesterol—or, better, the β-lipoprotein cholesterol—may give more reliable information about whether there is fat in the liver than is obtained by palpation. However, as Truswell points out, the concentration ranges of the plasma lipids are wide and there is considerable overlapping of these ranges between the various groups of patients graded according to the degree of fatty change in the liver (as assessed by the examination of biopsy specimens). If one considers also the other factors influencing plasma lipid concentrations, it is not to be expected that these measurements alone will be of clinical value except in a minority of cases. Nevertheless, according to Truswell, the presence of lipaemia during treatment, or the finding of pre-β-lipoprotein on paper electrophoresis of the serum proteins, or a rising concentration of serum cholesterol, all indicate that fat is coming out of the liver. During recovery from kwashiorkor, the concentration of plasma triglyceride increases rapidly, followed by β-lipoproteins a few days later, and albumin, cholesterol, and presumably α-lipoprotein, later still.

Serum enzymes in malnutrition

An increase in serum aspartate and alanine transaminases and isocitrate dehydrogenase in Nigerian children with kwashiorkor was reported by Baron (1960). These increases were considered to be due primarily to the release of enzymes from liver cells, with general tissue break-down, principally in the skeletal muscles, perhaps playing a part. In Jamaican children suffering from malnutrition a raised serum alanine transaminase activity, when associated with a raised serum bilirubin concentration, indicated a high probability of death; if serum isocitrate dehydrogenase activity was also raised, the probability of a fatal outcome was even higher (McLean, 1966).

On the other hand, in Uganda, Smith (1962) found no correlation between the serum aspartate or alanine transaminase activity and the severity of the kwashiorkor, and no consistent trend in individual children during treatment. Also in Uganda, lowered serum creatine kinase activity was found in many children with untreated kwashiorkor or marasmus (Balmer and Rutishauser, 1968), though in severely wasted children with kwashiorkor and in children with marasmus normal activities were sometimes found. It was suggested that this was the result of release of the enzyme from muscle, and in these children creatine kinase activity frequently fell during the first week of treatment before rising again slowly. In malnourished children who died, serum creatine kinase activity was frequently found to be raised just before death (Balmer and Rutishauser, 1968).

Serum activities of pseudocholinesterase, amylase and alkaline phosphatase were reported by Edozien (1961) to be reduced in kwashiorkor. Some, though not all, previous workers also found low serum alkaline phosphatase values in children with kwashiorkor; the various factors that might influence the level of this enzyme in the serum in kwashiorkor were discussed by Schwartz (1956).

Other enzyme changes in malnutrition were discussed by Waterlow and his collaborators (1960) and by Whitehead (1968).

PROTEIN TURNOVER RATES

The studies referred to above have mostly been concerned with essentially static measurements, i.e. measurements of protein concentrations at some point in time. However, changes in the amount or concentration of a protein are the result of changes in the rate of synthesis or catabolism, or both. Such changes may be undetectable by static measurements, and, in general, require the use of isotope tracer techniques. Experiments using such techniques have shown that in the malnourished child the rate of synthesis of albumin is greatly reduced (Picou and Waterlow, 1962; Cohen and Hansen, 1962), and that (as mentioned earlier in this chapter) the catabolic rate of albumin is also reduced (James and Hay, 1968). This change in the turnover rate of albumin is apparently brought about by a complex mechanism, synthesis altering rapidly with changes in the diet, and catabolism only after a time lag, possibly by a hormone-mediated control system.

These studies also reveal that even in states of severe protein deficiency a remarkable capacity for protein synthesis is maintained.

By the use of a technique involving continuous infusion of an isotopically labelled amino acid, Picou and Taylor-Roberts (1969) found that malnourished children have a normal net rate of protein synthesis but a considerably increased rate of nitrogen turnover. This can be explained by an increased efficiency of reutilization of amino acids in malnourished children, a greater proportion than normal of the amino acids released by the catabolism of protein being reincorporated into protein instead of being deaminated to form urea.

These and other studies on the turnover rates of plasma proteins in malnutrition have been critically reviewed by Garrow (1974).

LABORATORY INVESTIGATION OF PROTEINS IN MALNUTRITION

It may be helpful to attempt to draw a distinction between those biochemical changes that serve as 'markers' for malnutrition and those that appear to indicate some functional abnormality apart from a general lowering of protein synthesis. In the first group are the lowered concentrations of serum albumin, prealbumin, and so on. Although these may be important markers of nutritional status, it could be suggested that they often give little information of clinical value; thus Garrow (1974) comments that a low serum albumin concentration in a child with kwashiorkor 'tells us nothing that clinical examination would not have revealed'. (This is a view that many workers will disagree with. For example, reductions in the concentration of serum albumin have been regarded as having both diagnostic value (Whitehead *et al.*, 1973; Hay *et al.*, 1975) and clinical significance in relation to the development of oedema (Coward, 1975).) On the other hand, certain other observations, for example measurement of the plasma lipids, may suggest the presence of specific conditions or complications amenable to treatment, or, as in the case of certain enzyme estimations, provide information of prognostic value.

As far as defining nutritional status is concerned, it is clear that there are disadvantages in using plasma transferrin measurements for this purpose. Measurement of retinol will usually be impracticable, at least under field conditions; and retinol-binding protein is present only in very small concentrations in the plasma. Ingenbleek and his coworkers (1975b) suggest measurement of the serum prealbumin concentration as the most useful and accurate index available. Estimation of serum albumin may be useful in manifest malnutrition.

It is almost unnecessary to add that the investigation of proteins forms only a part of any assessment of malnutrition, which must also involve haematological investigations and take into account any deficiencies of potassium, vitamins, iron and so on, as well as the presence of dehydration; moreover, many cases are complicated by infections of various kinds which may considerably modify the clinical picture, as described earlier in this chapter. There is evidence also that altered hormonal balance, particularly of cortisol and insulin, can influence the type of protein–energy malnutrition that is likely to emerge (Whitehead *et al.*, 1978).

REFERENCES

Antia, A. U., H. McFarlane, and J. F. Soothill (1968), *Arch. Dis. Child.*, **43**, 459.

Arroyave, G. (1975) in *Protein Calorie Malnutrition* (Ed. R. E. Olson), Academic Press, New York and London, p. 343.

Awai, M., and E. B. Brown (1963), *J. Lab. Clin. Med.*, **61**, 363.

Axton, J. H. M. (1975), *Brit. Med. J.*, **iii**, 79.

Balmer, S. E., and I. H. E. Rutishauser (1968), *J. Pediat.*, **73**, 783.

Baron, D. N. (1960), *J. Clin. Path.*, **13**, 252.

Brock, J. F. (1961), *Recent Advances in Human Nutrition*, Little, Brown, Boston.

Chatterjee, K., and J. N. Chaudhuri (1961), *Indian J. Pediat.*, **28**, 195.

Cohen, S., and J. D. L. Hansen (1962), *Clin. Sci.*, **23**, 351.
Coward, W. A. (1975), *Brit. J. Nutr.*, **34**, 459.
Coward, W. A., and M. Fiorotto (1979), *Proc. Nutr. Soc.*, **38**, 51.
Coward, W. A., and R. G. Whitehead (1972), *Brit. J. Nutr.*, **27**, 383.
Coward, W. A., R. G. Whitehead, and P. G. Lunn (1977), *Brit. J. Nutr.*, **38**, 115.
Cravioto, J., C. L. de la Pena, and G. Burgos (1959), *Metabolism*, **8**, 722.
Crompton, D. W. T., S. Arnold, W. A. Coward, and P. G. Lunn (1978), *Trans. Roy. Soc. Trop. Med. Hyg.*, **72**, 195.
Dossetor, J. F. B., and H. C. Whittle (1975), *Brit. Med. J.*, **ii**, 592.
Edozien, J. C. (1961), *Pediatrics*, **27**, 325.
Fankhauser, S., J. Zeyer, D. Huber, and F. Reubi (1967), *J. Urol. Nephrol.*, **73**, 767.
FAO/WHO Recommendations (1975), *Food and Nutrition*, **1**, 11.
Gans, B. (1961), *W. African Med. J.*, **10**, 33.
Garib, M., M. F. S. El-Hawary, and J. J. El-Dali (1971), *J. Trop. Med. Hyg.*, **74**, 216.
Garrow, J. S. (1974), in *Structure and Function of Plasma Proteins* (Ed. A. C. Allison), vol. 1, Plenum Press, London, p. 283.
Gopalan, C. (1968) in *Calorie Deficiencies and Protein Deficiencies* (Eds. R. A. McCance and E. M. Widdowson), Churchill, London, p. 49.
Grant, D. B., J. Hambley, D. Becker, and B. L. Pimstone (1973), *Arch. Dis. Child.*, **48**, 596.
Hay, R. W., R. G. Whitehead, and C. C. Spicer (1975), *Lancet*, **ii**, 427.
Ingenbleek, Y., M. De Visscher, and Ph. De Nayer (1972), *Lancet*, **ii**, 106.
Ingenbleek, Y., H.-G. Van den Schrieck, Ph. De Nayer, and M. De Visscher (1975a), *Metabolism*, **24**, 633.
Ingenbleek, Y., H.-G. Van den Schrieck, Ph. De Nayer, and M. De Visscher (1975b), *Clin. Chim. Acta*, **63**, 61.
Jacobs, A., F. Miller, M. Worwood, M. R. Beamish, and C. A. Wardrop (1972), *Brit. Med. J.*, **iv**, 206.
James, W. P. T., and A. M. Hay (1968), *J. Clin. Invest.*, **47**, 1958.
Kluthe, R., G. Baumann, V. Bischoff, and H. Quirin (1971), *Medizin. Ernähr.*, **12**, 73.
Lipschitz, D. A., J. D. Cook, and C. A. Finch (1974), *New Engl. J. Med.*, **290**, 1213.
Masawe, A. E. J., and J. Rwabwogo-Atenyi (1973), *Arch. Dis. Child.*, **48**, 927.
McCance, R. A., and E. M. Widdowson (1966), *Lancet*, **ii**, 158.
McCance, R. A., and E. M. Widdowson (1968), *Calorie Deficiencies and Protein Deficiencies* (Eds.), Churchill, London.
McFarlane, H., M. I. Ogbeide, S. Reddy, K. J. Adcock, H. Adeshina, J. M. Gurney, A. Cooke, G. O., Taylor, and J. A. Mordie (1969), *Lancet*, **i**, 392.
McLean, A. E. M. (1966), *Clin. Sci.*, **30**, 129.
Müller, H., K. Roth, H. Quirin, N. Kleine, and R. Kluthe (1973), *Verh. deut. Ges. inn. Med.*, **79**, 719.
Muller, R. (1975), *Worms and Disease*, Heinemann, London.
Murphy, E. L. (1966), *Ghana Med. J.*, **5**, 58.
Ogbeide, M. J. (1971), *W. African Med. J.*, **20**, 313.
Olson, R. E. (1975), *Protein-Calorie Malnutrition* (Ed.), Academic Press, New York.
Olusi, S. O., H. McFarlane, B. O. Osunkoya, and H. Adesina (1975), *Clin. Chim. Acta*, **62**, 107.
Ooi, B. S., A. F. Darocy, and V. E. Pollak (1972), *Nephron*, **9**, 200.
Picou, D., and T. Taylor-Roberts (1969), *Clin. Sci.*, **36**, 283.
Picou, D., and J. C. Waterlow (1962), *Clin. Sci.*, **22**, 459.
Ramirez, G., W. Jubiz, C. F. Gutch, and W. J. Kolff (1972), *Trans. Amer. Soc. Artif. Internal Organs*, **18**, 244. (Cited by Wardle *et al.*, 1975.)
Rothschild, M. A., M. Oratz, J. Mongelli, L. Fishman, and S. S. Schreiber (1969), *J. Nutr.*, **98**, 395.
Schendel, H. E., J. D. L. Hansen, and J. F. Brock (1962), *S. African J. Lab. Clin. Med.*, **8**, 23.

Schwartz, R. (1956), *J. Clin. Path.*, **9**, 333.

Scrimshaw, N. S. (1975), in *Protein Calorie Malnutrition* (Ed. R. E. Olson), Academic Press, New York and London, p. 345.

Scrimshaw, N. S., C. E. Taylor, and J. E. Gordon (1968), *WHO Monograph Series*, No. 57.

Sidransky, H., D. S. R. Sarma, M. Bongiorno, and E. Verney (1968), *J. Biol. Chem.*, **243**, 1123.

Sirisinha, S. R. Suskind, R. Edelman, C. Charupatana, and R. E. Olson (1973), *Lancet*, **i**, 1016.

Smith, C. E. (1962), *J. Pediat.*, **61**, 617.

Smith, F. R., D. S. Goodman, M. S. Zaklama, M. K. Gabr, S. El Maraghy, and V. N. Patwardhan (1973), *Amer. J. Clin. Nutr.*, **26**, 973.

Truswell, A. S. (1975), in *Protein-Calorie Malnutrition* (Ed. R. E. Olson), Academic Press, New York, p. 119.

Truswell, A. S., and J. D. L. Hansen (1969), *S. African Med. J.*, **43**, 280.

Truswell, A. S., J. D. L. Hansen, C. E. Watson, and P. Wannenburg (1969), *Amer. J. Clin. Nutr.*, **22**, 568.

Wardle, E. N., D. N. S. Kerr, and H. A. Ellis (1975), *Clin. Nephrol.*, **3**, 114.

Waterlow, J. C. (1969), in *Mammalian Protein Metabolism* (Ed. H. N. Munro), Vol. 3, Academic Press, New York and London, p. 326.

Waterlow, J. C. (1975), in *Protein Calorie Malnutrition* (Ed. R. E. Olson), Academic Press, New York and London, p. 348.

Waterlow, J. C., J. Cravioto, and J. M. L. Stephen (1960), in *Advances in Protein Chemistry* (Eds. C. B. Anfinsen, Jr., M. L. Anson, K. Bailey, and J. T. Edsall), Vol. 15, Academic Press, New York and London, p. 131.

Whitehead, R. G. (1968), in *Calorie Deficiencies and Protein Deficiencies* (Eds. R. A. McCance and E. M. Widdowson), Churchill, London, p. 115.

Whitehead, R. G., W. A. Coward, and P. G. Lunn (1973), *Lancet*, **i**, 63.

Whitehead, R. G., W. A. Coward, P. G. Lunn, and I. Rutishauser (1977), *Trans. Roy. Soc. Trop. Med. Hyg.*, **71**, 189.

Wittmann, W., A. D. Moodie, S. A. Fellingham, and J. D. L. Hansen (1967), *S. African Med. J.*, **41**, 664.

Young, G. A., and F. M. Parsons (1970), *Clin. Chim. Acta*, **27**, 491.

Appendices

In these Appendices are included some of the commoner analytical procedures used in the analysis of body fluids for proteins. Most of these are in use in the writer's laboratory. No attempt has been made to describe the more complicated immunological tests, for details of which the reader should consult more specialized works.

APPENDIX 1

Collection and treatment of specimens for analysis

In general, specimens should be freshly collected and should be sent to the laboratory without delay. Many serum proteins are relatively stable at room temperature for a day or so, especially if a small amount of sodium azide (10 mg to every 2–5 ml of serum) is added; however, conditions of temperature during transportation over long distances cannot readily be controlled, unless the specimen is packed in a refrigerant. If complement conversion is to be assessed, special precautions must be taken (see Appendix 17). Particular care should be taken to preserve urine, especially if it is to be tested for Bence Jones protein: the addition of 25 mg of sodium azide or 2 drops of toluene to 25 ml of urine is recommended.

In the case of enzyme estimations, inhibitors of enzymic activity must be avoided, the specimen being kept cold and transported as rapidly as possible to the laboratory.

For most analyses, 1–2 ml of serum, urine, amniotic fluid, or cerebrospinal fluid is ample; the amount actually taken for analysis will usually be measured in microlitres, but it is desirable that larger amounts be sent. This has the effect of reducing errors due to evaporation and contamination, besides allowing repetition of the test, or the application of further tests, should this be necessary.

APPENDIX 2

Total protein in biological fluids

Of the substances in the body fluids that are determined for clinical purposes, proteins possess the greatest variety of structural features or constituents capable affording a basis for measurement. It is not surprising, therefore, that a great variety of methods have been proposed for their determination. The principal ones are listed in Table App. 2.1. Since the constituents measured by the different methods may vary independently in amount from one protein to another, it is to be expected that variations in the relative proportions of the proteins in a mixture will often lead to discrepancies when determinations are made by different methods. Equally, if a given method has been standardized by reference to a particular protein, estimations of another protein may be in error unless it happens to contain a similar proportion of the constituent that is, in effect, being measured.

One of the most widely used methods for the estimation of proteins, and the

Table App. 2.1. Methods proposed for the determination of total protein in plasma and other biological fluids

Principle	Selected references
Gravimetric	Robinson and Hogden, 1941
Specific gravity measurement	Phillips *et al.*, 1950; Van Slyke *et al.*, 1950
Measurement of refractive index	Naumann, 1964
Measurement of N content	Hiller *et al.*, 1948
Absorption in ultraviolet	Goldfarb *et al.*, 1951; Waddell, 1956; Tombs *et al.*, 1959
Biuret method	See text
Reaction with Folin–Ciocalteu reagent	Greenberg, 1936; Minot and Keller, 1936
Lowry method	See text
Sakaguchi reaction	Albanese *et al.*, 1946, 1947; Keyser, 1948
Turbidimetric method using sulphosalicylic acid or trichloroacetic acid	See text
Solution in HNO_3 and colour with NH_4OH	Hausdorf, 1950; Härtel, 1960
Formation of Cu–protein complex and determination of Cu	Goldberg, 1973; Doetsch and Gadsden, 1975
Dye binding	Pesce and Strande, 1973; Salo and Honkavaara, 1974; Bradford, 1976

one generally regarded as the method of choice, is based on the biuret reaction. This reaction depends upon the presence of peptide groups, approximately four amino acid residues being bound by chelation to each copper atom (Rising and Yang, 1932–33; Mehl *et al.*, 1949). Originally introduced by Riegler (1914), the biuret method has undergone innumerable modifications, among the most satisfactory of which is that of Weichselbaum (1946). His procedure is described below.

The low sensitivity of the biuret method, while adequate for most purposes, limits its use when the amount of material available is very small or its protein content low. Suggestions have been made for increasing its sensitivity (see e.g. Westley and Lambeth, 1960). However, when only small amounts of sample are available the method of Lowry and his coworkers (1951) is generally favoured. This very sensitive method involves reaction of the protein with copper in alkaline solution, followed by reduction of the phosphomolybdic–phosphotungstic reagent of Folin and Ciocalteu by the copper-treated protein. It should be noted that the 'colour values' for different proteins are not as constant for the Lowry as for the biuret method (Lowry *et al.*, 1951); the Lowry 'colour value' of a protein apparently depends upon its content of tryptophan and tyrosine (Daughaday *et al.*, 1952) and cysteine (Chou and Goldstein, 1960), and proteins vary considerably in their content of these amino acids. Another drawback associated with the Lowry method is its susceptibility to interference from non-protein substances, as when, for example, it is applied to the determination of protein in cerebrospinal fluid. The interference in this case is very considerable and, moreover, the great variability in the content of non-protein colour-producing substances from patient to patient renders the use of a fixed correction value, as recommended by Daughaday *et al.* (1952) and by Lous *et al.* (1956), unacceptable for the determination of protein in cerebrospinal fluid (Svensmark, 1958). Methods for the determination of protein in cerebrospinal fluid have been critically reviewed by Watson (1964) and are further discussed below.

Many of the non-protein substances referred to above as interfering in the Lowry determination are commonly encountered in biochemical work; they include Tris and other buffers, sulphydryl reagents, carbohydrates, chelating agents, and other substances (see Rej and Richards (1974) for references). One of the sulphydryl compounds that interfere is dithiothreitol, a substance widely used to protect thiol groups of enzymes and other proteins during isolation and purification; however, according to Heffron (1975) the interference can be allowed for at sufficiently low concentrations.

An extremely sensitive method has been proposed (Goldberg, 1973) in which copper is complexed to the protein and, after removal of excess copper by passage through a 'Sephadex' column, the complex is destroyed by digestion with hydrogen peroxide; addition of phenol and chloramine-T to the reaction mixture leads to a colour-producing reaction between the two compounds, catalysed by the copper. The method is very much more sensitive than that of Lowry.

Biuret method

Reagents

(1) *Stock biuret reagent* (Weichselbaum). Dissolve 45 g of sodium potassium tartrate in about 400 ml of 0.2 N sodium hydroxide. Add 15 g of finely powdered copper sulphate, $CuSO_4.5H_2O$, with stirring, and continue stirring until the crystals are completely dissolved. Then add 5 g of potassium iodide and dilute to 1 litre with 0.2 N sodium hydroxide.

(2) *Dilute biuret reagent.* Dilute 200 ml of the stock biuret reagent to 1 litre with 0.2 N sodium hydroxide containing 5 g of potassium iodide per litre.

(3) *Sodium hydroxide.* (a) 0.2 N and (b) 0.2 N containing 5 g of potassium iodide per litre. These solutions should be prepared from a carbonate-free concentrated solution of sodium hydroxide.

(4) *Tartrate–iodide solution* (for serum blank). Dissolve 9 g of sodium potassium tartrate in 0.2 N sodium hydroxide containing 5 g of potassium iodide per litre (Reagent 3 b) and dilute to 1 litre with this reagent.

(5) *Standard serum* of known protein content, or a solution of pure bovine or human serum albumin (Note 1).

Procedure

To 5 ml of dilute biuret reagent add 0.1 ml of serum and incubate at 30 °C (or 37 °C) for 10 min. (Note 2). After cooling to room temperature, measure the absorbance at 555 nm, or using a 540-nm filter, setting the zero with a blank consisting of 5 ml of the dilute biuret reagent plus 0.1 ml of water (Note 3). Treat the serum of known protein concentration in the same way (Note 4). For a serum blank determination add 0.1 ml of serum to 5 ml of the tartrate–iodide solution and read the absorbance, using tartrate–iodide solution for the zero setting. A similar blank should be performed for the standard.

Notes

(1) The standard may consist of a pool of normal sera, the protein content of which has been determined by the Kjeldahl method. The pooled serum should be distributed between a number of small tubes and stored in a deep freeze. Alternatively, pure bovine or human serum albumin may be used as standard; analytical criteria of purity are listed by Peters (1968). Accordingly to Finlayson (1965), purified albumin in 5 per cent sterile solution is stable for at least 5 years at 5 °C (except for minor changes in the state of aggregation). The use of bovine serum albumin as a primary standard for serum protein assays was also recommended by a Study Group of the Committee on Standards of the American Association of Clinical Chemists (Doumas, 1975).

(2) Weichselbaum suggested an incubation time of 30 min. The shorter

time here prescribed is preferred, since with some specimens a longer incubation causes an increase in turbidity (Reinhold, 1953).

(3) The serum blank is essential only when specimens are pigmented or oplaescent; however, accuracy is improved if blanks are included routinely.

(4) The linear response of the absorptiometer should be checked by testing a series of dilutions of the pooled serum. With a manual method linearity up to high values can readily be checked by the use of a somewhat greater volume of serum; however, with an automated method it is necessary to prepare a standard having a high concentration of protein. The protein concentration of the pool can be raised by treatment with dried acrylamide gel (Curtain, 1964; Keyser and Cawson, 1970), the undiluted serum serving to check the response at high protein concentrations; alternatively, when sera with increased protein concentration are available these can be tested both undiluted and diluted.

Lowry method

Reagents

(1) *Alkaline carbonate solution.* Dissolve 20.0 g of anhydrous sodium carbonate and 0.50 g of potassium sodium tartrate (Rochelle salt, $KNaC_4H_4O_6 . 4H_2O$) in 1 litre of 0.10 N sodium hydroxide. Store in a polyethylene bottle. This reagent is stable for at least 6 months.

(2) *Copper sulphate:* 0.10%. Dissolve 1.0 g of cupric sulphate ($CuSO_4.5H_2O$) in 1 litre of water. Store in a polyethylene bottle. This is stable for at least 3 months.

(3) *Working alkaline copper reagent.* Mix 45 ml of Reagent 1 with 5.0 ml of Reagent 2. This reagent should be prepared daily.

(4) *Folin—Ciocalteu reagent.* Obtainable from laboratory suppliers. Dilute so that 1.00 ml requires 9.0 ± 0.1 ml of 0.10 N NaOH to neutralize (phenolphthalein).

Procedure

In each of three 25-ml conical flasks place 10.0 ml of working alkaline copper reagent (Reagent 3). Add 0.1 ml of test fluid (suitably diluted if necessary) to the first, 0.1 ml of working protein standard to the second, and 0.1 ml of water to the third flask (this serves as the blank). Mix the contents of each flask and allow to stand at room temperature for 15 min. Then add rapidly, while swirling the flask, 1.0 ml of Folin–Ciocalteu reagent to each flask, with immediate mixing (Note 1), and allow to stand at room temperature for 30 min. Read the absorbances of test and standard at 700 nm (Note 2), setting the absorbance of the blank to zero. The colour is stable for about 15 min.

Notes

(1) Rapid mixing with the Folin–Ciocalteu reagent is essential, since at the pH of the copper-treated protein mixture the reagent is reactive for only a

short time (Folin and Denis, 1912; Knights *et al.*, 1962) and a delay of even a few seconds in complete mixing will lessen the amount of colour developed; nevertheless, colour development continues for several minutes after the reagent itself has become unreactive to freshly added protein (Lowry *et al.*, 1951).

(2) The wavelength of maximum absorbance for molybdenum blue is about 750 nm. However, the wavelength selected for the measurements is not critical, provided it is the same for tests and standards.

(3) As was emphasized by Lowry and his colleagues, various pure proteins give different extinction coefficients with the Folin reagent, trypsin, for example, having a chromogenicity three times that of gelatin. In the absence of copper much greater differences are found. This variation in chromogenicity must be kept in mind when the method is to be used for comparing different proteins; it is much less marked with mixtures of proteins as found in various tissues (Lowry *et al.*, 1951).

(4) The Folin–Ciocalteu phenol reagent reacts with numerous phenolic substances, and the possibility of interference by non-protein material must always be considered.

For a fuller discussion of these and other technical points the reader is referred to the article by Friedman (1965).

PROTEIN IN URINE AND CEREBROSPINAL FLUID

Protein in urine may be estimated by the biuret method, after preliminary precipitation. However, Bell and Baron (1968) have reported that, using trichloroacetic acid precipitation, recoveries of added albumin greater than 100% were obtained, apparently owing to the presence of protein-bound urinary pigments; a further disadvantage was that with low concentrations of protein incomplete precipitation was often obtained unless the urine–trichloroacetic acid mixture was allowed to stand overnight (Bell and Baron, 1968). Finally, a major difficulty is that the amount of protein precipitated by the reagents commonly employed (trichloroacetic acid, sulphosalicylic acid) varies according to the type of proteinuria; thus when glomerular permeability is increased, the bulk of the urinary proteins are precipitated by these reagents, whereas in tubular disorders, in which there is a preponderance of low molecular weight proteins, a relatively much smaller amount will be recovered. This difficulty would appear not to apply to the method proposed by Doetsch and Gadsden (1975, 1977), in which precipitation of the urinary protein is not involved, and in which, moreover, the high sensitivity of the Lowry method and the superior specificity of the biuret method are combined. In their procedure, protein is separated from interfering substances by gel filtration; a second, highly alkaline gel column is used to separate the protein–copper complex from excess cupric ions; and finally the copper stoichiometrically bound to peptide bonds is determined colorimetrically with diethyldithiocarbamate.

In another method that determines total urinary proteins (i.e. polypeptide substances with a molecular weight of over 10,000), the proteins are precipitated with a modified Tsuchiya's reagent (ethanolic hydrochloric acid–phosphotungstic acid) and the biuret reaction applied to the precipitate (Rice, 1975).

A sensitive method, applicable to both urine and cerebrospinal fluid, in which the proteins are precipitated by trichloroacetic acid together with a proportional amount of Ponceau S dye, and the red precipitate subsequently dissolved in sodium hydroxide to give a voilet-coloured solution, has been described (Pesce and Strande, 1973).

Other methods have been described by Yatzidis (1977) and by Meola and his coworkers (1977).

Total protein in cerebrospinal fluid

As mentioned above, the extremely sensitive *Lowry method* is unsuitable for the estimation of protein in cerebrospinal fluid on account of its susceptibility to interference by non-protein substances. Measurement of the ultraviolet absorption at 205–210 nm, the wavelengths at which the absorption of proteins in solution is mainly due to the peptide bonds (Goldfarb *et al.*, 1951) and at which the specific absorption of most proteins is many times the value at 280 nm, is also highly sensitive, but the necessity for preliminary dialysis of cerebrospinal fluid renders the method unsuitable for routine use (Pennock *et al.*, 1968). The *biuret method*, as usually performed, has a relatively low sensitivity and it is generally necessary to concentrate the proteins in the cerebrospinal fluid by means of precipitation before applying the colour reaction; however, in a modification proposed by Bürgi and his coworkers (1967) advantage is taken of the high spectral absorbance of the protein–copper complex in the near-ultraviolet region, readings being made at 334 nm. As little as 0.1 ml of cerebrospinal fluid will suffice for the analysis. Some caution is, however, necessary in applying the biuret reaction directly to cerebrospinal fluid in this way; Goa (1953), who also measured the absorbance of the complex in the near-ultraviolet region (330 nm), recommended precipitation of the proteins before applying the biuret reaction, because he found that some non-protein nitrogenous compounds occurring in cerebrospinal fluid also react. Possibly the most convenient method for the routine measurement of protein in cerebrospinal fluid is the *turbidimetric method* of Meulemans (1960) using a sulphosalicylic acid–sodium sulphate precipitating fluid. The incorporation of sodium sulphate in the reagent leads to the production of similar degrees of turbidity by equal amounts of albumin and γ-globulin; if it is omitted, the result is considerably dependent on the albumin:globulin ratio of the specimen. Trichloroacetic acid precipitation has also been used, but it has been reported that the accuracy of the method is not very high (Henry *et al.*, 1956) and that reproducibility is poor (Pennock *et al.*, 1968), though other investigators have apparently obtained satisfactory results (Rice, 1965).

Two methods are described here: the sulphosalicylic acid method and the Ponceau S-trichloroacetic acid method mentioned above.

Sulphosalicylic acid method

Reagent

A 3 per cent w/v solution of sulphosalicylic acid in 7 per cent w/v sodium sulphate, Na_2SO_4.

Procedure

To 1 ml of cerebrospinal fluid add 3 ml of reagent, allow to stand for 10 min. and measure the turbidity at 680 nm with a spectrophotometer. As standard, treat a solution of human serum albumin in the same way.

Notes

(1) A linear relationship holds between total protein concentration and turbidity up to a protein concentration of 2.5 g/l.
(2) Pennock and his coworkers (1968) found that turbidity increases by 1 per cent for each degree C rise in temperature. For the most accurate results, therefore, temperature control is necessary.

Trichloroacetic acid–Ponceau S method (Pesce and Strande, 1973)

Reagents

(1) *Ponceau S:* 40 g in 1 litre of distilled water.
(2) *Trichloroacetic acid:* 300 g in 1 litre of distilled water.
(3) *Working reagent:* Dilute 2 ml of Reagent 1 and 98 ml of Reagent 2 with distilled water to 1 litre.
(4) *Sodium hydroxide:* 8 g/l in distilled water.
(5) *Protein stock standard* containing 80 g protein/l.
(6) *Protein working standards:* 400 and 800 mg/l.
(7) '*Albustix*' *strips* (Ames Co.).

Procedure

Determine the approximate protein content of the sample with an 'Albustix' strip. If the reading indicates:

(a) less that 1 g/l, take 50 μl of sample for the test (Note 1);
(b) between 1 and 3 g/l, take 25 μl;
(c) over 3 g/l, take 5μl.

To the appropriate amount of sample (Note 2) or standard add 500 μl of working reagent (Reagent 3), mix well, and centrifuge for 10 min. at 3500 r/min. Completely remove the supernatant fluid with a Pasteur pipette. To the red precipitate add 1 ml of Reagent 4, mix, and read at 560 nm against water (Note 3). Allowance must be made in the calculation for the amount of sample taken.

Notes

(1) For samples having protein concentrations of less than 100 mg/l, modify the procedure by taking 2 ml of sample and 0.2 ml of working reagent.

(2) It is important that specimens be well spun or filtered, to remove particles.

(3) The colour is stable for 6 h at room temperature.

If desired, quantities of sample and reagents can be increased so as to give a larger final volume of solution.

REFERENCES

Albanese, A. A., V. Irby, and B. Saur (1946), *J. Biol. Chem.*, **166**, 231.
Albanese, A. A., B. Saur, and V. Irby (1947), *J. Lab. Clin. Med.*, **32**, 296.
Bell, J. L., and D. N. Baron (1968), *Proc. Assoc. Clin. Biochem.*, **5**, 63.
Bradford, M. M. (1976), *Analyt. Biochem.*, **72**, 248.
Bürgi, W., R. Richterich, and M. Briner (1967), *Clin. Chim. Acta*, **15**, 181.
Chou, S. C., and A. Goldstein (1960), *Biochem. J.*, **75**, 109.
Curtain, C. (1964), *Nature*, **203**, 1380.
Daughaday, W. H., O. H. Lowry, N. J. Rosebrough, and W. S. Fields (1952), *J. Lab. Clin. Med.*, **39**, 663.
Doetsch, K., and R. H. Gadsden (1975), *Clin. Chem.*, **21**, 778.
Doetsch, K., and R. H. Gadsden (1977), *Clin. Chem.*, **23**, 1186.
Doumas, B. T. (1975), *Clin. Chem.*, **21**, 1159.
Finlayson, J. S. (1965), *J. Clin. Invest.*, **44**, 1561.
Folin, O., and W. Denis (1912), *J. Biol. Chem.*, **12**, 239.
Friedman, H. S. (1965), in *Standard Methods of Clinical Chemistry*, Vol. 5 (Ed. S. Meites), Academic Press, New York and London, p. 223.
Goa, J. (1953), *Scand. J. Clin. Lab. Invest.*, **5**, 218.
Goldberg, M. I. (1973), *Analyt. Biochem.*, **51**, 240.
Goldfarb, A. R., L. J. Saidel, and E. Mosovich (1951), *J. Biol. Chem.*, **193**, 397.
Greenberg, D. (1936), *J. Lab. Clin. Med.*, **21**, 431.
Härtel, A. (1960), *Röntgen-Praxis*, **13**, 167; see *Chem. Abs.*, 1961, **55**, 9525f.
Hausdorf, G. (1950), *Med. Klin.*, **45**, 1375.
Heffron, J. J. A. (1975), *S. African J. Med. Sci.*, **40**, 57.
Henry, R. J., G. Sobel, and M. Segalove (1956), *Proc. Soc. Exp. Biol.*, **92**, 748.
Hiller, A., J. Plazin, and D. D. Van Slyke (1948), *J. Biol. Chem.*, **176**, 1401.
Keyser, J. W. (1948), *Biochem. J.*, **43**, 488.
Keyser, J. W., and M. Cawson (1970), *Clin. Chem.*, **16**, 147.
Knights, E. M., Jr., R. P. MacDonald, and J. Ploompuu (1962), *Ultramicro Methods for Clinical Laboratories*, 2nd edn., Grune and Stratton, New York, p. 151.
Lous, P., C. M. Plum, and M. Schou (1956), *Nord. Med.*, **55**, 693.
Lowry, O. H., N. J. Rosebrough, A. L. Farr, and R. J. Randall (1951), *J. Biol. Chem.*, **193**, 265.
Mehl, J. W., E. Pacovska, and R. J. Winzler (1949), *J. Biol. Chem.*, **177**, 13.
Meola, J. M., M. A. Vargas, and H. H. Brown (1977), *Clin. Chem.*, **23**, 975.
Meulemans, O. (1960), *Clin. Chim. Acta*, **5**, 757.

Minot, A. S., and M. Keller (1936), *J. Lab. Clin. Med.*, **21**, 743.

Naumann, H. N. (1964), in *Serum Proteins and the Dysproteinemias* (Eds. F. W. Sunderman and F. W. Sunderman), Lippincott, Philadelphia, p. 86.

Pennock, C. A., L. P. Passant, and F. G. Bolton (1968), *J. Clin. Path.*, **21**, 518.

Pesce, M. A., and C. S. Strande (1973), *Clin. Chem.*, **19**, 1265.

Peters, T., Jr. (1968), *Clin. Chem.*, **14**, 1147.

Phillips, R. A., D. D. Van Slyke, P. B. Hamilton, V. P. Dole, K. Emerson, Jr., and R. M. Archibald (1950), *J. Biol. Chem.*, **183**, 305.

Reinhold, J. G. (1953), in *Standard Methods of Clinical Chemistry, Vol. 1* (Ed. M. Reiner), Academic Press, New York, p. 88.

Rej, R., and A. H. Richards (1974), *Analyt. Biochem.*, **62**, 240.

Rice, E. W. (1965), in *Standard Methods of Clinical Chemistry, Vol. 5* (Ed. S. Meites), Academic Press, New York and London, p. 231.

Rice, E. W. (1975), *Clin. Chem.*, **21**, 398.

Riegler, E. (1914), *Z. anal. Chem.*, **53**, 242.

Rising, M. M., and P. S. Yang (1932–33), *J. Biol. Chem.*, **99**, 755.

Robinson, H. W., and C. G. Hogden (1941), *J. Biol. Chem.*, **140**, 853.

Salo, E. J., and E. I. Honkavaara (1974), *Scand. J. Clin. Lab. Invest.*, **34**, 283.

Svensmark, O. (1958), *Scand. J. Clin. Lab. Invest.*, **10**, 50.

Tombs, M. P., F. Souter, and N. F. Maclagan (1959), *Biochem. J.*, **73**, 167.

Van Slyke, D. D., A. Hiller, R. A. Phillips, P. B. Hamilton, V. P. Dole, R. M. Archibald, and H. A. Eder (1950), *J. Biol. Chem.*, **183**, 331.

Waddell, W. J. (1956), *J. Lab. Clin. Med.*, **48**, 311.

Watson, D. (1964), *Clin. Chem.*, **10**, 412.

Weichselbaum, T. E. (1946), *Amer. J. Clin. Path.*, **16**, Tech. Sect. 10, 40.

Westley, J., and J. Lambeth (1960), *Biochim. Biophys. Acta*, **40**, 364.

Yatzidis, H. (1977), *Clin. Chem.*, **23**, 811.

APPENDIX 3

Albumin in biological fluids

Many of the chemical methods for total protein mentioned in Appendix 2 have been applied to the determination of albumin, after preliminary fractionation of the proteins, and the same qualifications as to their accuracy apply. However, in the determination of an individual protein, such as albumin, an additional problem arises from the need either to select a reaction that is specific for this protein or to effect a preliminary separation from the other proteins present before applying one of the many less specific reactions. The application to whole serum of methods that are not specific must inevitably lead to errors, at least with some abnormal sera. Nevertheless, dye-binding methods have been widely used, and one employing bromocresol green (Bartholomew and Delaney, 1964, 1966; Rodkey, 1964, 1965; Northam and Widdowson, 1967) appears to be satisfactory for serum albumin concentrations in the normal range;* with lower concentrations the albumin is over-estimated (Webster *et al.*, 1974), on account of the presence of certain α- and β-globulin fractions in the serum that react with bromocresol green (Webster, 1974), and in these circumstances a specific immunoprecipitation method is to be preferred. The use of bromocresol purple (Louderback *et al.*, 1968; Carter, 1970; Pinnell and Northam, 1978) may overcome this difficulty. Serum albumin may also be determined after electrophoresis, by measurement of the dye uptake—preferably by comparison with a standard of known albumin content, run at the same time and treated in precisely the same way (Keyser and Stephens, 1962; Keyser, 1968). The immunoprecipitation method of Schultze and Schwick (1959), in an ultramicro-modification suggested by Hölzer and Binzus (1963), has been used successfully by the writer (Keyser, 1968). As little as 25 μl of 1–400 dilution of serum produces, with suitable antisera, a satisfactory degree of turbidity for optical measurement with a sensitive spectrophotometer. When large numbers of sera are to be tested, however, an automated procedure will generally be preferred.

Specific immunochemical methods are applicable to urine and cerebrospinal fluid as well as to serum.

In this section a manual method using bromocresol green is described. The

*In the writer's experience this is the case when pooled normal human serum is used for the standardization (see Note 2). According to Wegfahrt and his colleagues (1970) and Ferreria and Price (1974), who used purified human serum albumin as the standard, the bromocresol green method gives somewhat higher results than those given by immunoprecipitation. The latter authors found a mean difference of about 5 g/l. Presumably the use of normal serum as standard compensates for the small amounts of bromocresol-green-binding proteins that are normally present.

'rocket' technique may also be used (see Appendix 10) or automated immunoprecipitation (Appendix 13).

DETERMINATION OF SERUM ALBUMIN WITH BROMOCRESOL GREEN

Several procedures have been published for measuring serum albumin with bromocresol green, either manually or using automated equipment (Rodkey, 1965; Bartholomew and Delaney, 1966; Hernandez *et al.*, 1967; Dow and Pinto, 1969; Doumas *et al.*, 1971; Doumas and Biggs, 1972).

Manual method (Doumas and Biggs, 1972)

Reagents

(1) *Succinic acid:* 5 g in 100 ml water.
(2) *Sodium hydroxide:* 10 g in 100 ml water.
(3) *Succinate buffer:* 0.10 M, pH4.15. Dissolve 11.8 g of succinic acid and 100 mg of sodium azide in 800 ml of water, adjust the pH to 4.15 with sodium hydroxide (10g/1), and dilute to 1 litre with water.
(4) *Bromocresol green stock solution:* 0.60 mmol/l. Dissolve 432 mg of bromocresol green (sodium salt) and 100 mg of sodium azide in water to 1 litre. (Alternatively, dissolve 419 mg of the free acid in 10 ml of 0.1 N sodium hydroxide, add 100 mg of sodium azide, and dilute to 1 litre as before.)
(5) *Working dye solution.* Mix one volume of stock bromocresol green solution with three volumes of 0.10 M succinate buffer, add 4 ml of 30% 'Brij-35' (obtainable from B. D. H. Chemicals Ltd., Poole, Dorset, U. K.) per litre and carefully adjust the pH to 4.20 ± 0.05. Should the pH be above 4.25, use succinic acid (5 g/100 ml) for the adjustment.
(6) *Albumin stock standard solution:* 100 g/l. Dissolve 10 g of human serum albumin (corrected for moisture content) and 50 mg of sodium azide in water to 100 ml. Store in a refrigerator.
(7) *Albumin working standards:* 20, 30, 40, 50, and 60 g/l. Prepare by diluting the stock standard with an aqueous solution of sodium azide (50 mg/100 ml). Store the solutions in a refrigerator.

Procedure

To 5 ml of the working dye solution add 25 μl of serum, mix and allow to stand at room temperature for 10 min. Measure the absorbance of the solution at 628 nm after adjusting the instrument to zero absorbance with the working dye solution. Treat in the same way 25-μl amounts of the working standards. If a sample is more than moderately lipaemic determine a serum blank, using 25 μl of serum and 5 ml of 0.075 M succinate buffer, pH 4.20; the absorbance, with water as reference, is subtracted from the test reading.

Notes

(1) The reagents containing azide are stable at room temperature for at least 5 months; albumin solutions prepared as described above and kept in the refrigerator remain sterile for at least 6 months (Doumas and Biggs, 1972).

(2) Although the authors recommend pure albumin for preparing the standards, pooled normal human serum is satisfactory. The albumin concentration in the serum is determined by fractionation with 26% sodium sulphate (Na_2SO_4), followed by determination of the protein nitrogen in the filtrate, with use of the factor 6.25 for conversion to protein. Although it is recognized that fractionation in this way does not sharply separate the albumin from the globulins, it has nevertheless been shown that the protein-nitrogen content of the filtrate does correlate remarkably well with the albumin as determined electrophoretically, except in certain diseases (Majoor, 1942, 1946, 1947; Milne, 1947); and the present writer has generally found good agreement between albumin results obtained by dye-binding procedures standardized in this way, by cellulose acetate electrophoresis, and by an immunoprecipitation procedure (Keyser, 1968).

Using two different dyes (2-(4′-hydroxybenzeneazo)-benzoic acid (HABA) and methyl orange), Watson and Nankiville (1964) found that standardization with electrophoretically pure albumin led to overestimation of the albumin concentration of normal plasmas to the extent of 10–20 g/l, indicating some loss of dye-binding power in the albumin preparation used as standard. Such an effect does not appear to have been reported for bromocresol green.

3. Moderate lipaemia is stated to have no influence on the results; excessive haemolysis should be avoided.

4. Heparin and EDTA do not interfere with the analysis.

5. Sodium salicylate does not interfere, even at a concentration of 600 mg/l.

For a more detailed discussion of the method the reader is referred to the paper by Doumas and Biggs (1972).

REFERENCES

Bartholomew, R. J., and A. Delaney (1964), *Proc. Austral. Assoc. Clin. Biochemists*, **1**, 64.

Bartholomew, R. J., and A. Delaney (1966), *Proc. Austral. Assoc. Clin. Biochemists*, **1**, 214.

Carter, P. (1970), *Microchem. J.*, **15**, 531.

Doumas, B. T., and H. G. Biggs (1972), in *Standard Methods of Clinical Chemistry*, *Vol. 7* (Ed. G. R. Cooper), Academic Press, New York and London, p. 175.

Doumas, B. T., W. A. Watson, and H. G. Biggs (1971), *Clin. Chim. Acta*, **31**, 87.

Dow, D., and P. V. C. Pinto (1969), *Clin. Chem.*, **15**, 1006.

Ferreria, P., and C. P. Price (1974), *Clin. Chim. Acta*, **55**, 259.

Hernandez, O., L. Murray, and B. Doumas (1967), *Clin. Chem.*, **13**, 701 (abstr.).

Hölzer, K. H., and G. Binzus (1963), *7th International Congress of Internal Medicine, Munich, 1962*, Vol. 2, Thieme, Stuttgart, p. 536.

Keyser, J. W. (1968), *Clin. Chem.*, **14**, 360.
Keyser, J. W., and B. T. Stephens (1962), *Clin. Chem.*, **8**, 526.
Louderback, A., E. H. Mealy, and N. A. Taylor (1968), *Clin. Chem.*, **14**, 793.
Majoor, C. L. H. (1942), Ph.D. Thesis, Amsterdam, cited by Majoor (1946).
Majoor, C. L. H. (1946), *Yale J. Biol. Med.*, **18**, 419.
Majoor, C. L. H. (1947), *J. Biol. Chem.*, **169**, 583.
Milne, J. (1947), *J. Biol. Chem.*, **169**, 595.
Northam, B., and G. M. Widdowson (1967), *Assoc. Clin. Biochemists Tech. Bull. 11.*
Pinnell, A. E., and B. E. Northam (1978), *Clin. Chem.*, **24**, 80.
Rodkey, F. L. (1964), *Clin. Chem.*, **10**, 643.
Rodkey, F. L. (1965), *Clin. Chem.*, **11**, 478.
Schultze, H. E., and G. Schwick (1959), *Clin. Chim. Acta*, **4**, 15.
Watson, D., and D. D. Nankiville (1964), *Clin. Chim. Acta*, **9**, 359.
Webster, D. (1974), *Clin. Chim. Acta*, **53**, 109.
Webster, D., A. H. C. Bignell, and E. C. Attwood (1974), *Clin. Chim. Acta*, **53**, 101.
Wegfahrt, P. F., M. B. Fish, F. B. Aldana, and S. B. Aronson (1970), in *Adv. Autom. Anal., Technicon Int. Congr.* (Eds. E. C. Barton *et al.*), Thurman Assoc., Miami, Fla., p. 113.

APPENDIX 4

Electrophoresis

The phenomenon of electrophoresis—the movement of charged particles in a liquid medium under the influence of an electric field—has been known since the early years of the last century, but it was not until Tiselius introduced his now classical apparatus in 1937 that the technique of electrophoresis became a practical tool for the analysis of mixtures of biological compounds.

The principles of the Tiselius 'moving boundary' method of electrophoresis are described in numerous publications (see, for example, Schultze and Heremans, 1966), and its many biological and medical applications provided scope for a substantial review (Luetscher, 1947) only 10 years after its introduction. The technique is, however, complex and time-consuming, and the equipment expensive, and an important advance came with the introduction of supporting media, such as filter paper, in which the electrophoretic migration took place. In fact, the use of filter paper as a supporting medium in electrophoretic analysis was first described by König in 1937 and Klobusitzky and König in 1939, for the separation of dyeing agents and snake toxins, but their work did not attract much attention; and it was not until the work of Tiselius that this simple method was further developed, almost simultaneously and independently of each other, by Wieland and Fischer (1948, 1949), Turba and Enenkel (1950), and Durrum (1950), and, immediately afterwards, by Grassmann and Hannig (1950) and by Cremer and Tiselius (1950) (see Grassmann, 1956).

Other supporting media besides filter paper have been used, notably cellulose acetate (Kohn, 1957a, b) and agar gel. Agar gel as an electrophoretic medium was first used by Kendall and his collaborators during the period 1923–1926 (see Kendall, 1928). The electrophoretic fractionation of proteins in this material, however, was apparently first described by Gordon and his collaborators (1949).

In all these cases the material used functions simply as a stabilizing or supporting medium. Certain other materials, *viz.* starch gel (Smithies, 1955) and acrylamide gel (Ornstein, 1959; Davis and Ornstein, 1959; Raymond and Weintraub, 1959), provide in addition a 'sieve' or 'molecular filtration' effect (Smithies, 1955), the interstices in the material having dimensions comparable with those of the protein molecules themselves.

The choice of supporting medium depends on the object of the analysis. For most clinical diagnostic purposes cellulose acetate or agar gel is preferable to filter paper; indeed, using filter paper it is possible for very faint paraprotein bands, which show up distinctly on cellulose acetate, to remain undetected.

Cellulose acetate also has several other advantages, notably in allowing more rapid and complete separation than occurs with filter paper, and in the elimination of background staining. A method using cellulose acetate is described below.

For further information on electrophoretic techniques the reader is referred to Ivor Smith (1976).

Method

Reagents

(1) *Barbitone buffer:* pH 8.6, 0.075M.

(2) *Ponceau S:* 5 g Ponceau S and 75 g trichloroacetic acid in water to 1 litre.

(3) *Acetic acid:* 5% v/v.

Method

Wet a strip of cellulose acetate in the buffer by floating it on the surface (Note 1). Remove excess buffer by gently blotting with filter paper, connect the ends of the strip to the buffer compartments in suitable apparatus by means of filter paper pads, and apply a suitable quantity—usually about 0.3 μl—of serum in a neat line across the strip but finishing at least 5 mm from the edges (Note 2). Pass a current of 0.4–0.5 mA/cm width of strip for 30–120 min (Note 3). At the end of the run immerse the strip in dye solution for 10 min, then rinse out the excess of dye with several changes of 5% acetic acid, i.e. until the background is white. Finally allow the strip to dry.

Evaluation of pattern

For most purposes visual examination of strips is adequate, photometric scanning or measurement of the various fractions by elution of the dye rarely being necessary. When measurements are made, it is common practice to calculate the concentrations of the various fractions from the proportions of the dye bound by those fractions as compared with the total amount of dye bound on the strip; however, using Ponceau S staining it was found that this method of calculation often gave results somewhat different from those obtained by running in parallel a standard of known albumin content and comparing the amounts of albumin-bound dye in test and standard (Keyser and Watkins, 1972).

For a discussion of the many points of technique influencing results, the reader is referred to the detailed account by Kohn (1968).

Notes

(1) Immersion of the strip before the buffer has soaked into it will result in trapping of air and production of opaque spots.

(2) It is essential to apply the serum evenly. Application may be with a fine capillary, which is moved along a straight edge placed across the tank; alternatively a sample applicator may be used. The position of the starting line—i.e. whether it is central or to one end of the strip—will influence the separation pattern obtained, and should be determined experimentally for the particular conditions employed; endosmotic flow, which is more pronounced with cellulose acetate than with filter paper, results in improved separation of the serum proteins. Kohn (1968) recommends that with most brands of cellulose acetate the serum sample be applied between a third and half way along the strip from the edge of the filter paper pad at the cathode end.

The amount of serum applied will depend on the method of evaluation to be employed, elution requiring a larger amount than scanning. Another consideration is that if the strip is to be stained for glycoproteins or lipoproteins, larger samples will be necessary than for simple protein staining.

(3) If a trace of saturated bromophenol blue is added to one of the serum samples, the progress of the separation can be followed (the dye forms a complex with the albumin).

REFERENCES

Cremer, H. D., and A. Tiselius (1950), *Biochem. Z.*, **320**, 273.

Davis, B. J., and L. Ornstein (1959), paper read at meeting of The Society for the Study of Blood (New York Academy of Medicine).

Durrum, E. L. (1950), *J. Amer. Chem. Soc.*, **72**, 2943.

Gordon, A. H., B. Keil, and K. Šebesta (1949), *Nature*, **164**, 498.

Grassmann, W. (1956), in *Ciba Foundation Symposium on Paper Electrophoresis* (Eds. G. E. W. Wolstenholme and E. C. P. Millar), Churchill, London, p. 1.

Grassmann, W., and G. Hannig (1950), *Naturwissenschaften*, **37**, 496.

Kendall, J. (1928), *Science*, **67**, 163.

Keyser, J. W., and G. L. Watkins (1972), *Clin. Chem.*, **18**, 1541.

Klobusitzky, D.v., and P. König (1939), *Arch. exp. Path. Pharmak.*, **192**, 271.

Kohn, J. (1957a), *Biochem. J.*, **65**, 9.

Kohn, J. (1957b), *Clin. Chim. Acta*, **2**, 297.

Kohn, J. (1968), in *Chromatographic and Electrophoretic Techniques, Vol. 2: Zone Electrophoresis* (Ed. I. Smith), Heinemann, London, p. 84.

König, P. (1937), *Actas e trabalhos Congresso Sul-Americano de Chimica, Rio de Janeiro e Sao Paulo*, **2**, 334. (Cited by Grassmann, 1956.)

Luetscher, J. A., Jr. (1947), *Physiol. Rev.*, **27**, 621.

Ornstein, L. (1959), in published discussion following paper by B. J. Davis, L. Ornstein, P. Taleporos, and S. Koulish, *J. Histochem. Cytochem.*, **7**, 291.

Raymond, S., and L. S. Weintraub (1959), *Science*, **130**, 711.

Schultze, H. E., and J. F. Heremans (1966), *Molecular Biology of Human Proteins*, Vol. 1, Elsevier, Amsterdam.

Smith, I. (1976), Ed., *Chromatographic and Electrophoretic Techniques, Vol. 2: Zone Electrophoresis*, 4th edn., Heinemann, London.

Smithies, O. (1955), *Biochem. J.*, **61**, 629.

Tiselius, A. (1937), *Trans. Faraday Soc.*, **33**, 524.

Turba, F., and A. J. Enenkel (1950), *Naturwissenschaften*, **37**, 93.

Wieland, Th., and E. Fischer (1948), *Naturwissenschaften*, **35**, 29.

Wieland, Th., and E. Fischer (1949), *Liebigs Ann.*, **564**, 152.

APPENDIX 5

Paraprotein estimation

Measurement of the plasma concentration of paraproteins is important in allowing, in most cases, an assessment of the size of the tumour and in monitoring the progress of patients and the response of their tumours to therapy. Radial immunodiffusion is generally unsuitable for these measurements, and the method generally used is electrophoretic separation of the plasma proteins and determination of the amount of dye bound by the paraprotein. Daniels and his coworkers (1975) investigated three methods—electrophoresis, radial immunodiffusion, and electroimmunodiffusion—and found that they yield divergent results; it was concluded that serum protein electrophoresis offers the most reliable and reproducible means of measuring paraproteins for the monitoring of patients with monoclonal gammopathies. The procedure described below is that of Hobbs (1965).

Method

Reagents

These are as for cellulose acetate electrophoresis (Appendix 4) and, in addition, the following:

(1) *Amidoschwartz 10B:* 0.25% in methanol, containing 3% trichloroacetic acid (Note 1).
(2) *Methanol–glacial acetic acid mixture:* 9 : 1 parts by vol.
(3) *Methanol.*

Procedure

Take a suitable quantity of the serum (Note 2) and separate the proteins electrophoretically on cellulose acetate (see Appendix 4). Place the strips, one at a time, surface downwards, in the dye solution and leave for 5 min. Wash twice with methanol–glacial acetic acid mixture for about 5 min to remove excess of dye, then rinse twice in methanol and dry flat between sheets of blotting paper. Finally scan the electrophoretic patterns with a suitable densitometer (Note 3), and calculate the paraprotein concentration from the percentage of dye taken up by the paraprotein (Note 4).

Notes

(1) Ponceau S (see Appendix 4) may be used instead.

(2) It is essential to work within the range of linearity of dye uptake, the limit often being set by the narrow band of paraprotein: application of too much serum will lead to underestimation of the paraprotein concentration. This point can be checked by running strips with decreasing amounts of serum until the calculated percentage of paraprotein becomes constant (Hobbs, 1967).

(3) In the writer's laboratory the electrophoretic separation is done on Gelman Hawksley 'Sepraphore X' membranes and the patterns scanned with a 'Quick-Scan Junior' (Helena Instrument Co., Beaumont, Texas, USA) after clearing with an aqueous solution containing 32.0% dimethylformamide and 20.0% 'Triton' X-405 by volume (Gelman Instrument Co., Ann Arbor, Michigan).

(4) According to Hobbs (1967), IgG, IgA, and IgD paraproteins can be calculated from dye binding and total protein as determined by the biuret method (bovine albumin being used as standard); however, since the biuret method underestimates IgM paraproteins by 12%, he prefers to use the specific gravity gradient tube method of Lowry and Hunter (1945) for determining the total protein in such cases.

The estimation of paraprotein by this method is based on the assumption that changes in the relative amounts of the other proteins do not affect the result—in other words, that all the major protein fractions have the same dye-binding power. In spite of this objection, the method has given useful results in practice.

REFERENCES

Daniels, J. C., T. M. Vyvial, W. C. Levin, and S. E. Ritzmann (1975), *Clin. Chem.*, **21**, 243.

Hobbs, J. R. (1965), *Nature*, **207**, 292.

Hobbs, J. R. (1967), *Brit. Med. J.*, **iii**, 699.

Lowry, O. H., and T. H. Hunter (1945), *J. Biol. Chem.*, **159**, 465.

APPENDIX 6

Immunoelectrophoresis and immunofixation

IMMUNOELECTROPHORESIS

Immunoelectrophoresis is a combination of electrophoresis and immunodiffusion in a unified technique (Grabar and Williams, 1953). Electrophoretic separation of the proteins of blood serum, or other biological fluid, is followed by double diffusion against an antiserum contained in a trough parallel to the axis of electrophoretic migration: where antigens and their corresponding antibodies meet at equivalence points, precipitates are formed. As a result of the preliminary electrophoretic separation these precipitates are arranged in a characteristic system of arcs between the electrophoretic zones and the trough, each antigen producing an independent arc as it precipitates with its specific antibody (Figure 2.2). The method is generally used in the form of a microtechnique introduced by Scheidegger (1955). There are many slight variations of technique; the procedure outlined below will generally be found satisfactory.

Method

Reagents

(1) *Barbitone buffer:* pH 8.2, 0.025 M.

(2) *Gel for electrophoresis.* Prepare sufficient of a 1% w/v solution of agar (Oxoid 'Ionagar' or Difco 'Agar Noble') in barbitone buffer (ionic strength 0.025) to serve for the preparation of a number of slides (see below).

(3) *Antisera.* A good quality anti-human serum, and in addition specific antisera to IgG, IgA, and IgM and to kappa and lambda light chains (free and bound).

(4) *Ponceau S*: 5 g Ponceau S and 75 g trichloroacetic acid in water to 1 litre (Note 1).

(5) *Acetic acid:* 2%.

Preparation of slides

Clean thoroughly a number of microscope slides (7.5 × 2.5 cm) and treat each slide as follows. Warm the slide and smear it evenly with a drop of hot, molten 3% agar, and then dry it on a hot plate or in a hot-air oven (Note 2). Place the slide on a level surface and run 2.0 ml of the hot buffered 1% agar

(Reagent 2) evenly over its surface. After the gel has cooled and solidified, cut a well with the aid of a suitable cutter (1.5 mm external diameter) and remove the agar plug by gentle suction (Note 3).

Electrophoresis

Fill the well with the test sample (Note 4), using a length of fine glass capillary tubing. Place the slide in a suitable electrophoresis tank and made connexion with the buffer compartments. Using the buffer recommended, and a current of 8 mA per slide, good separation is obtained in about 45 min (Note 5).

Application of antiserum

At the end of the run, remove the slide from the tank and cut a trough, or a pair of troughs (Figure 2.2), to receive the antiserum. The troughs should be about 60 mm long, 1 mm wide and about 3–5 mm from the antigen well, and exactly parallel to the axis of electrophoretic migration. Fill the troughs with antiserum with the aid of a fine Pasteur pipette. In investigating paraproteins it is often useful to employ specific antisera to IgG, IgA, and IgM and antisera to bound kappa and lambda chains.

Development of precipitin pattern

Place the slide in a moist chamber on a level surface and leave it at room temperature for 18–24 hours (Note 6).

Drying and staining

If it is necessary to stain the precipitin lines, remove the excess of unprecipitated protein by washing in saline (or phosphate-buffered saline, pH 7.5) for 2–3 days, the saline being changed daily. Then cover the slide with a piece of thick filter paper and allow the agar to dry at 37 °C. Remove the filter paper carefully and stain the slide with Ponceau S (Reagent 4) for 10 min, wash with 2% aqueous acetic acid to remove excess stain, and allow to dry.

Evaluation of immunoelectrophoretic pattern

Although with practice it is quite easy to obtain excellent precipitin patterns, their interpretation may on occasion demand considerable experience. It is useful to build up a reference 'library' of stained slides, obtained both with normal sera and with sera giving typical abnormal patterns. For illustrations and interpretations of immunoelectrophoretic patterns in disease the reader is referred to Grabar and Burtin (1964) and to Arquembourg and his coworkers (1970).

Notes

(1) Other stains can be used. Some workers prefer to use a mixture of stains, to allow for differential staining by the various proteins.

(2) Some workers omit the preliminary coating with 3% agar. In the writer's experience, omission of this stage often results in separation of the gel from the slide during the washing process.

(3) The cutting operations are greatly facilitated by the use of precision gel punches, which cut out holes and troughs at the same time. It is usually recommended that the gel in the troughs be removed only *after* the electrophoretic run.

(4) It is advisable to test the sample both neat and diluted, since abnormalities may be obscured in the presence of an excess of protein. In the writer's laboratory the serum is examined neat and also diluted 1:3 and 1:6 with buffer.

(5) Addition of a small amount of bromophenol blue to the serum allows visual control of the length of the run, the dye binding to and migrating with the albumin.

(6) It is important to remember that free light chains diffuse much faster than the larger immunoglobulin molecules, such as IgG, and indeed they may produce precipitin arcs in less than an hour; furthermore, in the presence of a large excess of antigen the precipitate can be redissolved and disappear. When urine is being examined for the presence of Bence Jones protein the slide should be observed at half-hourly intervals up to about 3 h after the addition of antiserum to the trough.

IMMUNOFIXATION

A new technique, *immunofixation electrophoresis*, was described by Alper and Johnson in 1969 for the study of microheterogeneity of protein antigens.

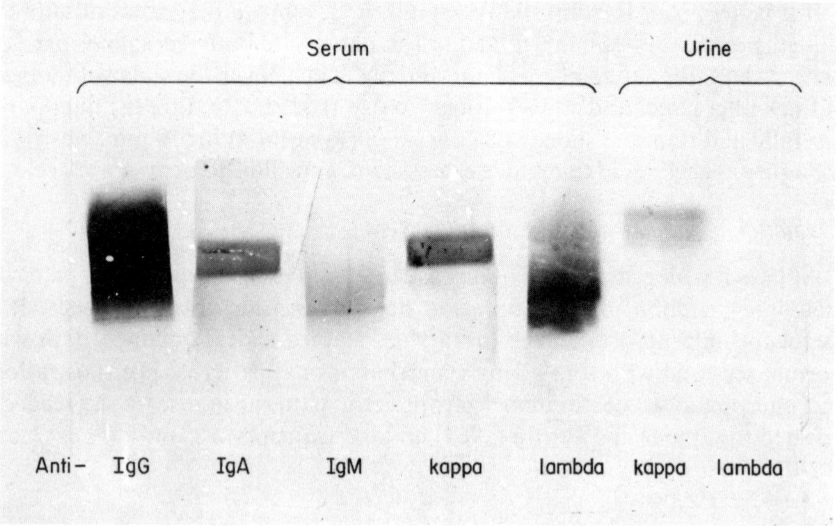

Figure App. 6.1. Patterns obtained by immunofixation electrophoresis of serum and urine from a patient with IgA (kappa-type) paraproteinaemia. (Kindly supplied by Dr. J. Whicher.)

After electrophoretic separation of the proteins in agarose gel or other suitable medium, exposure to an appropriate antiserum allows the protein to be fixed with virtually no interfering diffusion. In this way the degree of resolution is much improved, and extremely small bands can be demonstrated and characterized. The antiserum may be applied either by layering on the gel, as described in the original procedure (Alper and Johnson), or by the application of strips of cellulose acetate impregnated with antiserum (Ritchie and Smith, 1976a,b).

The amounts of specimen and antiserum used depend on the circumstances. In general, serum samples should be diluted to give an antigen concentration of 1–2 g/l; urine samples should contain 0.1–0.2 g/l. Excess moisture on the surface of the gel where samples are to be applied is first removed by means of a 2.5-cm strip of cellulose acetate placed smoothly over the application area for 10–15 s. The diluted sample (100 μl) is then applied to the gel through a slotted mask used as a guide to positioning and allowed to diffuse into the gel for 2–5 min, after which any excess is removed with a piece of filter paper. After electrophoresis, the area of gel containing the protein under investigation is overlaid with a strip of cellulose acetate impregnated with antiserum of the appropriate concentration (which must be determined by experiment), and the gel left in a moist chamber for 1 h. The gel is then placed under a filter paper and a number of dry absorbent towels and the whole covered with a plate of glass or plastic and a 2-kg weight. After 10–15 min the absorbent pads are carefully removed and the plate washed in saline. The pressing process is repeated and the gel dried in a stream of warm air and stained with Amido Black or Coomassie Brilliant Blue in the usual way.

Some workers add polyethylene glycol (PEG) to the antiserum (cf. Appendix 13), at a final concentration of 4 per cent. This is conveniently done by mixing equal volumes of antiserum and an 8 per cent solution of PEG in saline.

A number of different antisera may be applied to the same sample on a single plate, or a number of samples may be fixed with the same antiserum.

The details of the technique may have to be modified for special purposes. For example, in the investigation of cryoproteins, electrophoresis at higher temperatures than are usually employed may be necessary if these proteins are to migrate satisfactorily. For further details the original publications should be consulted.

REFERENCES

Alper, C. A., and A. M. Johnson (1969), *Vox Sang.*, **17**, 445.

Arquembourg, P. C., J. E. Salvaggio, and J. N. Bickers (1970), *Primer of Immunoelectrophoresis*, Ann Arbor-Humphrey, London.

Grabar, P., and P. Burtin (1964), Eds., *Immuno-electrophoretic Analysis*, Elsevier, Amsterdam.

Grabar, P., and C. A. Williams, Jr. (1953), *Biochim. Biophys. Acta.*, **10**, 193.

Ritchie, R. F., and R. Smith (1976a), *Clin. Chem.*, **22**, 497.

Ritchie, R. F., and R. Smith (1976b), *Clin. Chem.*, **22**, 1982.

Scheidegger, J. J. (1955), *Int. Arch. Allergy Appl. Immunol.*, **7**, 103.

APPENDIX 7

Detection of Bence Jones protein

The various screening tests for Bence Jones proteinuria were investigated by Hobbs (1966a). The best of them proved to be simple layering of the urine over concentrated hydrochloric acid (Bradshaw, 1906), a test that detected 13 out of 15 cases with concentrations of 10–50 mg of Bence Jones protein per litre of urine. The surest method, however, was found to be electrophoresis or gel filtration of the concentrated urine followed by immunoprecipitation (Hobbs, 1966b). Occasionally Bence Jones protein can be detected in unconcentrated urine.

Method

Pass the urine through two 'Millipore' membranes, the first excluding particles of diameter 1.0 μm and the second those of 0.2 μm (Note 1). Concentrate the urine 200- to 300-fold by using a Sartorius collodion shell inside a Buchner flask attached to a vacuum pump. Take a portion of the concentrated urine and subject it to electrophoresis on cellulose acetate alongside the patient's serum. Take another portion for immunoelectrophoresis, using antisera specific to free kappa and lambda chains, respectively (Note 2).

Immunoelectrophoresis using antisera to kappa and lambda chains may also be applied to serum (Figure App. 7.1).

Notes

(1) By using two filter membranes in this way it is possible to re-use the 0.2-μm membrane a number of times. Filtration is necessary to remove particles which might block the collodion membrane and bacteria which are capable of destroying the protein. Amicon filters may be used instead of 'Millipore'; they permit the rapid processing of large numbers of specimens.

(2) It is essential to observe the slide at short intervals for the appearance of light-chain precipitin arcs, which may be formed in less than an hour and which may disappear if much antigen is present.

Interpretation

Light chains occur normally in the urine at concentrations of about 2.5 mg/l; however, these normal B-chains show diffuse electrophoretic mobility (ranging

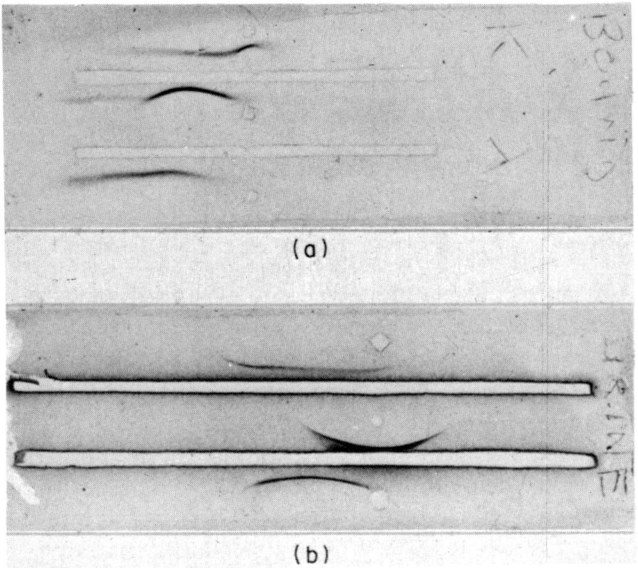

Figure App. 7.1. Detection of Bence Jones protein: (a) kappa type, in a specimen of serum, and (b) lambda type, in urine (different patients). On each slide, the middle well contained the specimen, and the top and bottom wells contained, respectively, type kappa and type lambda control serum; the upper trough was filled with antiserum to kappa chains, and the lower with antiserum to lambda.

from the α_2- to the slow γ-globulin region), reflecting the distribution of the normal immunoglobulins, and antigenically both kappa and lambda classes are present (70 per cent and 30 per cent respectively). By contrast, Bence Jones proteins have a relatively restricted mobility (usually different from that of the serum paraprotein), and are composed of either kappa or lambda chains but not both. Some typical results are illustrated in Figure App. 7.1.

REFERENCES

Bradshaw, T. R. (1906), *Brit. Med. J.*, **ii**, 1442.

Hobbs, J. R. (1966a), *Biochem. J.*, **99**, 15P.

Hobbs, J. R. (1966b), in *Scientific Basis of Medicine, Annual Reviews*, Athlone Press, London, p. 106.

APPENDIX 8

Quantitative immunoelectrophoresis

In the immunoelectrophoretic procedure described in Appendix 6, no attempt is made to measure quantitatively the concentrations of the various proteins, but gross variations from the normal may be detected. Some workers have measured the areas of the main immunoprecipitates, these areas being related linearly to the amount of the corresponding antigen (Afonso, 1964; Bogdanikowa *et al.*, 1966). In a variation of the 'rocket' technique described in Appendix 10 the proteins are first separated electrophoretically in one dimension and are then 'forced' electrophoretically at right angles into an antiserum-containing gel (Ressler, 1960; Clarke and Freeman, 1967, 1968). However, in this case the antiserum used is a polyvalent one, and each specimen produces a series of peaks, corresponding to the various immunologically distinct proteins present in the specimen. By this method Clarke and Freeman were able to demonstrate more than 50 immunologically distinct peaks, though not all the antigens have yet been identified. Quantitative measurement is based upon comparison of the area of each peak with that of the corresponding peak obtained with a suitable reference standard—usually a pool of normal human serum. Modifications of the technique have been introduced (Firestone and Aronson, 1969; Versey, 1970; Davies *et al.*, 1971; Afonso, 1974; Bradwell and Burnett, 1975a, b). The literature on quantitative immunoelectrophoretic methods has been surveyed by Verbruggen (1975).

The procedure described here is essentially the modification by Davies and his coworkers (1971) of Clarke and Freeman's method. It incorporates a number of modifications found to be necessary or helpful (Fuller and Keyser, 1972; Miss J. Fuller, private communication; Bradwell and Burnett, 1975a, b,c.).

Method

Reagents

(1) *Barbitone buffer:* 0.06 M, pH 8.6.

(2) *Agarose:* 2% w/v in water. Make a 2% solution of agarose (L'Industrie Biologique Française S. A., 35–39, Quai au Moulin de Cage, Gennevilliers (Seine), France) in water in a glass bottle by heating in a boiling water bath. Allow the bottle to cool somewhat and then place it in a water bath at 50 °C.

(3) *Coomassie Brilliant Blue:* 2 g/l in a mixture of methanol, glacial acetic acid, and water (4:1:6 by volume).

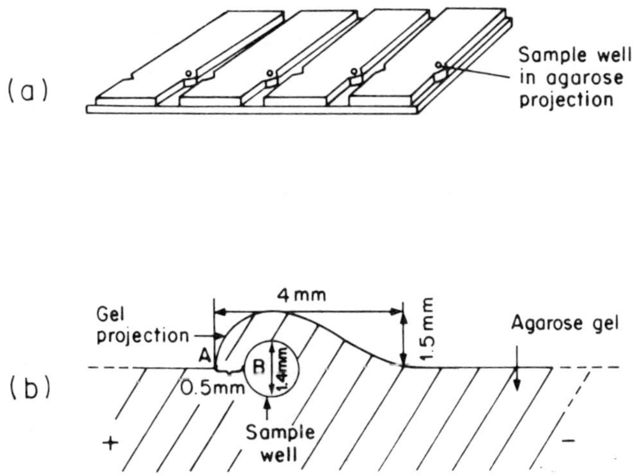

Figure App. 8.1. (a) First-dimension gels with wells placed in a small agarose projection. (b) Diagram of sample well placed in first-dimension gel. (Reproduced from A. R. Bradwell and D. Burnett, *Clin. Chim. Acta*, 1975, **62**, 457, by permission of Elsevier/North-Holland Biomedical Press and the authors.)

Procedure

Preparation of plates for electrophoretic separation

Take a glass slide (5 × 5 cm), previously cleaned with ethanol, and place it on a level surface. Add 2 ml of 2% agarose (at 50 °C) to 2 ml of 0.06 M barbitone (also at 50 °C), mix the two solutions by swirling and pour onto the plate. After about 5 min cut the gel into four portions, using a cutter that produces a small projection as shown in Figure App. 8.1. Then punch a sample well of the dimensions and in the position shown in Figure App. 8.1 (Note 1). Remove the plugs of agarose and any excess of fluid, and apply the samples (Note 2). Include a pooled reference serum on each plate.

Electrophoretic separation

Apply a potential difference of 10 V/cm to the gel for 30 min, making electrical connexion with the buffer by means of double layers of absorbent lint (Note 3), and cooling with water (Note 4).

Preparation of slides for second run

While the electrophoretic separation is in progress, prepare the antiserum-containing agarose by mixing a suitable quantity of the antiserum (anti-whole human serum) with a 10 g/l solution of agarose in the diluted barbitone buffer (0.03 M, pH 8.6) (Note 5). This should be done at such a time that the interval between the first and second runs is kept to a minimum and does not exceed 30 min. At the end of the first run, place each strip along one side of a clean slide so that the original sample hole is in the lower right-hand corner of the slide but away from the edge. Then cover the rest of the slide with 3 ml of antiserum in buffered agarose, again on a level surface.

Electrophoresis into antiserum

Reverse the electrodes and replace the lint connexions with fresh ones. (These should first be thoroughly wetted with 0.03 M buffer and then squeezed to

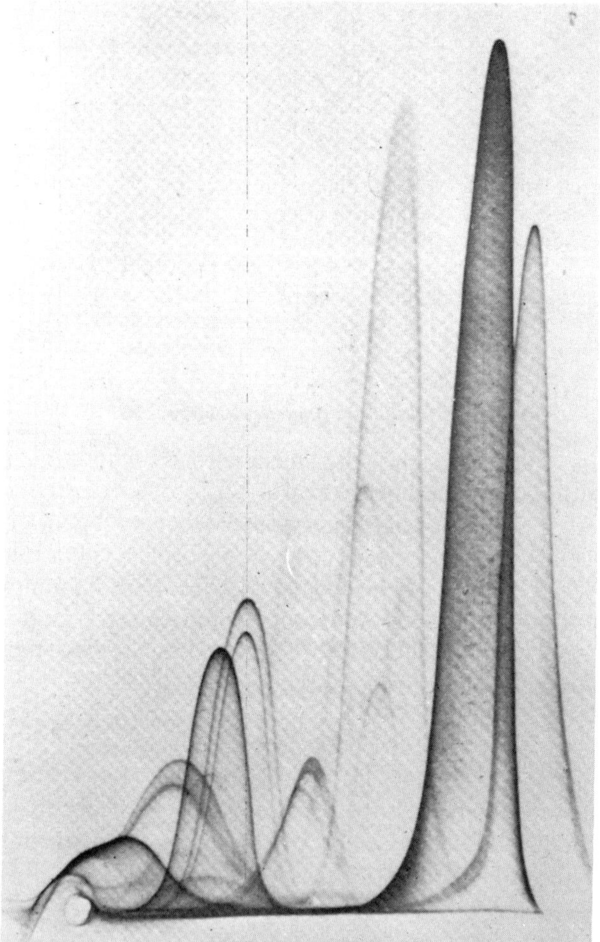

Figure App. 8.2. Example of pattern obtained with method of quantitative immunoelectrophoresis described. (Reproduced from A. R. Bradwell and D. Burnett, *Clin. Chim. Acta*, 1975, **62**, 457, by permission of Elsevier/North-Holland Biomedical Press and the authors.)

remove excess.) Place the plate in the tank and pass a current at right angles to the direction of the first separation; apply a potential difference of 10 V, measured across the gel itself, for at least 17 h (again with water cooling). At the end of the run remove the plate and place it on a flat surface. Cover the gel with a layer of filter paper, soaked in saline, taking care to exclude air bubbles, and cover this in turn with several layers of dry cellulose paper (paper towels) and a weight. After a few minutes remove the paper towels, and, without removing it from the gel, soak the filter paper again in saline for a few minutes, place dry paper towels on top, and repeat the process. After three or four changes of the paper all the excess protein will have been absorbed from the gel. Finally dry the plate by removing all but the filter paper and exposing it to a stream of warm air: the filter paper can then be lifted off and the proteins stained (Note 6).

Evaluation of pattern

With the aid of a photographic enlarger project the stained pattern onto a sheet of white paper and draw the enlarged peaks as accurately as possible (Note 7). Draw a straight baseline and measure the areas of the peaks with a planimeter.

The identification of the peaks can be difficult, and specific stains may be used to help; e.g. lipoproteins may be identified with Sudan Black (Uriel, 1964), caeruloplasmin with potassium ferrocyanide (Schen and Rabinovitz, 1966), haptoglobin with benzidine (Northam *et al.*, 1963), and transferrin by autoradiography using added ^{59}Fe ferrous citrate (Thorbecke *et al.*, 1971). Another aid to identification is measurement of the distance of migration, the mobility of each protein being compared with that of albumin (Fuller and Keyser, 1972). A study by Weeke (1970b) provides examples of methods for identifying known serum proteins and characterizing unnamed ones. With practice it is possible to recognize certain peaks by their characteristic appearance and position in the pattern; other peaks may then be provisionally identified by their relationship to these 'reference' peaks.

Notes

(1) The sample well should be placed so that not more than half is in the gel projection, otherwise some protein will not migrate out of the well; and there should be between 0.5 and 1.0 mm of gel between points A and B (Figure App. 8.1b) to prevent rupture of the edge of the well on application of the sample (Bradwell and Burnett, 1975b).

(2) Generally 1 μl of serum is taken. With cerebrospinal fluid the volume is adjusted so that 30–35 μg of protein is applied, up to a maximum volume of 10 μl; larger volumes require too long for absorption by the gel, and diffusion may give rise to unsatisfactory patterns and interference with adjacent samples. It is generally best to apply cerebrospinal fluid samples before serum samples, so that the latter do not have time to diffuse excessively.

If the test samples are available in sufficient volume, a known amount of acetylated albumin may be added to each so that a correction may subsequently be made for variations in the volumes applied. This is rarely possible with cerebrospinal fluid, on account of the limited amounts available. In any case, acetylated albumin has almost double the mobility of albumin itself, so that only about half of the antibody-containing gel is utilized. Versey and Slater (1973) have suggested using transferrin as the internal standard, so that no material need be added. This gives a greater degree of accuracy than do procedures involving the addition of a standard. The transferrin concentration in the specimen must of course be measured by an alternative method, e.g. 'rocket' electrophoresis. Yet another proposal is to use carbamylated transferrin (Weeke, 1970a); this produces a peak overlapping that of prealbumin, so the gel is full utilized (cf. acetylated albumin).

(3) Some varieties of lint may be unsuitable. Absorbent lint (BPC) (Johnson and Johnson) was found to be satisfactory.

(4) Various types of apparatus incorporate a water-cooled plate on which the slides are placed.

(5) The amount of antiserum necessary will depend upon its titre. Using antiserum (prepared in rabbits) obtained from Wellcome Reagents Ltd. (Beckenham, Kent, UK), it has been found necessary to use 0.25 ml per plate for serum and 0.1 ml for cerebrospinal fluid analysis.

(6) The method of removing excess protein is that described by Bradwell and Burnett (1975c).

(7) Alternatively, the enlarged image can be focussed on photographic paper ('Ilfoprint DR4.5L', matt, single weight, from Ilford Ltd., Basildon, Essex, UK, is suitable) and the peaks on the developed prints measured. This procedure eliminates the errors associated with manual outlining of the peaks; however, it was found to be unsatisfactory with patterns given by cerebrospinal fluid, the photographs showing poor resolution and the disappearance of certain peaks that were visible to the naked eye when the projection was made onto white paper.

A semi-automated two-dimensional immunoelectrophoretic method has been developed by Versey and his coworkers (1973).

REFERENCES

Afonso, E. (1964), *Clin. Chim. Acta*, **10**, 114.
Afonso, E. (1974), *Clin. Chim. Acta*, **54**, 123.
Bogdanikowa, B., J. Drozd, L. Dubinska, and T. Bogdanik (1966), *Clin. Chim. Acta*, **14**, 807.
Bradwell, A. R., and D. Burnett (1975a), *Clin. Chim. Acta*, **58**, 283.
Bradwell, A. R., and D. Burnett (1975b), *Clin. Chim. Acta*, **62**, 457.
Bradwell, A. R., and D. Burnett (1975c), *Clin. Chem.*, **21**, 637.
Clarke, H. G. M., and T. Freeman (1967), in *Protides of the Biological Fluids: Proceedings of 14th Colloquium, Bruges, 1966* (Ed. H. Peeters), Elsevier, Amsterdam, p. 503.
Clarke, H. G. M., and T. Freeman (1968), *Clin. Sci.*, **35**, 405.

Davies, D. R., E. D. Spurr, and J. B. Versey (1971), *Clin. Sci.*, **40**, 411.
Firestone, H. J., and S. B. Aronson (1969), *Amer. J. Clin. Path.*, **52**, 615.
Fuller, J. M., and J. W. Keyser (1972), *Clin. Chem.*, **18**, 625.
Northam, B. E., D. S. Rowe, and N. E. Winstone (1963), *Lancet*, **i**, 348.
Ressler, N. (1960), *Clin. Chim. Acta*, **5**, 795.
Schen, R. J., and M. Rabinovitz (1966), *Clin. Chim. Acta*, **13**, 537.
Thorbecke, G. J., G. M. Hochwald, and C. A. Williams (1971), in *Methods in Immunology and Immunochemistry* (Eds. C. A. Williams and M. W. Chase), Vol. 3, Academic Press, New York, p. 352.
Uriel, J. (1964), in *Immuno-electrophoretic Analysis* (Eds. P. Grabar and P. Burtin), Elsevier, Amsterdam, p. 30.
Verbruggen, R. (1975), *Clin. Chem.*, **21**, 5.
Versey, J. M. B. (1970), *Biochem. J.*, **118**, 57P.
Versey, J. M. B., and L. Slater (1973), *Ann. Clin. Biochem.*, **10**, 1.
Versey, J. M. B., L. Slater, and J. R. Hobbs (1973), *J. Immunol. Methods*, **3**, 63.
Weeke, B. (1970a), *Scand. J. Clin. Lab. Invest.*, **25**, 161.
Weeke, B. (1970b), *Scand. J. Clin. Lab. Invest.*, **25**, 269.

APPENDIX 9

Crossed immunoelectrophoresis

An ingenious electrophoretic technique (Bussard, 1959; Libich, 1959) for demonstrating precipitin reactions depends on the fact that as a result of electroendosmotic flow the antibodies (contained in the γ-globulin fraction) move towards the cathode, whereas many antigens move towards the anode, at the alkaline pH generally used. This technique, which is known as counter-current, crossed, or cross-over immunoelectrophoresis, or counter electrophoresis, can be performed on filter paper or cellulose acetate or in agar gel. The antibody-containing specimen is placed on the anode side and the antigen-containing specimen on the cathode side, on the same electrophoretic axis and separated by a small distance, e.g. 5–10 mm. On passage of an electric current the reactants move towards each other and produce a line of precipitation between the sites of application.

The method has been used to demonstrate precipitating antibodies in the serum of patients with Hashimoto's thyroiditis, and for the detection of hepatitis-associated or Australia antigen, hydatid disease (Kelkar and Kotwal, 1975; Sorice *et al.*, 1975), and a variety of bacterial antigens (McIllmurray, 1976; *Lancet*, 1976).

A technique has been suggested for detecting both Australia antigen and antibody in a single experiment, by placing the test specimen in a well between the laboratory control antiserum (on the anode side) and antigen (on the cathode side); however, this procedure is not recommended, in view of the report by Alter and his coworkers (1971) that under certain conditions the control antigen may migrate past the central well and precipitate with the control antibody to produce a false positive reaction.

Crossed immunoelectrophoresis has been widely used for the detection of α-fetoprotein in the diagnosis of primary hepatoma, though in laboratories that routinely estimate this protein quantitatively by radioimmunoassay such screening techniques are falling into disuse.

In testing biological fluids for specific antigens by the method of crossed immunoelectrophoresis in agar gel or in agarose, it is usually necessary to set up one or more dilutions of the test material, since an excess of antigen may produce a false negative result. As an alternative, Kohn (1970, 1973) has proposed testing different sample volumes in adjacent wells of different size against the one antiserum—an arrangement of wells which also permits identification of the precipitation lines by means of a reaction of immunological identity with a positive control. Some of the pitfalls associated with the use of these techniques for the detection of Australia antigen have been discussed by Kohn and Morgan (1971).

Two procedures are described here: the first is Kohn's, using cellulose acetate and applying two samples of different size; and in the second the need for making dilutions of the test fluid is obviated by the use of opposed triangular or tapered troughs, which ensure a large excess of antigen at one end and of antibody at the other, with a continuous change in the proportion in between (Libich, 1959; Keyser and Lewis, 1973).

Method using cellulose acetate membrane (Kohn, 1973; Kohn and Kahan, 1976)

Cut sheets of cellulose acetate membrane to the desired size and shape to accommodate the required number of tests. Mark the membrane with a non-diffusible ink, impregnate with buffer, and make depressions of suitable size and shape (to retain the samples during application) by pressing the impregnated sheet gently against a plastic template (Notes 1 and 2). Blot lightly, apply the samples and antiserum to the appropriate depressions and pass a current not exceeding 0.5 mA per cm width of membrane. Treat a positive control in the same way as the test serum. After a suitable time (usually 40–60 min) remove the membrane, place it in an eluting fluid (e.g. 3% sodium chloride with a trace of detergent) and agitate gently for about 15 min. Then stain for about an hour or more in Nigrosin (0.02% in 5% acetic acid) (Note 3) until the precipitation lines of the positive control are clearly visible, rinse under running tap water, and allow to dry. Examine the uncleared membrane against a strong source of light.

To demonstrate the presence of antibody, carry out the same procedure using a known antigen solution.

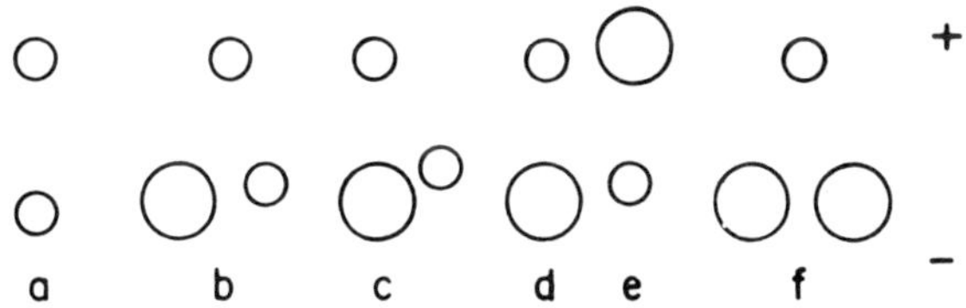

Figure App. 9.1. Application patterns for crossed immunoelectrophoresis on cellulose acetate membrane. (a) Conventional, equal volumes; (b) screening pattern, general purpose; (c) high sensitivity, wide range; (d) for weak antigens; (e) for weak antibody; (f) specificity check. Approx. diam. of 'wells': large, 4 mm; medium, 3 mm; small, 2 mm. If exceptionally wide range expected, (c) or combination of (d) and (e) is recommended. (Reproduced from J. Kohn and M. Kahan, *J. Immunol. Methods*, 1976, **11**, 303, by permission of Elsevier/North-Holland Biomedical Press and the authors.)

Notes

(1) It is not essential to make these depressions, but they facilitate application of the samples. It is important to make the wells *before* blotting the membrane.

(2) The actual application pattern depends on the conditions of the test and must be selected for each antigen–antibody system investigated. For demonstrating the presence of antigen Kohn (1976) suggests: (i) conventional pattern with equal volumes, 3–5 μl, of antigen and antibody (Figure App. 9.1a); (ii) screening pattern (Figure App. 9.1b): two test samples, 1–2 μl and 5–7 μl respectively, are applied 2 mm apart on the cathode side, and 3–4 μl of the antiserum or antibody-containing fluid are placed on the anode side 6–10 mm from the test samples; (iii) for weak antigens a larger sample volume is recommended (Figure App. 9.1d), and if weak antibody is expected a large application on the anode side will increase the sensitivity (Figure App. 9.1e).

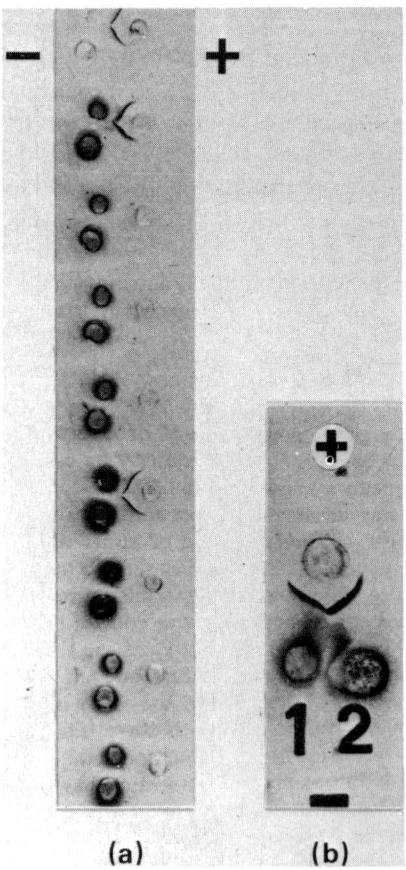

Figure App. 9.2. (a) Results of typical screening test for presence of α-fetoprotein. Note the shape of the precipitation lines in positive tests. (b) Specificity check: (1) positive control; (2) test sample. (Reproduced from J. Kohn and M. Kahan, *J. Immunol. Methods*, 1976, **11**, 303, by permission of Elsevier/North-Holland Biomedical Press and the authors.)

(3) For rapid staining Kohn recommends using an alcoholic solution of Nigrosin (1 vol. of saturated Nigrosin, 10 vols. of 50% methanol, and 1 vol. of glacial acetic acid). The membrane is left for 5–10 min in this solution and then rinsed in tap water as above and allowed to dry.

The sensitivity of the technique is very high. In the case of α-fetoprotein it is of the order of 200 ng/ml (Kohn and Weaver, 1974).

Method of using triangular troughs

Cover a slide with a 1-mm layer of 1% agar in barbitone buffer of pH 8.2, ionic strength 0.05, and cut tapered troughs with either a fine scalpel or a gel punch. Troughs with the dimensions shown in Figure App. 9.3 have proved to be satisfactory. Dilute the antiserum and test serum respectively with one-third volume of a 1% solution of agar in the buffer, kept molten at 40–45 °C, and rapidly transfer the mixtures to the appropriate troughs, where gelling will occur. Make connexion with the buffer in the tank in the usual way with filter paper and pass a constant current of about 1.4 mA per cm width of agar plate. Under these conditions visible precipitin lines are produced within about one to two hours.

Figure App. 9.4 shows a reaction for α-fetoprotein obtained with cord blood serum examined both neat and diluted in order to illustrate the principle of the method. By observing the extent and strength of the precipitin lines, and their distances from the two troughs, one can make a semiquantitative assessment of the amount of antigen present. The method would appear to be generally applicable.

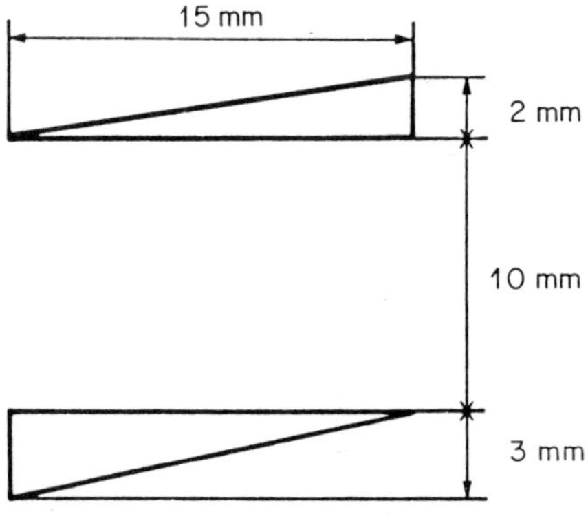

Figure App. 9.3. Pattern of antigen (lower) and antibody troughs. (Reproduced, with permission, from J. W. Keyser and K. Lewis, *J. Clin. Path.*, 1973, **26**, 160.)

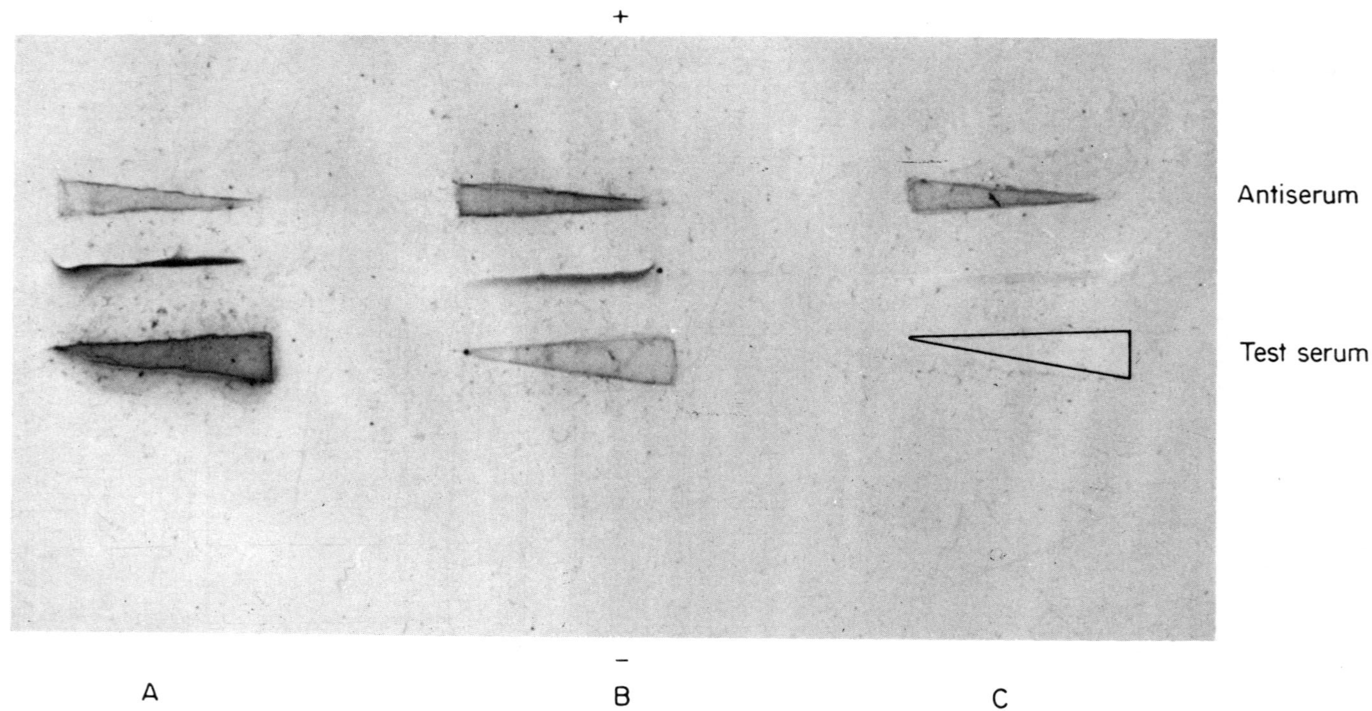

Figure App. 9.4. Precipitin line obtained by the method of Libich with specimen of cord blood serum and anti-α-fetoprotein serum. A, undiluted specimen; **B**, specimen diluted 1 : 10; C, specimen diluted 1 : 50. In this experiment the specimens (undiluted and diluted) were mixed with an equal volume of 1% agar. Stained with Coomassie Brilliant Blue. (Reproduced, with permission, from J. W. Keyser and K. Lewis, *J. Clin. Path.*, 1973, **26**, 160.)

REFERENCES

Alter, H. J., P. V. Holland, and R. H. Purcell (1971), *J. Lab. Clin. Med.*, **77**, 1000.
Bussard, A. (1959), *Biochim. Biophys. Acta*, **34**, 258.
Kelkar, S. S., and S. E. Kotwal (1975), *Lancet*, **i**, 755.
Keyser, J. W., and K. Lewis (1973), *J. Clin. Path.*, **26**, 160.
Kohn, J. (1970), *J. Clin. Path.*, **23**, 733.
Kohn, J. (1973), *Tumor Res.*, **8**, 42.
Kohn, J., and M. Kahan (1976), *J. Immunol. Methods*, **11**, 303.
Kohn, J., and J. R. Morgan (1971), *J. Clin. Path.*, **24**, 673.
Kohn, J., and P. C. Weaver (1974), *Lancet*, **ii**, 334.
Lancet (1976), *Annotation*, **ii**, 890.
Libich, M. (1959), *Folia Biol.*, **5**, 71.
McIllmurray, M. B. (1976), *Lab-Lore* (Welcome Reagents Ltd.), **7**, 401.
Sorice, F., S. Delia, and L. Castagnari (1975), *Lancet*, **ii**, 617.

APPENDIX 10

'Rocket' immunoelectrophoresis

A method of estimating proteins by electrophoresis into an antibody-containing gel was described by Laurell (1966). The method is applicable to most proteins with anodic migration at pH 8.6, and even to cathodically migrating proteins after suitable treatment (p. 282). As the protein migrates into the gel, antigen–antibody complexes are produced, and these form a visible precipitate at the point of equivalence. For best results the concentration of antibody in the gel, and the amount of test serum taken, should be adjusted so that antibody concentrations are kept to a minimum and peak heights range from 1–4 cm.

Method

Reagents

(1) *Barbitone buffer:* pH 8.6, 0.025 M (Note 1). This buffer is used both for preparing the gel and for the electrophoresis tank.

(2) *Agarose:* 1.0–1.2% in 0.025 M barbitone buffer (Reagent 1) (Note 2).

(3) *Specific antiserum.*

(4) *Staining solution:* Coomassie Blue, 2 g/l, in a mixture of methanol, acetic acid, and water (4:1:6 by volume).

(5) *Destaining solution:* a mixture of methanol, acetic acid, and water as above.

(6) *Standards.*

Procedure

Preparation of gel

The volume of antiserum required will depend on the titre of the batch used; the exact amount required must be determined by experiment.

Melt a suitable volume of the agarose solution (Reagent 2) and allow it to equilibrate in a water bath at 52 °C. Add the appropriate amount of antiserum and mix thoroughly. Pour the mixture onto a warm glass plate (10 × 10 cm) resting on a horizontal surface, taking care to avoid the formation of bubbles and ensuring that the agarose is spread evenly over the whole plate. After 15–20 min punch wells about 5 mm apart and 1.5 cm from the cathodal side of the plate, with the aid of a stainless steel gel punch having an external diameter of about 1.7 mm, and remove the gel plugs by suction. The row of wells should not extend to within 10 mm of the edges of the plate.

Place the prepared plate in the electrophoresis chamber and make electrical contact with the buffer by means of absorbent lint wicks 10 cm wide. Start water cooling.

Application of samples and standards

Apply the appropriate volume of test samples and standards to the origin wells with a micropipette.

Electrophoresis

Apply a voltage of 10–12 V/cm and allow migration to proceed to completion (Note 3).

Drying and staining

Remove the plate from the tank and wash it for about $\frac{1}{2}$ h in saline. Remove from the saline, cover the gel with a piece of filter paper, then add several cellulose paper layers and apply a light weight for 15 min. Remove the papers, wash the plate briefly in saline, and allow to dry in a warm oven.

Immerse the plate in staining solution for a few minutes and then remove excess stain by washing in destaining solution.

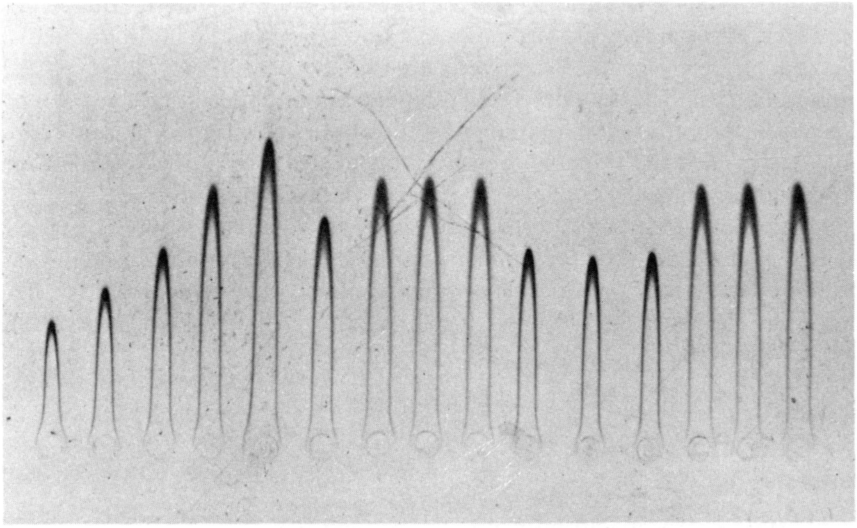

Figure App. 10.1 Electroimmunodiffusion.

Measurement

Measure the heights of the precipitin peaks (from the anodal border of the origin well to the tip of the peak). Construct a standard curve from the peak heights of the standards, and read the concentrations of the test samples from this curve.

Notes

(1) Various concentrations of buffer are used by different workers; the exact concentration is not critical. In general, the lower the ionic strength of the buffer the faster the rate of electrophoretic migration.

(2) A number of commercially available agarose preparations are suitable, including those from L'Industrie Biologique Française, Miles Laboratories, and Behringwerke.

(3) Electrophoresis must be allowed to go to completion, i.e. until the highest standards show no further increase in peak height. This should be established by experiment. Usually 3–4 h will suffice.

IgG, IgA, and IgM BY MODIFIED LAURELL IMMUNOELECTROPHORESIS

The unmodified Laurell 'rocket' technique as described above is unsuitable for the estimation of polyclonal IgG and IgM since in agarose at pH 8.6 these proteins exhibit both anodic and cathodic migration; moreover, the double peaks formed are wide and their height cannot be measured accurately. Weeke (1968) increased the surface negative charge of the proteins by treatment with potassium cyanate, the carbamylated proteins migrating towards the positive pole and forming single peaks. (IgA will travel anodally without this treatment.) However, at room temperature carbamylation takes about 6 h. An alternative method of increasing the negative charge of the proteins, by reaction with β-propiolactone, has been described (Stephan and Frahm, 1971); but the most convenient procedure for routine purposes would appear to be that of Teppo (1973), in which the proteins are simply incubated with formaldehyde. This procedure produces the same result as carbamylation and requires only a 20-min incubation at room temperature. Although, as mentioned above, treatment of IgA is not necessary for anodal migration, the formylated protein does produce taller, narrower peaks which are more accurately measured. The procedure described here follows the directions of Slater (1975, and private communication).

Method

Reagents

(1) *Antisera:* sheep anti-human IgA, IgG, and IgM.

(2) *Formaldehyde solution:* 36%.

(3) *Agarose:* 15 g/l in distilled water.
(4) *Barbitone buffer:* 0.04 M and 0.02 M, both pH 8.6.
(5) *Saline:* nephelometric grade, with 'Tween' 20 added (0.15 ml/l).
(6) *Coomassie Brilliant Blue:* as on p. 280.
(7) *Destaining solution:* as on p. 280.

Procedure

Preparation of plates

Prepare either small or large plates (Note 1), using agarose–buffer mixture in the following amounts:

	Plate size (cm)	*Vol. of buffer (ml)*	*Vol. of agarose (ml)*
Small plate	8 × 8	5.5	5.5
Large plate	10 × 20	13.5	13.5

(The amount of antiserum required must be determined by experiment.)

Pour the agarose–buffer–antiserum mixture onto small plates on a level surface. For large plates, clip two plates together on either side of a U-shaped perspex mould-former, pour in the agarose–buffer mixture and allow bubbles to rise to the surface and disperse; when the gel is partially set, transfer it to a refrigerator for at least 20 min, then remove the clips, slide the plates apart and lift off the mould former.

Cut wells in the gel as described above, except that in the case of IgA and IgM the cutter should have a diameter of 2.5 mm instead of 1.7 mm.

Preparation of standards and samples

Make 1-in-100 and 1-in-10 dilutions of the stock formaldehyde solution in 0.02 M barbitone buffer, to give 0.36% and 3.6% solutions (Note 2). Prepare standards from a serum pool as follows:

S1: 1-in-4 dilution in 3.6% formaldehyde;
S2: 1-in-5 dilution in 0.36% formaldehyde;
S3: 1-in-10 dilution in 0.36% formaldehyde;
S4, S5, and S6: doubling dilutions of S3 in barbitone buffer (after 20-min incubation period).

Test sera are diluted 1-in-10 in 0.36% formaldehyde. Cerebrospinal fluid and urine are diluted with 1/9th volume of 3.6 per cent, formaldehyde (i.e. 9 parts of sample plus 1 part of formalin).

Standards 1–3 and all samples are incubated with formaldehyde at room temperature for at least 20 min.

Application of sample, etc.

This is done as described above. After application increase the voltage to 10–12 V/cm for fast runs (4 h) or 1–2 V/cm for slow runs (overnight).

Process the plate and measure the heights of the peaks as described above.

Notes

(1) The plates should be cleaned with methanol.

(2) The stock formaldehyde solution loses strength on keeping. This can be allowed for by decreasing slightly its dilution for use.

REFERENCES

Laurell, C.-B. (1966), *Analyt. Biochem.*, **15**, 45.
Slater, L. (1975), *Ann. Clin. Biochem.*, **12**, 19.
Stephan, W., and U. Frahm (1971), *Z. klin. Chem. klin. Biochem.*, **9**, 224.
Teppo, A.-M. (1973), at *9th International Congress of Biochemistry*, Stockholm.
Weeke, B. (1968), *Scand. J. Clin. Lab. Invest.*, **21**, 351.

APPENDIX 11

Detection of heavy-chain diseases by 'rocket immunoselection'

Free heavy-chain proteins have been detected by immunoelectrophoretic and double-diffusion methods, but the interpretation of the precipitin patterns is often complicated by the presence of normal immunoglobulins. An immunoselection technique was introduced by Rádl (1970) for the light-chain typing of immunoglobulins in small samples of biological material, and this formed the basis of a method for the detection of heavy chains proposed by Gale and his coworkers (1974). The sample is subjected to electrophoresis in an agarose plate containing kappa and lambda antisera in the lower section and the appropriate heavy-chain antiserum (γ-, α-, or μ-chain) in the upper section: light chains and immunoglobulins containing light chains are precipitated in the lower section, and free heavy chains migrate into the upper, where they are precipitated as a separate 'rocket' (Figures App. 11.2 and App. 11.3).

Method

Reagents

(1) *Agarose.* Dissolve 15 g agarose (Miles Laboratories Ltd., Stoke Poges, Slough, Bucks., UK) in water to 1 litre.

(2) *Electrophoresis buffer:* sodium barbitone, pH 8.6, 0.02 M.

(3) *Working buffer:* sodium barbitone, pH 8.6, 0.04 M.

(4) *Antisera* to kappa and lambda chains, and to γ-, α-, and μ-chains (Note 1).

(5) *Formaldehyde:* see Appendix 10.

(6) *Staining solution:* see Appendix 10.

(7) *Washing solution:* see Appendix 10.

Procedure

Pour plates with a mixture of agarose and buffer in three sections as indicated in Figure App. 11.1 (Note 2), using the following quantities:

Section 1: 2 ml of agarose and 2 ml of 0.04 M buffer mixed with 0.2 ml of light-chain antiserum (i.e. kappa and lambda antisera mixed in equal volumes) (Note 3).

Section 2: 1.5 ml of agarose + 1.5 ml of 0.04 M buffer.

Section 3: 2 ml of agarose +2 ml of 0.04 M buffer mixed with the appropriate volume of heavy-chain antiserum (Note 4).

Formylate test samples as follows:

γ- and α-chain investigations: Dilute the formaldehyde with 0.04 M buffer in the proportion of 3.6 ml of formaldehyde to 1 litre of buffer. Dilute test samples 100-fold and allow to stand at room temperature for 30 min.

μ-chain investigations: Dilute test samples 50-fold with the same solution and allow to stand at room temperature for 30 min.

Place the slide in the electrophoresis apparatus and apply a voltage of 10 V/cm for a few hours, then dry and stain the slides as described in Appendix 10.

Typical results are illustrated in Figures App. 11.2 and App. 11.3. On account of electroendosmosis the bases of the heavy-chain peaks are not situated at the junction between the middle and upper sections (i.e. sections 2 and 3 of Figure App. 11.1), but at some distance into the plain agarose section.

Notes

(1) Only certain types of antisera are suitable for this test. Dakopatts antisera have proved satisfactory. The light-chain antisera must have been prepared with the use of insoluble immunoabsorbents, since absorption by addition of the opposite light chain will result in co-precipitation on subsequent admixture of the kappa and lambda antisera, and absorption with heavy chains would interfere with the subsequent tests.

(2) This is done with the aid of a divider, which is used to contain the agarose within each section in turn, the divider being removed after the agarose has solidified.

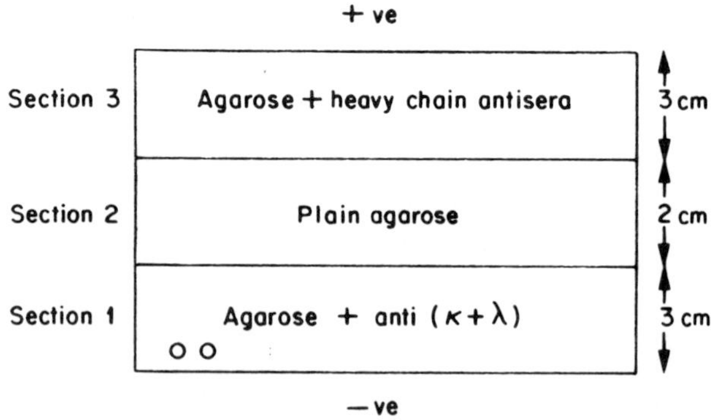

Figure App. 11.1. Plan of plate for 'rocket immunoselection'. (Reproduced from D. J. S. Gale, J. M. B. Versey, and J. R. Hobbs, *Clin. Chem.*, 1974, **20**, 1292, with the permission of the authors and the American Association for Clinical Chemistry.)

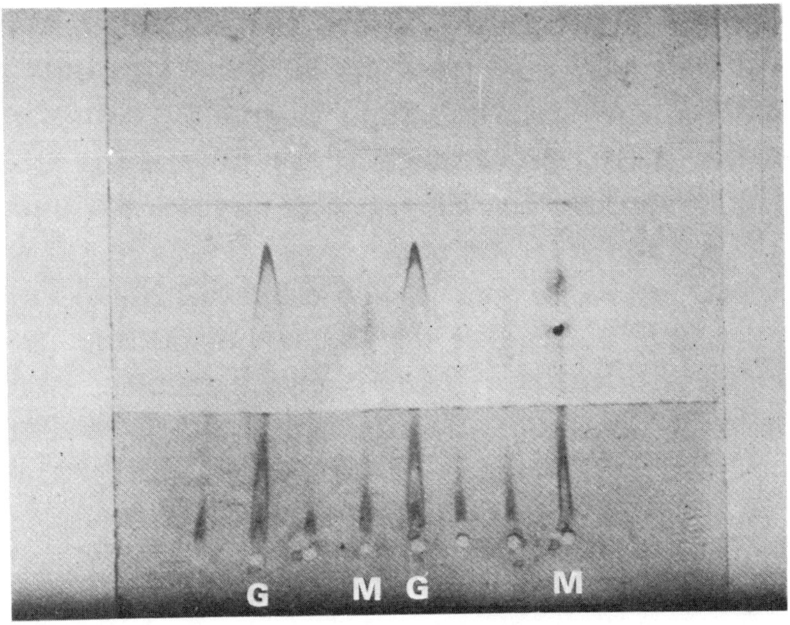

Figure App. 11.2. Results of investigation for γ-chain disease. M indicates sera from patients with IgG myelomatosis, one of which contained 60 g of $\gamma_2\lambda_2$ paraprotein per litre; its peak gained the mid-zone. The peaks from two sera from patients with known γ-chain disease are clearly seen in the mid-zone. The remaining wells contained polyclonal IgG at concentrations of 20–40 g/l. (Reproduced from D. J. S. Gale, J. M. B. Versey, and J. R. Hobbs, *Clin. Chem.*, 1974, **20**, 1292, with the permission of the authors and the American Association for Clinical Chemistry.)

(3) This amount of antiserum (Dakopatts) is stated to be sufficient to precipitate all monoclonal immunoglobulins bearing light chains, in concentrations up to 30 /gl. If larger amounts of immunoglobulin are present the sample should be diluted to a greater extent or a larger amount of light-chain antiserum should be used.

(4) For Dakopatts γ-, α- and μ-antisera 50 μl is a suitable quantity.

There are several possible sources of error. Positive results may be obtained if the sample has been stored for a long period, as certain classes of immunoglobulins—notably IgG_3—are degraded on storage. It has also been reported that paraproteinaemias may show free heavy chains or heavy-chain fragments in the serum (Bhoopalam *et al.*, 1971); and certain types of immunoglobulins can apparently possess light chains in which the determinants are structurally inaccessiblc (Osterland and Chaplin, 1966) and which could thus escape precipitation by the anti-kappa and anti-lambda antisera in the test. Such proteins could show a reaction with the heavy-chain antisera. However, the presence of such immunoglobulins in serum has been questioned (Gale *et al.*, 1974).

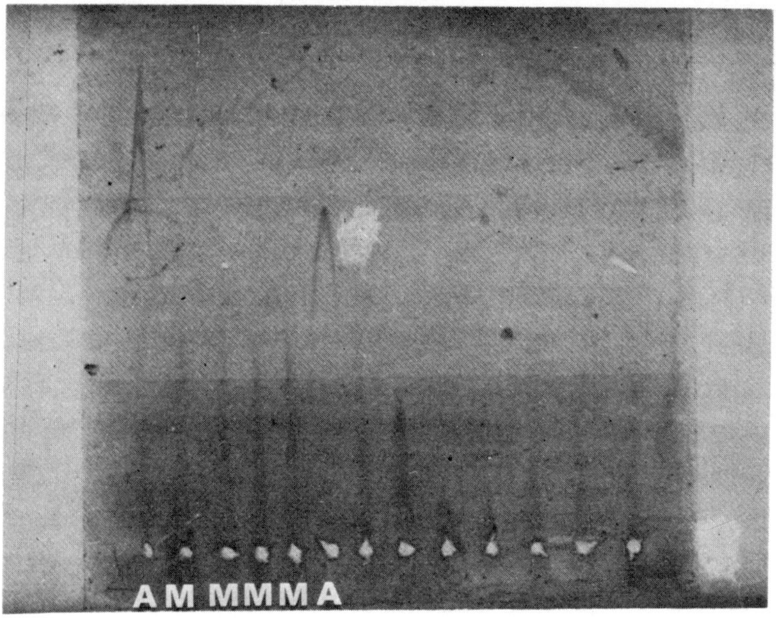

Figure App. 11.3. Results of investigation for α-chain disease. Sera from two known patients showed the peaks in the upper zones. The wells marked M contained known IgA myeloma sera. The remainder contained polyclonal IgA at concentrations of 4–12 g/l. (Reproduced from D. J. S. Gale, J. M. B. Versey, and J. R. Hobbs, *Clin. Chem.*, 1974, **20**, 1292, with the permission of the authors and the American Association for Clinical Chemistry.)

REFERENCES

Bhoopalam, N., B. M. Lee, V. J. Yakulis, and P. Heller (1971), *Arch. Int. Med.*, **128**, 437.
Gale, D. J. S., J. M. B. Versey, and J. R. Hobbs (1974), *Clin. Chem.*, **20**, 1292.
Osterland, C. K., and H. Chaplin (1966), *J. Immunol.*, **96**, 842.
Rádl, J. (1970), *Immunology*, **19**, 137.

APPENDIX 12

Radial immunodiffusion

This type of precipitin reaction is performed by incorporating one of the two reactants—usually the antibody—in agar gel spread on a flat surface and allowing the other reactant to diffuse into it from a well. Ring-shaped precipitation bands form and migrate outwards concentrically around the holes until the equivalence point has been reached. Originally developed by Petrie (1932) for qualitative comparative purposes, the technique was subsequently used in various forms for the semiquantitative measurement of antigens (Ouchterlony, 1949; Feinberg, 1957; Hayward and Augustin, 1957; Crowle, 1960). It was placed on a firm quantitative basis by Mancini and his colleagues (1964, 1965), who showed that a linear relationship exists between the area bounded by the ring and the concentration of antigen, provided that diffusion is allowed to go to completion. In a convenient modification introduced by Fahey and McKelvey (1965) a shorter diffusion time is used.

Immunodiffusion plates for the determination of a wide range of antigens are obtainable commercially; however, some workers prefer to prepare their own. A detailed description of the preparation of plates and of conducting the determination is given by Hobbs (1970). In the case of commercially produced plates, the manufacturer's instructions should, in general, be followed.

Method

Place the recommended amount of test solution or standard, suitably diluted if necessary, in each hole, and cover the plate and allow it to stand at room temperature until diffusion is complete.

Using oblique illumination from underneath, and viewing the plate against a matt black background, measure the diameters of the rings as accurately as possible (Note 1). On semilogarithmic paper plot the concentrations of the standards vertically on the log scale against precipitin diameters on the linear scale (Note 2).

Notes

(1) If the rings are faint they may be made easier to see by treatment with 5 per cent acetic acid (for 1 min only) or, alternatively, by staining with Ponceau S or Nigrosin after washing in repeated changes of saline for 24–36 h to remove soluble proteins.

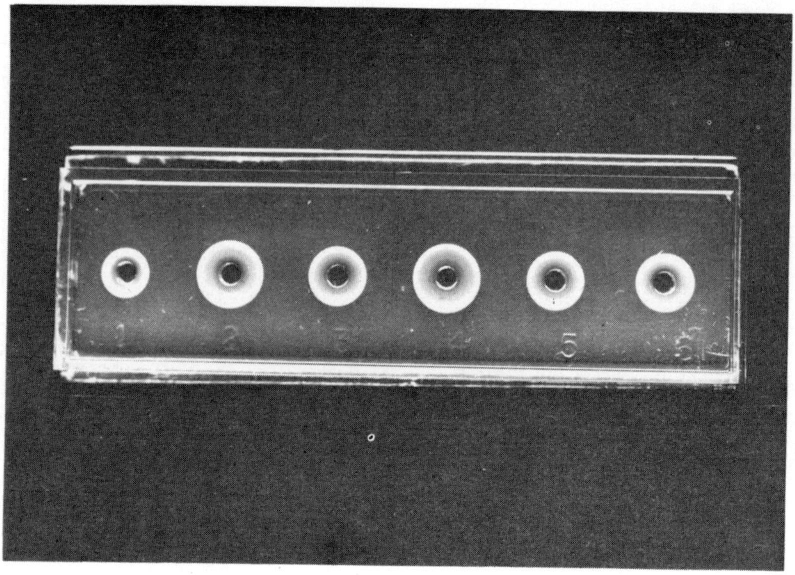

Figure App. 12.1. Single radial immunodiffusion.

(2) Straight lines are not always obtained, readings often falling on a smooth curve.

Errors

Apart from obvious sources of error, such as irregular edges to the wells or the presence of residual pieces of agar in them (i.e. with home-made plates), inaccurate filling of the wells, and so on, a major sources of error lies in the use of unsuitable antisera or standards. The antisera should be monospecific for the test antigens and should produce one sharp precipitin ring at the concentration employed. (The formation of two precipitation rings in commercially available agar gels containing rabbit antiserum to human IgM heavy chains is apparently due to the presence of both high and low molecular weight IgM which differ partly in antigenic determinants (Mulder *et al.*, 1972). The presence of low molecular weight IgM will lead to overestimation of 19S IgM. Double-ring formation has been seen with other proteins also, notably C3.) In the case of immunoglobulins it is essential that parallel calibration curves should be given by pooled normal serum and the test serum; monoclonal immunoglobulins cannot be accurately measured by comparison with pooled normal serum as standard, as they often exist in polymeric form or show idiotypic antigenicity (Hobbs *et al.*, 1966).

REFERENCES

Crowle, A. J. (1960), *J. Lab. Clin. Med.*, **55**, 593.
Fahey, J. L., and E. M. McKelvey (1965), *J. Immunol.*, **94**, 84.

Feinberg, J. G. (1957), *Int. Arch. Allergy*, **11**, 129.
Hayward, B. J., and R. Augustin (1957), *Int. Arch. Allergy*, **11**, 192.
Hobbs, J. R. (1970), Association of Clinical Pathologists Broadsheet 68.
Hobbs, J. R., G. M. J. Slot, C. H. Campbell, G. P. Clein, J. T. Scott, D. Crowther, and H. T. Swan (1966), *Lancet*, **ii**, 614.
Mancini, G., J. P. Vaerman, A. O. Carbonara, and J. F. Heremans (1964), in *Protides of the Biological Fluids: Proceedings of 11th Colloquium, Bruges, 1963* (Ed. H. Peeters), Elsevier, Amsterdam, p. 370.
Mancini, G., A. O. Carbonara, and J. F. Heremans (1965), *Immunochemistry*, **2**, 235.
Mulder, J., L. C. E. Sloots, and M. A. T. Verhaar (1972), *J. Immunol. Methods*, **2**, 89.
Ouchterlony, Ö. (1949), *Acta Path. Microbiol. Scand.*, **26**, 516.
Petrie, G. F. (1932), *Brit. J. Exp. Path.*, **13**, 38.

APPENDIX 13

Nephelometric techniques

AUTOMATED IMMUNOPRECIPITATION

In this method, which was developed by Kahan and Sundblad (1967), Eckman and his coworkers (1970), Killingsworth and his coworkers (1971), and others, suitable dilutions of test serum or standard and of antiserum are allowed to react in an automated system and the resulting turbidity is measured by means of a nephelometer. The precipitin reaction was found by Hellsing and Laurent (1964) to be enhanced in the presence of certain polymers; the one generally employed in automated immunoprecipitation is polyethylene glycol. Continuous-flow nephelometric analysis for specific proteins using Technicon Auto-Analyzer equipment was described by Ritchie and his coworkers (1973).

Details of the operation of the equipment will be found in the manufacturer's instructions and are not given here.

It is important to note that all samples, standards, and reagents must be free from particulate matter, and nephelometric grade saline (prepared by passage through a 2-μm filter) is used for all dilutions. The technique requires monospecific antisera of high avidity and high titre.

LASER NEPHELOMETRY

The high intensity of light that can be achieved in a laser beam allows a substantial increase in sensitivity in the detection of weak light scattering, as compared with 'conventional' nephelofluorimetry; and the highly monochromatic nature of the light makes it ideal for light-scattering techniques. A number of instruments have appeared on the market which incorporate a laser as a radiation source and measure the amount of forward light scatter. These instruments, which are either manually operated or automated discrete analysers, have a high degree of sensitivity and a wide range of measurement (Caputo, 1976; Deaton *et al.*, 1976); similar nephelometric systems have been incorporated into centrifugal analysers (Buffone *et al.*, 1975a, b).

An evaluation of one of these instruments has recently appeared (Whicher *et al.*, 1978).

Laser nephelometric measurement of proteins will undoubtedly become more widely used, chiefly on account of its speed and sensitivity.

REACTION RATE NEPHELOMETRY

As its name implies, this is a method of nephelometric analysis in which the rate of development of antigen–antibody complexes is measured. Such kinetic measurements offer considerable advantages over 'end-point' procedures, because corrections for turbidity in the sample are eliminated and the speed of analysis may be increased.

For details of the theory of kinetic measurement of light scattering the reader is referred to the original publications (Anderson, 1970; Tiffany *et al.*, 1974; Buffone *et al.*, 1974a, b, 1975a, b; Sternberg, 1977).

REFERENCES

Anderson, N. G. (1970), *Amer. J. Clin. Path.*, **52**, 778.

Buffone, G. J., J. Savory, and R. E. Cross (1974a), *Clin. Chem.*, **20**, 1320.

Buffone, G. J., R. E. Cross, J. Savory, and C. Soodak (1974b), *Analyt. Chem.*, **46**, 2047.

Buffone, G. J., J. Savory, R. E. Cross, and J. E. Hammond (1975a), *Clin. Chem.*, **21**, 1731.

Buffone, G. J., J. Savory, and J. Hermans (1975b), *Clin. Chem.*, **21**, 1735.

Caputo, M. J. (1976), in *Protides of the Biological Fluids: Proceedings of the 24th Colloquium, Bruges, 1976* (Ed. H. Peeters), Pergamon Press, Oxford, p. 677.

Deaton, C. D., K. W. Maxwell, R. S. Smith, and R. L. Creveling (1976), *Clin. Chem.*, **22**, 1465.

Eckman, I., J. B. Robbins, C. J. A. Van den Hamer, J. Lenz, and I. H. Scheinberg (1970), *Clin. Chem.*, **16**, 558.

Hellsing, K., and T. C. Laurent (1964), *Acta Chem. Scand.*, **18**, 1303.

Kahan, J., and L. Sundblad (1967), in *Automation in Analytical Chemistry II: Technicon Symposium, Paris, 1966*, p. 361.

Killingsworth, L. M., J. Savory, and P. O. Teague (1971), *Clin. Chem.*, **17**, 374.

Ritchie, R. F., C. A. Alper, J. Graves, N. Pearson, and C. Larson (1973), *Amer. J. Clin. Path.*, **59**, 151.

Sternberg, J. C. (1977), *Clin. Chem.*, **23**, 1456.

Tiffany, T. O., J. M. Parella, W. F. Johnson, and C. A. Burtis (1974), *Clin. Chem.*, **20**, 1055.

Whicher, J. T., D. E. Perry, and J. R. Hobbs (1978), *Ann. Clin. Biochem.*, **15**, 77.

APPENDIX 15

Thin-layer chromatography of proteins

In 1962 Determann introduced a thin-layer method of gel filtration analogous to thin-layer chromatography, which has since been used for the qualitative analysis of serum proteins (Johansson and Rymo, 1962; Andrews, 1964; Morris, 1964; Grant and Everall, 1965; Williamson and Allison, 1967; Carter and Hobbs, 1971). The procedure described here is that of Williamson and Allison (1967), which is based on the system of Morris (1964). A procedure using columns is described by Thompson and Stokes (1977).

Method

Reagents

(1) *Saline:* 0.5 M sodium chloride in water.

(2) *'Sephadex' G-200 'Superfine'.*

(3) *Dye:* saturated solution of amido black 10B in methanol–water–glacial acetic acid (5:4:1 by volume).

(4) *Destaining solution:* dye solvent as above.

Discarded photographic half-plates (approx. 12 × 16 cm), freed from the emulsion coating, carefully cleaned, and scribed with a diamond transversely 3 cm from one end, are used as support for the gel ('Sephadex' G-200 'Superfine'), which is applied on the unscribed side in a 0.25-mm layer by means of a Stahl-type spreader (Stahl, 1958) (obtainable from Desaga, Heidelberg, and Camlab, Cambridge). Transparent polystyrene food boxes (13.5 × 22.5 × 8 cm), with tightly fitting lids, are used as containers to set up the plates (Figure App. 15.1). Flow of eluant is stopped, while the sample is being applied, by means of a support placed under one end so that the plate is horizontal.

Apply 1 μl of each of the test samples to the origin (indicated by the scribed line, visible through the gel), taking care to avoid damage to the gel surface and applying no sample nearer than 1.5 cm to the edge of the gel. Remove the cork, and allow the saline to flow through the gel at a rate sufficient to move a haemoglobin marker 1.4–1.6 cm/h. After 4 or 5 h remove the plate and dry at 50–60 °C for 15–30 min. Immerse the plate in amido black 10B dye for 5–10 min, and then remove excess stain with dye solvent (5–10 min in each of two successive wash-baths).

The position and intensity of the stained proteins can be determined accurately by transmission-densitometric scanning.

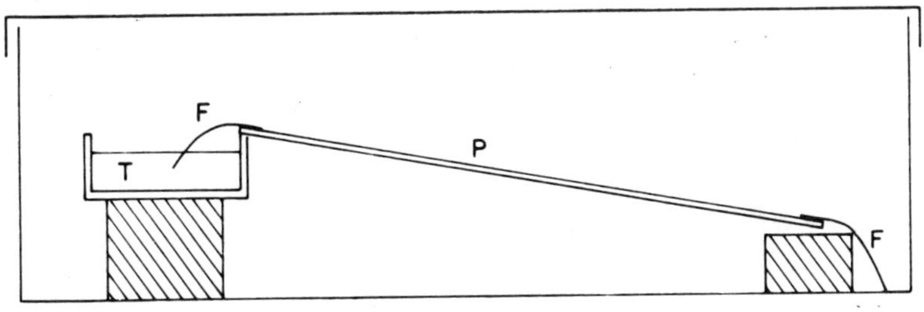

Figure App. 15.1. Apparatus for thin-layer 'Sephadex' chromatography of proteins. (After C. J. O. R. Morris, *J. Chromat.*, 1964, **16**, 167, by permission of Elsevier Scientific Publishing Co., Amsterdam, and Prof. Morris.)

The protein constituents can also be revealed by immunodiffusion. After the chromatographic separation, and while the gel is still wet, apply to the plate a strip of Whatman 3MM paper, 16 cm long and 3–5 mm wide, marked off in pencil in numbered 1-cm or 0.5-cm divisions, placing the strip in such a way that it extends from the top edge and along the line of run of the sample. Leave the strip in place until it is visibly damp (1–2 min), remove it carefully, and place it on the surface of a thin layer of agar or agarose gel on a glass slide (Note). Soak a similar strip of filter paper, 2 mm wide, in antiserum and place it on the gel, parallel to the first strip and about 3 mm from it. Leave the slide in a moist chamber until precipitin lines form (usually, overnight).

Note

For most purposes 1.5 ml of 1 per cent high-quality agar (Oxoid 'Ionagar') or 0.5 per cent agarose gel (Industrie Biologique Française S.A., Gennevilliers (Seine), France) on an ordinary 7.5 × 2.5-cm microscope slide is satisfactory.

REFERENCES

Andrews, P. (1964), *Biochem. J.*, **91**, 222.
Carter, P. M., and J. R. Hobbs (1971), *Brit. Med. J.*, **ii**, 260.
Determann, H. (1962), *Experientia*, **18**, 430.
Grant, G. H., and P. H. Everall (1965), *J. Clin. Path.*, **18**, 654.
Johansson, B. G., and L. Rymo (1962), *Acta chem. scand.*, **16**, 2067.
Morris, C. J. O. R. (1964), *J. Chromat.*, **16**, 167.
Stahl, E. (1958), *Chemikerzeitung*, **82**, 323.
Thompson, R. A., and R. P. Stokes (1977), in *Techniques in Clinical Immunology* (Ed. R. A. Thompson), Blackwell, Oxford, p. 25.
Williamson, J., and A. C. Allison (1967), *Lancet*, **ii**, 123.

APPENDIX 16

Detection of cryoglobulins

The following procedure is based on numerous publications (Peetoom and Van Loghem-Langereis, 1965; Cawley, 1969; Nakamura, 1974; etc.).

Method

Take the blood into a warmed syringe and allow it to clot by keeping it at 37 °C for 1–2 h. Centrifuge at 37 °C.

Remove a portion of the serum and keep it at 4 °C for 24 h or longer (Note 1).

Centrifuge at 4 °C.

If there is a cryoglobulin precipitate, wash it four times by resuspending it in ice-cold buffered saline (pH 7.4) and recentrifuging each time (Note 2).

Finally redissolve in saline or barbitone buffer (pH 8.6, i.s. 0.05) at 37 °C (1 ml for every 1 ml of serum originally taken), and subject the redissolved precipitate to immunoelectrophoresis, using appropriate antisera.

Notes

(1) Another portion of the serum can be removed for comparison with the supernatant fluid obtained from the specimen centrifuged at 4 °C. Careful measurement, in triplicate, of the immunoglobulin concentrations can indicate how much IgA, IgG, or IgM has been removed in the precipitate; according to Hobbs (1971) this gives a better measure than the 'cryocrit' and is superior also to immunoelectrophoresis of the cryoprecipitate, owing to contamination of the latter by trapped plasma proteins.

(2) A more stringent purification of the cryoglobulin is described by Wang and his coworkers (1974). They dissolve the precipitate in warm buffered saline solution (pH 8.0) at 37 °C, then reprecipitate at 4 °C. This procedure is repeated at least three times, the cryoprotein being washed three times with chilled saline after each precipitation.

To detect cryofibrinogenaemia, take the blood into a warm syringe as before, and place it immediately in a warm tube containing citrate or EDTA. Separate the plasma at 37 °C and incubate a portion at 4 °C overnight. Centrifuge at 4 °C. Wash any cryoprecipitate in cold saline containing EDTA, and dissolve at 37 °C as above. Subject the redissolved precipitate to immunochemical analysis, using an antifibrin antiserum.

REFERENCES

Cawley, L. P. (1969), *Electrophoresis and Immunoelectrophoresis*, Little, Brown, Boston.
Hobbs, J. R. (1971), *Adv. Clin. Chem.*, **14**, 219.
Nakamura, R. M. (1974), *Immunopathology: Clinical Laboratory Concepts and Methods*, Little, Brown, Boston, p. 190.
Peetoom, F., and E. Van Loghem-Langereis (1965), *Vox Sang.*, **10**, 281.
Wang, A. C., J. V. Wells, H. H. Fudenberg, and J. Gergely (1974), *Immunochemistry*, **11**, 341.

APPENDIX 17

Complement studies

Total haemolytic complement

This is assessed by estimating the amount of serum required as a source of complement to produce lysis of 50 per cent of a standard amount of sensitized (i.e. antibody-coated) sheep red cells. Since the curve relating the volume of serum to the amount of lysis approaches 100 per cent lysis asymptotically, the total lytic unit of complement (CH_{100}), can be estimated only approximately, so it is usual to determine the point at which 50 per cent lysis has occurred (CH_{50}). Full details, including a discussion of the factors that influence the haemolytic action of complement, are given in Mayer's extensive account (1961). Details of the test are also given by Lachmann and his coworkers (1973), Hudson and Hay (1976), and Brown and Hobart (1977).

Individual components

The individual components of the complement system are measured more often than total haemolytic complement. Radial immunodiffusion, Laurell 'rocket' electrophoresis, automated immunoprecipitation, or laser nephelometry may be used. It is also possible to measure individual complement components by functional haemolytic assays (Rapp and Borsos, 1970).

The limitations of immunochemical assays of complement proteins have been discussed by Whicher (1978). Activation of components may result in the generation of conversion products that may cross-react in the assay system, and the conversion products themselves may show subtle differences depending on the cause of activation. Differences in antisera and standards have also been responsible for variation in results from one laboratory to another, especially in the case of C3. In the investigation of inherited deficiencies of complement components, functional assays are essential as deficiencies may arise from functionally defective proteins which are immunologically cross-reactive with their normal counterparts.

The evaluation of complement measurements is also complicated by a number of *in vivo* factors, also summarized by Whicher (1978). C3, C4, and factor B (C3 proactivator, glycine-rich β-glycoprotein, GBG) behave as 'acute-phase reactants', and serum concentrations are increased in most conditions associated with inflammation. The release of proteolytic enzymes from various tissues as a result of ischaemia, necrosis, or intravascular coagulation may produce cleavage of complement components similar to that occurring in immune activation; this may result in lowered complement concentrations and the production of fragments indistinguishable from activation products. Yet another complication is found in the production of immune complexes in 'showers' of short duration that probably occurs in some conditions; this may result in there being no evidence of immune-complex activity at the time when the clinical features are most evident.

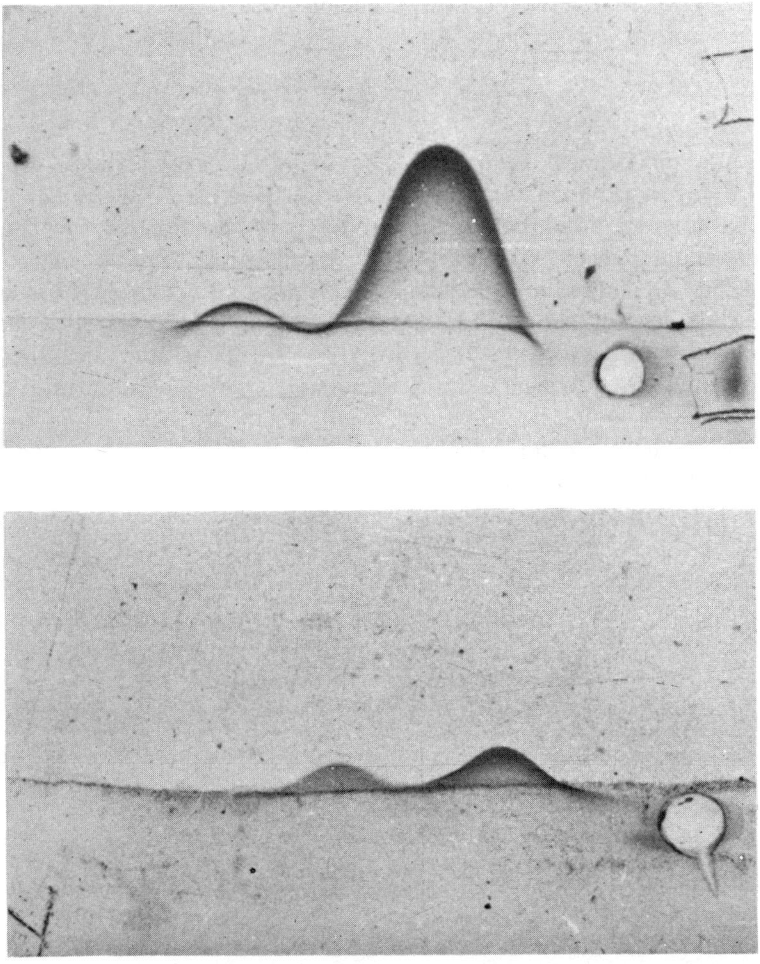

Figure App. 17.1. Demonstration by quantitative immunoelectrophoresis of complement components and their respective conversion products. Above, C3 and C3c; below, C4 and C4a. In each case the conversion product is on the left.

Complement activation

The finding of a lowered concentration of any of several complement components in the serum affords some evidence of complement activation. A better method of demonstrating this, however, is the demonstration of activation products of low molecular weight. The conversion products of C3, C4, and Factor B, *viz.* C3c, C4a, and $\bar{B}$, can be separated from the native molecule on the basis of their different molecular size and charge; they can therefore be detected by immunoelectrophoresis or counter immunoelectrophoresis (Arroyave and Tan, 1976) and measured by quantitative immunoelectrophoresis (Versey, 1973). Figure App. 17.1 shows patterns obtained by the method of quantitative immunoelectrophoresis, demonstrating C3 and C4 and their respective conversion products.

Collection of specimens

For immunochemical estimations, 2 ml of freshly taken serum to which is added 10 mg of sodium azide as preservative is despatched in a clean container to the laboratory. If complement conversion is to be estimated, care must be taken to avoid trauma to the vein, since this causes release of tissue proteases, and the first 3–4 ml of blood should be discarded so as to eliminate tissue activators; the blood is then placed in a bottle containing EDTA, which chelates the calcium, causing dissociation of the C1qrs complex; after centrifugation, which should be performed as soon as possible and preferably within 15–30 min, the plasma should be frozen and dispatched in 'dry ice'.

Functional tests of complement require fresh serum that has been separated from the clot after 1–2 h at room temperature; the serum may be stored at $-20°$ C for a week, or at $-70°$ C or lower for an indefinite period, before being tested (Thompson, 1978).

REFERENCES

Arroyave, C. M., and E. M. Tan (1976), *J. Immunol. Methods*, **13**, 101.

Brown, D., and M. J. Hobart (1977), in *Techniques in Clinical Immunology* (Ed. R. A. Thompson), Blackwell, Oxford, p. 65.

Hudson, L., and F. C. Hay (1976), *Practical Immunology*, Blackwell, Oxford, p. 134.

Lachmann, P. J., M. J. Hobart, and W. P. Aston (1973), in *Handbook of Experimental Immunology, Vol. 1: Immunochemistry* (Ed. D. M. Weir), Blackwell, Oxford, p. 5.1.

Mayer, M. M. (1961), in *Experimental Immunochemistry*, 2nd edn., by E. A. Kabat and M. M. Mayer, Thomas, Springfield, Ill., p. 133.

Rapp, H. J., and T. Borsos (1970), *Molecular Basis of Complement Action*, Appleton–Century–Crofts, New York, 1970.

Thompson, R. A. (1978), *The Practice of Clinical Immunology*, 2nd edn., Arnold, London, p. 122.

Versey, J. M. B. (1973), *Ann. Clin. Biochem.*, **10**, 100.

Whicher, J. T. (1978), *Clin. Chem.*, **24**, 7.

APPENDIX 18

α-Fetoprotein by radioimmunoassay

For the detection of grossly raised serum concentrations of α-fetoprotein in patients with primary carcinoma of the liver crossed immunoelectrophoresis (Appendix 9) may be used; and for the quantitative estimation of α-fetoprotein in amniotic fluid the 'rocket' technique (Appendix 10) is suitable. However, when it is a question of estimating the minute amounts of α-fetoprotein present in serum in conditions other than those associated with gross increases, these techniques do not possess the requisite sensitivity and some form of radioimmunoassay is usually necessary. The method described here is that of Ruoslahti and Seppälä, which employs a second antibody for the separation stage. Other published assay procedures, such as that of Leek and Chard (1974), use polyethylene glycol instead of a second antibody.

An immunoenzymic assay has been proposed for the measurement of serum α-fetoprotein (Alpert *et al.*, 1974; see also Alpert, 1975), but this has barely adequate sensitivity and is not suitable for use when large numbers of specimens have to be tested.

Method (After Ruoslahti and Seppälä, 1971; Monk and Goldie, 1976)

Reagents

(1) *Phosphate buffers:* 0.5 M, 0.1 M, and 0.05 M, pH 7.5.

(2) *Phosphate-buffered saline:* 1 vol. 0.05 M phosphate buffer, 4 volumes saline (9 g NaCl/l), and human serum albumin 0.05 per cent.

(3) *α-Fetoprotein:* 0.5 mg/ml in 0.05 M phosphate buffer (pH 7.5). Dispense suitable amounts into plastic containers and store at − 70 °C.

(4) *$Na^{125}I$:* obtainable from The Radiochemical Centre, Amersham.

(5) *Chloramine-T:* dissolve 20 mg in 4 ml 0.5 M phosphate buffer. Prepare just before use.

(6) *Sodium metabisulphite:* dissolve 25 mg in 2 ml 0.1 M phosphate buffer. Prepare just before use.

(7) *'Sephadex' G 25*, coarse (Note 1).

(8) *Antibody to α-fetoprotein:* prepared in rabbit.

(9) *Rabbit serum:* diluted 1 : 50.

(10) *Anti-rabbit serum.*

(11) *α-Fetoprotein standard* (Note 2).

(12) *Sodium iodide:* 200 mg in 5 ml of 0.1 M phosphate buffer, pH 7.5.

Procedure

Preparation of 'Sephadex' column (Note 1)

Allow 20 g of 'Sephadex' G25 to soak overnight in 200 ml of 0.05 M phosphate buffer. The day before the iodination, prepare a column of overall length up to about 9 cm, in a glass tube plugged with glass wool. Saturate the column with 0.5 ml of human serum albumin (2 % in 0.05 M phosphate buffer), and wash off the excess with 0.05 M phosphate buffer.

Preparation of ^{125}I-α-fetoprotein label (Note 3)

To 5 μl of solution containing 2.5 μg of α-fetoprotein add 0.5 mCi $Na^{125}I$ contained in 10 μl, followed by 20 μl of chloramine-T. Mix for 10–20 s, and then immediately add 20 μl of metabisulphite and mix. Add 100 μl of sodium iodide.

Add the iodination mixture to the column and elute with phosphate buffer (0.1 M, pH 7.5) (20 ml). Collect the eluate in fractions, each of about 0.5 ml, in tubes containing 50 μl of 0.5 per cent human serum albumin in phosphate buffer.

Measure the radioactivity in each fraction and plot the number of counts against the fraction number. Two peaks of radioactivity should be obtained, the first one corresponding to the labelled α-fetoprotein. From the tubes corresponding to the first peak, pool the two fractions giving the highest count. Store at −20 °C in 50-μl portions.

For use, dilute the solution with phosphate-buffered saline containing human serum albumin so that, using the quantities prescribed in the assay, the amount of labelled α-fetoprotein in each tube is approximately 1 ng.

Determination of optimum dilutions of first and second antibodies

The optimum dilutions of the first and second antibodies (using a fixed quantity, approx. 1 μl, of carrier serum) must be determined by experiment, the concentration of each in turn being kept constant while that of the other is varied. For the first antibody, a dilution is chosen that will give a percentage binding of about 60–70%: too high a concentration of antibody will result in an insensitive assay.

As the concentration of *second* antibody is increased, the amount of radioactivity in the precipitate increases up to a plateau and then declines sharply: the dilution corresponding to a point a little way along the plateau is selected for routine use.

Procedure for assay

Set up diluent blank, tests, standards, and quality control specimens, in duplicate, adding the solutions in the order shown in Table App. 18.1, *viz.*

Table App. 18.1. Showing amounts of samples and reagents in procedure described (see text)

	Buffer (μl)	Sample or standard (μl)	Label (μl)	Diluted antiserum (μl)
Diluent blank	900	—	100	—
Zero	800	—	100	100
Standards	700	100	100	100
Samples	700	100	100	100
Total counts	—	—	100	—

buffer, sample or standard, label, diluted antiserum. Shake the tubes on a vortex mixer and incubate overnight at 4 °C.

Next day, to every tube except the one labelled 'total counts' add 50 μl of diluted rabbit serum and 50 μl of diluted anti-rabbit serum, shake on a vortex mixer, and incubate at 37 °C for 2 h. Centrifuge at 4000 r/min. for 40 min. Aspirate the supernatant fluid and count the radioactivity in the precipitate by means of a gamma counter.

Plot per cent binding against concentration of α-fetoprotein, on semilogarithmic paper. From this curve, read off the concentrations of α-fetoprotein in the test and quality control specimens.

Notes

(1) Ion exchange resin tubes (Bio-Rad) may be used instead.

(2) This may be a pure preparation of α-fetoprotein or, preferably, a reference serum such as 72/227 (obtainable from the National Institute for Biological Standards and Control, Holly Hill, London, NW3). If the latter is used, results may be expressed in units/1. A weight value in terms of mg α-fetoprotein per litre has been assigned to this preparation (Keyser *et al.*, 1976). In either case, dilutions of the reference preparation should be prepared in α-fetoprotein-free human serum.

(3) Alternatively, ^{125}I-labelled α-fetoprotein may be obtained commercially.

REFERENCES

Alpert, E. (1975), *Lancet*, **i**, 807.
Alpert, E., R. Coston, and J. Perrotto (1974), *Lancet*, **i**, 626.
Keyser, J. W., J. Kohn, and A. M. Ward (1976), *Lancet*, **i**, 1015.
Leek, A. E., and T. Chard (1974), in *L'Alpha-foeto-protéine* (Ed. R. Masseyeff), Editions INSERM, Paris, p. 563.
Monk, A. M., and D. J. Goldie (1976), *Brit. J. Obstet. Gynaec.*, **83**, 845.
Ruoslahti, E., and M. Seppälä (1971), *Int. J. Cancer*, **8**, 374.

APPENDIX 19

IgE by radioimmunoassay

The technique of radial immunodiffusion (Appendix 12) is not sufficiently sensitive for measuring serum IgE unless the concentration is grossly raised. An autoradiographic modification using ^{125}I-labelled antiglobulin in a second stage (Rowe, 1969) is relatively time consuming and has not proved satisfactory for measurements at the lower part of the normal range. A method widely used at present is the solid-phase radioimmunosorbent test (RIST). Labelled and unlabelled IgE compete for binding to anti-IgE attached to 'Sephadex' particles; the 'Sephadex' is then washed and the radioactivity measured in a gamma counter. The method was developed by Johansson and his coworkers (1968), and a kit containing the necessary reagents is marketed by Pharmacia. The procedure is not described here as full instructions are supplied with the kit. It may be noted, however, that the use of half volumes throughout (for reasons of economy) gives quite acceptable results.

A 'sandwich' method was developed by Ceska and Lundkvist (1972), in which the test serum is incubated with a filter paper disk to which anti-IgE antibody has been coupled; IgE in the serum becomes bound to the antibody, and on subsequent incubation with ^{125}I-labelled antiserum the latter is in turn bound in proportion to the amount of IgE on the disk. A kit based on this method is also available from Pharmacia. Greater sensitivity in measuring IgE concentrations at the lower end of the normal range is obtained with this method than with the solid-phase radioimmunosorbent test (RIST).

REFERENCES

Ceska, M., and U. Lundkvist (1972), *Immunochemistry*, **9**, 1021.
Johansson, S. G. O., H. Bennich, and L. Wide (1968), *Immunology*, **14**, 265.
Rowe, D. S. (1969), *Bull. Wld. Hlth. Org.*, **40**, 613.

APPENDIX 20

Standards for immunoglobulin estimations

It is well known that normal ranges obtained for plasma immunoglobulins by different laboratories have not agreed closely, even for comparable populations. That the differences were usually due mainly to technical reasons rather than to variations in the populations studied is suggested by comparisons such as those made by Buckley and her coworkers (1968), who showed that the results obtained for a single serum specimen by several well-established laboratories could differ by a factor of three. Discrepancies of this magnitude are presumably the result of differences between the standards and/or antisera employed. For valid comparison the standard should be qualitatively identical with the substance being determined; however, it is probable that the heterogeneity of the immunoglobulins will vary from one individual to another, and in different diseases, so that this ideal is unlikely to be attained. The question of variations in antisera is discussed below.

With the object of improving the agreement between laboratories, a freeze-dried preparation of diluted human serum which had been examined by a number of laboratories was accepted by the World Health Organisation as the International Reference Preparation for IgG, IgA, and IgM (Rowe *et al.*, 1970; Anderson *et al.*, 1971).

One batch, designated 67/86, was divided into two portions. One portion was established as the British research standard (now designated the 1st British Standard) for human serum immunoglobulins G, A, and M. The other portion was established by the WHO as the 1st International Reference Preparation for human serum immunoglobulins G, A, and M. The unit was defined as the activity of a given weight of freeze-dried preparation, but for all practical purposes the activity per ampoule is 100 units (Rowe *et al.*, 1970, 1973).

The International Reference Preparation, the British Standard and preparations related to it may be requested from the National Institute for Biological Standards and Control, Holly Hill, Hampstead, London NW3. In the Americas the related preparation 67/95 may be requested from the NCI Immunodiagnostic Reference Centre, 6715 Electronic Drive, Springfield, Va. 22151, USA. Workers elsewhere should request Preparation 67/97 from the WHO International Reference Centre for Immunoglobulins, 21, rue du Bugnon, 1011 Lausanne, Switzerland.

The International Reference Preparation 67/86 is available only in limited amounts and, in general, is reserved for the calibration of national standards.

The MRC Research Standard for IgD (67/37) and the 1st British Standard for

IgE (75/502) may be requested from the National Institute for Biological Standards and Control. (The International Reference Preparation for IgE, 68/341, has been shown to contain hepatitis B antigen (private communications from Dr. S. G. Anderson and Dr. F. T. Perkins).)

The importance of using a uniform standard was demonstrated by the results obtained when a group of sera were analysed in ten highly reputable laboratories (Rowe *et al.*, 1972). When each laboratory expressed its results with reference to its own standard, the ratio of the highest to the lowest value obtained by the ten laboratories for a single serum specimen was 2.2 for IgG, 3.2 for IgA, and 5.0 for IgM. In contrast, when the International Reference Preparation was used as standard the corresponding ratios were 1.36, 1.17, and 1.31 respectively. These results clearly establish the value of using a common standard.

Immunoglobulin concentrations are most precisely expressed in units; but some workers may prefer to express concentrations in terms of weight per unit volume. Conversion factors, based on the best available estimates, have been published by Humphrey and Batty (1974).

Although, as mentioned above, the collaborative results obtained with the WHO reference preparations showed relative uniformity, some divergence was noted. Attention has been drawn to the possibility that since antisera are usually raised against proteins that are antigenically heterogeneous they may give inconsistent results even when used in comparative assays of highly purified immunoglobulins (Lea and Ward, 1972).

The problems involved in the standardization of immunoglobulin measurements have been reviewed by Reimer and Maddison (1976).

Finally, it should be noted that the inter-laboratory comparisons of immunoglobulin estimations using WHO standards were based on the use of an immunodiffusion technique—usually single radial diffusion. More recent experience has demonstrated that these preparations are less suitable as standards in automated immunoprecipitation techniques, on account of the turbidity that is present when the material is reconstituted.

REFERENCES

Anderson, S. G., D. R. Bangham, I. Batty, W. Becker, B. Cinader, M. van der Giessen, F. Hymes, D. Long, F. Peetom, K. Pondman, M. Raynaud, C. B. Reimer, D. S. Rowe, H. G. Schwick, and S. Vrancheva (1971), *Ann. Inst. Pasteur*, **121**, 629.

Buckley, R. H., S. C. Dees, and W. M. O'Fallon (1968), *Pediatrics*, **41**, 600.

Humphrey, J. H., and I. Batty (1974), *J. Immunol.*, **113**, 428.

Lea, D. J., and D. J. Ward (1972), *Lancet*, **ii**, 770.

Reimer, C. B., and S. E. Maddison (1976), *Clin. Chem.*, **22**, 577.

Rowe, D. S., S. G. Anderson, and B. Grab (1970), *Bull. Wld. Hlth. Org.*, **42**, 535.

Rowe, D. S., B. Grab, and S. G. Anderson (1972), *Bull. Wld. Hlth. Org.*, **46**, 67.

Rowe, D. S., B. Grab, and S. G. Anderson (1973), *Bull. Wld. Hlth. Org.*, **49**, 320.

APPENDIX 21

Normal values for some plasma proteins

The following ranges, which are taken from various sources, must be regarded as a rough guide only; in general, they apply to healthy, non-pregnant adults who are not receiving medication. Certain ranges (e.g. those for immunoglobulins) are markedly different for children; many vary slightly with age in adults, and in some cases there are sex differences.

Protein	Range*
α_1-Acid glycoprotein	0.5–1.0
Albumin	35–48
Antithrombin III	0.17–0.30 (serum) 0.22–0.39 (plasma)
α_1-Antitrypsin	1.8–3.0
C3	0.7–1.6
C4	0.13–0.50
Caeruloplasmin	0.2–0.45
C1-esterase inhibitor	0.15–0.35
Carcinoembryonic antigen	< 0.1–20 μg/l
C-reactive protein	< 10 mg/l
α-Fetoprotein	< 20 μg/l
Fibrinogen	2.0–4.5
Haemopexin	0.5–1.1
IgA, IgG, IgM	See Chapter 1
α_2-Macroglobulin	1.5–4.5
β_2-Microglobulin	1–2.5 mg/l
Prealbumin	0.2–0.4
Pregnancy-associated α_2-glycoprotein	Usually < 50 mg/l
Retinol-binding protein	30–60 mg/l
Transferrin	2.0–4.0

*g/l unless otherwise stated

Index

Note: Page numbers of figures and tables are in *italic* type.